MR Imaging of Head and Neck Cancer

Editor

AHMED ABDEL KHALEK ABDEL RAZEK

MAGNETIC RESONANCE IMAGING CLINICS OF NORTH AMERICA

www.mri.theclinics.com

Consulting Editors
SURESH K. MUKHERJI
LYNNE S. STEINBACH

February 2022 • Volume 30 • Number 1

ELSEVIER

1600 John F. Kennedy Boulevard • Suite 1800 • Philadelphia, Pennsylvania, 19103-2899

http://www.mri.theclinics.com

MRI CLINICS OF NORTH AMERICA Volume 30, Number 1
February 2022 ISSN 1064-9689, ISBN 13: 978-0-323-83566-4

Editor: John Vassallo (j.vassallo@elsevier.com)
Developmental Editor: Arlene Campos

Magnetic Resonance Imaging Clinics of North America (ISSN 1064-9689) is published quarterly by Elsevier Inc., 360 Park Avenue South, New York, NY 10010-1710. Months of issue are February, May, August, and November. Business and Editorial Offices: 1600 John F. Kennedy Blvd., Ste. 1800, Philadelphia, PA 19103-2899. Customer Service Office: 3251 Riverport Lane, Maryland Heights, MO 63043. Periodicals postage paid at New York, NY and additional mailing offices. Subscription prices are $408.00 per year (domestic individuals), $1053.00 per year (domestic institutions), $100.00 per year (domestic students/residents), $455.00 per year (Canadian individuals), $1069.00 per year (Canadian institutions), $573.00 per year (international individuals), $1069.00 per year (international institutions), $100.00 per year (Canadian students/residents), and $275.00 per year (international students/residents). International air speed delivery is included in all *Clinics* subscription prices. All prices are subject to change without notice. **POSTMASTER:** Send address changes to *Magnetic Resonance Imaging Clinics*, Elsevier Health Sciences Division, Subscription Customer Service, 3251 Riverport Lane, Maryland Heights, MO 63043. Customer Service (orders, claims, online, change of address): Elsevier Health Sciences Division, Subscription **Customer Service, 3251 Riverport Lane, Maryland Heights, MO 63043. Tel:1-800-654-2452 (U.S. and Canada); 314-447-8871 (outside U.S. and Canada). Fax: 314-447-8029. E-mail: journalscustomerservice-usa@elsevier.com (for print support); journalsonlinesupport-usa@elsevier.com (for online support).**

Reprints. For copies of 100 or more of articles in this publication, please contact the Commercial Reprints Department, Elsevier Inc., 360 Park Avenue South, New York, NY 10010-1710. Tel.: 212-633-3874; Fax: 212-633-3820; E-mail: reprints@elsevier.com.

Magnetic Resonance Imaging Clinics of North America is covered in the *RSNA Index of Imaging Literature, MEDLINE/PubMed (Index Medicus)*, and *EMBASE/Excerpta Medica*.

Contributors

CONSULTING EDITORS

SURESH K. MUKHERJI, MD, MBA, FACR
Clinical Professor, Marian University, Director
of Head and Neck Radiology, ProScan
Imaging, Regional Medical Director, Envision
Physician Services, Carmel, Indiana, USA

LYNNE S. STEINBACH, MD, FACR
Emeritus Professor of Radiology on Full Recall,
Department of Radiology and Biomedical
Imaging, University of California, San
Francisco, San Francisco, California, USA

EDITOR

**AHMED ABDEL KHALEK ABDEL RAZEK,
MD**[†]
Professor and Head, Department of Diagnostic
Radiology, Faculty of Medicine, Mansoura
University, Mansoura, Egypt

AUTHORS

**AHMED ABDEL KHALEK ABDEL RAZEK,
MD**[†]
Professor and Head, Department of Diagnostic
Radiology, Faculty of Medicine, Mansoura
University, Mansoura, Egypt

TOUGAN TAHA ABDELAZIZ, MD
Department of Diagnostic Radiology, Ain
Shams Faculty of Medicine, Cairo, Egypt

AMRO ABDELKHALEK, MD
Internship at Mansoura University Hospital,
Mansoura Faculty of Medicine, Mansoura, Egypt

ASHLEY H. AIKEN, MD
Department of Radiology and Imaging
Sciences, Emory University School of
Medicine, Atlanta, Georgia, USA

KRISTEN L. BAUGNON, MD
Department of Radiology and Imaging
Sciences, Emory University School of
Medicine, Atlanta, Georgia, USA

MINERVA BECKER, MD
Diagnostic Department, Professor, Division of
Radiology, Unit of Head and Neck and

Maxillo-facial Radiology, Geneva University
Hospitals, University of Geneva, Geneva,
Switzerland

CLAUDIO DE VITO, MD, PhD
Diagnostic Department, Division of Clinical
Pathology, Geneva University Hospitals,
Geneva, Switzerland

ADEL T. DENEVER, MD
Faculty of Medicine, Department of
Surgery, Mansoura University, Mansoura,
Egypt

AYMAN EL-BAZ, PhD
BioImaging Laboratory, Department of
Bioengineering, J.B. Speed School of
Engineering, University of Louisville, Louisville,
Kentucky, USA

ALI H. ELMOKADEM, MD
Department of Diagnostic Radiology,
Mansoura University Faculty of Medicine,
Mansoura, Egypt

[†]Deceased

NERMEEN A. ELSEBAIE, MD
Department of Radiology, Alexandria Faculty
of Medicine, Alexandria, Egypt

ELLIOTT FRIEDMAN, MD
Department of Neuroradiology, Associate
Professor, The University of Texas Health
Science Center at Houston, Houston, Texas,
USA

OMNEYA A. GAMALELDIN, MD
Department of Radiology, Alexandria Faculty
of Medicine, Alexandria, Egypt

DANIEL THOMAS GINAT, MD, MS
Department of Radiology, University of
Chicago, Pritzker School of Medicine, Chicago,
Illinois, USA

EMAN HELMY, MD
Department of Diagnostic Radiology, Faculty
of Medicine, Mansoura University, Mansoura,
Egypt

BENJAMIN Y. HUANG, MD, MPH
Department of Radiology, UNC School of
Medicine, Chapel Hill, North Carolina, USA

ELSHARAWY KAMAL, MD
Faculty of Medicine, Department of
Otorhinolaryngology Head and Neck Surgery,
Mansoura University, Mansoura, Egypt

JORDAN KEMME, MD
Department of Radiology and Imaging
Sciences, Emory University School of
Medicine, Atlanta, Georgia, USA

REEM KHALED, MD
Department of Diagnostic Radiology, Faculty
of Medicine, Mansoura University, Mansoura,
Egypt

ANN D. KING, MBChB, FRCR, MD
Professor, Department of Imaging and
Interventional Radiology, The Chinese University
of Hong Kong, Prince of Wales Hospital, Shatin,
New Territories, Hong Kong SAR, China

MANAR MANSOUR, MD
Faculty of Medicine, Department of Diagnostic
Radiology, Mansoura University, Mansoura,
Egypt

YANN MONNIER, MD, PhD
Department of Clinical Neurosciences, Clinic of
Otorhinolaryngology, Head and Neck Surgery,

Unit of Cervicofacial Surgery, Geneva
University Hospitals, Geneva, Switzerland

SURESH K. MUKHERJI, MD, MBA, FACR
Clinical Professor, Marian University, Director
of Head and Neck Radiology, ProScan
Imaging, Regional Medical Director, Envision
Physician Services, Carmel, Indiana, USA

AHMED NAGLAH, PhD
BioImaging Laboratory, Department of
Bioengineering, J.B. Speed School of
Engineering, University of Louisville, Louisville,
Kentucky, USA

MARIA OLGA PATINO, MD
Associate Professor, Department of
Neuroradiology, The University of Texas Health
Science Center at Houston, Houston, Texas,
USA

JUSTIN D. RODRIGUEZ, MD
Department of Radiology, Duke University,
Durham, North Carolina, USA

GEHAD A. SALEH, MD
Faculty of Medicine, Department of Diagnostic
Radiology, Mansoura University, Mansoura,
Egypt

A. MORGAN SELLECK, MD
Department of Otolaryngology–Head and Neck
Surgery, University of North Carolina Hospitals,
Chapel Hill, North Carolina, USA

MOSAD SOLIMAN, MD
Department of Vascular Surgery, Mansoura
University Faculty of Medicine, Mansoura,
Egypt

AHMED M. TAWFIK, MD
Associate Professor of Radiology, Faculty of
Medicine, Department of Diagnostic and
Interventional Radiology, Mansoura University
Hospital, Mansoura, Egypt

XIN WU, MD
Department of Radiology and Imaging
Sciences, Emory University School of
Medicine, Atlanta, Georgia, USA

COLIN ZUCHOWSKI, MD
Department of Radiology and Imaging
Sciences, Emory University School of
Medicine, Atlanta, Georgia, USA

Contents

> Routine and advanced MR imaging sequences are used for locoregional spread, nodal, and distant staging of head and neck squamous cell carcinoma, aids treatment planning, predicts treatment response, differentiates recurrence for postradiation changes, and monitors patients after chemoradiotherapy.

> Nasopharyngeal carcinoma is endemic in parts of the world such as southern China and Southeast Asia. It is predominantly an undifferentiated carcinoma with a strong genetic basis and a close association with the Epstein-Barr virus. The ability of MR imaging to depict the boundaries of the primary tumor and its relationship with the complex structures of the skull base makes it the technique of choice for imaging of this disease in the head and neck. This article describes the MR imaging findings pertinent to staging and management and a new role of MR imaging in early cancer detection, in addition to a brief discussion of differential diagnoses.

> MR imaging is the modality of choice in the evaluation of oral cavity and oropharyngeal cancer. Routine postcontrast MR imaging is important for the accurate localization and characterization of the locoregional extension of oral cavity and oropharyngeal cancers. The anatomy of the oral cavity and oropharynx is complex; accurate interpretation is vital for description of the extension of the masses. Understanding the new changes in the eighth edition of the American Joint Committee on Cancer staging system. MR imaging is the imaging modality of choice for detection of perineural spread.

> State-of-the-art MR imaging of the larynx and hypopharynx with high-resolution surface coils, parallel imaging techniques, and DWI has several advantages over CT for assessing submucosal tumor spread, in particular neoplastic involvement of the paraglottic space, laryngeal cartilages, and extralaryngeal soft tissues. Current

surveillance protocoling and reviews treatment approaches, common posttreatment changes, and pearls for identifying disease recurrence in a subsite-based approach.

Head and neck reconstructive surgical techniques are complex; now the microvascular free tissue transfer is the most frequently used. The postreconstruction imaging interpretation is challenging due to the altered anatomy and flap variability. We aim to improve radiologists' knowledge with diverse methods of flap reconstruction for an accurate appreciation of their expected cross-sectional imaging appearance and early detection of tumor recurrence and other complication.

Neoplasms of the salivary glands are characterized by their marked histologic diversity giving them nonspecific imaging findings. MR imaging is the best imaging modality to evaluate salivary gland tumors. Multiparametric MR imaging combines conventional imaging features, diffusion-weighted imaging, and perfusion imaging to help distinguish benign and low-grade neoplasms from malignant tumors; however, a biopsy is often needed to establish a definitive histopathologic diagnosis. An awareness of potential imaging pitfalls is important to prevent mistakes in salivary neoplasm imaging.

This article reviews soft tissue tumors of the head and neck following the 2020 revision of *WHO Classification of Soft Tissue and Bone Tumours*. Common soft tissue tumors in the head and neck and tumors are discussed, along with newly added entities to the classification system. Salient clinical and imaging features that may allow for improved diagnostic accuracy or to narrow the imaging differential diagnosis are covered. Advanced imaging techniques are discussed, with a focus on diffusion-weighted and dynamic contrast imaging and their potential to help characterize soft tissue tumors and aid in distinguishing malignant from benign tumors.

Soft tissue vascular anomalies show a wide heterogeneity of clinical manifestations and imaging features. MR imaging has an important role in the diagnosis and management of vascular lesions of the head and neck. MR angiography is mandatory in cases of arteriovenous and combined malformations to assess the high-flow nature/component of the lesions and plan therapy. Infantile hemangiomas can be differentiated from congenital hemangiomas by clinical course. Reactive vascular tumors have nonspecific features similar to infantile hemangiomas. Locally malignant and malignant vascular tumors have irregular borders, infiltration of different tissue planes, and lower apparent diffusion coefficient values than benign vascular tumors.

MAGNETIC RESONANCE IMAGING CLINICS OF NORTH AMERICA

SERIES OF RELATED INTEREST

Advances in Clinical Radiology
Available at: www.advancesinclinicalradiology.com

Neuroimaging Clinics of North America
Available at: www.neuroimaging.theclinics.com

Radiologic Clinics of North America
Available at: www.radiologic.theclinics.com

VISIT THE CLINICS ONLINE!
Access your subscription at:
www.theclinics.com

PROGRAM OBJECTIVE

The goal of Magnetic Resonance Imaging Clinics of North America is to keep practicing physicians up to date with current clinical practice by providing timely articles reviewing the state of the art in patient care.

TARGET AUDIENCE

All practicing physicians and healthcare professionals who provide patient care utilizing findings from Magnetic Resonance Imaging.

LEARNING OBJECTIVES

Upon completion of this activity, participants will be able to:

1. Review the importance of imaging in the detection of recurrent tumors and monitoring patients after treatments.
2. Discuss MR imaging and the detection of early cancers that are difficult to detect by other means.
3. Recognize the use of AI in medical imaging to guide radiologists to more accurate image interpretation and diagnosis.

ACCREDITATION

DISCLOSURE OF CONFLICTS OF INTEREST

UNAPPROVED/OFF-LABEL USE DISCLOSURE

TO ENROLL

METHOD OF PARTICIPATION

CME INQUIRIES/SPECIAL NEEDS

Tribute

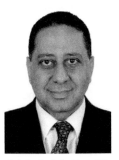

Ahmed Abdel Khalek Abdel Razek, MD

While in the final stages of editing this issue, Dr Abdel Razek passed away suddenly. He had previously edited the May 2018 *Neuroimaging Clinics*, and we appreciate his knowledge and insight with this latest issue. We mourn his loss and offer our sincere condolences to his family, friends, and colleagues.

Suresh Mukherji, Consulting Editor
Lynne Steinbach, Consulting Editor
John Vassallo, Publisher

IN MEMORY OF THE LATE DR AHMED ABDEL RAZEK (1961-2021)

For his family, friends, and those who knew him well, the loss of Dr Abdel Razek is greater than what words could describe; perhaps they can find solace in the great memories he left for us all. For those who never met him, I hope these brief words can give you a glimpse of his life and character.

Dr Abdel Razek was born on September 9, 1961. He studied medicine in Mansoura in the Nile Delta of Egypt and graduated from medical school in 1984. He started practicing in Mansoura University Hospital as a resident of diagnostic and interventional radiology and obtained a master's degree in Radiology in 1989, followed by a doctoral degree in 1994. He was promoted to Professor of Radiology in 2004. He was appointed the head of the Radiology Department in 2018.

I have known him as a mentor and a teacher since 2003, and then as coauthor and senior colleague since 2012. During this whole long journey with all its phases, I have never, not even a single time, seen him without his genuine, warm smile and the welcoming look on his face. He dealt with everyone with impeccable manners and handled every issue with reason and wisdom.

Abdel Razek was a scientist by definition. He had an unequalled passion for learning, teaching, and research. He was simply in love with the whole process. From reading new articles, to reviewing articles for journals, to collecting research data, to writing and editing manuscripts—he never felt bored or stopped working. Dr Abdel Razek would look so quiet and peaceful, but his mind was always busy with ideas and preparing for the next research project. His work, as lead author, was published in more than 200 articles in peer-reviewed high-impact journals. He contributed several book chapters and lectured more than 250 times at national and international congresses (eg, RSNA, ECR, ASNR, ASHNR, and ARRS). He was a reviewer for more than 20 high-impact journals, and a member of the editorial board of a number of international journals and societies. He was awarded several state awards and other

Magn Reson Imaging Clin N Am 30 (2022) xi–xii
https://doi.org/10.1016/j.mric.2021.10.001
1064-9689/22/© 2021 Published by Elsevier Inc.

mri.theclinics.com

scientific awards from RSNA and ECR during his career.

Dr Abdel Razek was known for his helpful attitude. He supervised over one hundred Master's and PhD candidates, with whom he loved to share knowledge and to set an example as the supportive team leader. No matter how busy he was, he always found time for those who needed his help or advice.

I am so proud and grateful to know such a great scientist and noble person. May his soul rest in peace.

Ahmed M. Tawfik, MD
Department of Diagnostic and
Interventional Radiology
Mansoura University Hospital
60 Elgomhoreya Street
Mansoura 35516, Egypt

E-mail address:
ahm_m_tawfik@hotmail.com

Foreword
MR Imaging of Head and Neck Cancer

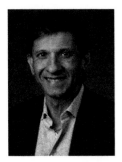

Suresh K. Mukherji, MD, MBA, FACR
Consulting Editor

Writing a foreword for an issue of *Magnetic Resonance Imaging Clinics of North America* is usually a happy occasion, as I have a chance to personally congratulate and thank the editors and authors for their wonderful contributions.

Unfortunately, Dr Ahmed Abdel Razek unexpectedly passed away during the final stages of publication of this issue on head and neck cancer. I have known Dr Abdel Razek for 20+ years, and he was a thoughtful, generous, and talented individual who had an unbridled passion for head and neck radiology. He was an incredibly gifted radiologist, but I will remember him most for his kindness and humility.

I would encourage you to read the beautiful tribute to Dr Ahmed Abdel Razek by Dr Ahmed Tawfik. It is clear the world has lost a talented radiologist, exemplary physician-scientist, and a "born leader." I have lost a wonderful colleague and friend whom I will dearly miss.

Suresh K. Mukherji, MD, MBA, FACR
Marian University
Head and Neck Radiology
ProScan Imaging
Carmel, IN, USA

E-mail address:
sureshmukherji@hotmail.com

Magn Reson Imaging Clin N Am 30 (2022) xiii
https://doi.org/10.1016/j.mric.2021.11.001
1064-9689/21/© 2021 Published by Elsevier Inc.

Role of MR Imaging in Head and Neck Squamous Cell Carcinoma

Ahmed Abdel Khalek Abdel Razek, MD[a,†], Nermeen A. Elsebaie, MD[b],
Omneya A. Gamaleldin, MD[b], Amro AbdelKhalek, MD[c],
Suresh K. Mukherji, MD, MBA, FACR[d,*]

KEYWORDS

• Head and neck cancer • Squamous cell carcinoma • MR imaging • Diffusion • Perfusion • Staging

KEY POINTS

- Squamous cell carcinoma is the most common tumor in the head and neck region.
- Routine precontrast and postcontrast studies are used for the initial evaluation of patients with head and neck cancer.
- MR imaging is important for locoregional spread and staging of head and neck cancer.
- Advanced MR imaging such as diffusion-weighted imaging and perfusion MR imaging are used for initial diagnosis and follow-up of patients with head and neck cancer.
- Imaging is important for the detection of recurrent tumors and monitoring patients after therapy.

BASIC BACKGROUND

Squamous cell carcinoma (SCC) accounts for about 95% of all cancers in the head and neck (HN) region and is the sixth most common cancer worldwide. It can originate from the mucosal epithelial lining of the oral cavity, pharynx, larynx, and sinonasal tract or the skin. Different risk factors lie behind the development of head and neck squamous cell carcinoma (HNSCC) including tobacco and alcohol consumption, exposure to environmental pollutants as well as viral infections namely human papillomavirus (HPV) and Epstein Bar virus (EBV). Infection with HPV is increasingly recognized as a common risk factor for HNSCC mainly arising in the oropharynx. More than 70% of oropharyngeal cancers are associated with an HPV infection with HPV-16 being the primary causative subtype. EBV is a known risk factor for HNSCC arising from the nasopharynx. Currently, significant changes have been made to the WHO classification of HNSCC based on HPV or EBV tumor status. HNSCC is generally more common in men, about 3 to 6 times more than women. The median age of diagnosis for nonvirally associated HNSCC is 66 years. HPV-associated oropharyngeal cancer and Epstein–Barr virus (EBV)-associated nasopharyngeal cancer can present at a relatively younger age, with the median age of diagnosis is about 53 and 50 years, respectively.[1–5]

HNSCC can originate from subsites within the oral cavity (44%), larynx (31%), or pharynx (25%). Clinical presentation of HNSCC varies according to the site of the primary tumor. Cancers of the oral cavity classically present early with a nonhealing ulcer and so they usually present at an early stage. Primary tumors of the oropharynx typically become symptomatic at a later stage, because of their hidden anatomic location. Symptoms include

[a] Department of Diagnostic Radiology, Mansoura University, Elgomheryia Street, Mansoura 35512, Egypt;
[b] Department of Radiology, Alexandria Faculty of Medicine, Champollion Street, El-Khartoum Square, El Azareeta Medical Campus, Alexandria 21131, Egypt; [c] Internship at Mansoura University Hospital, Mansoura Faculty of Medicine, 60 Elgomheryia Street, Mansoura 35512, Egypt; [d] Marian University, Head and Neck Radiology, ProScan Imaging, Carmel, IN, USA
[†] Deceased
* Corresponding author.
E-mail address: sureshmukherji@hotmail.com

Magn Reson Imaging Clin N Am 30 (2022) 1–18
https://doi.org/10.1016/j.mric.2021.08.001
1064-9689/22/© 2021 Elsevier Inc. All rights reserved.

dysphagia, odynophagia, or otalgia. Patients with HPV-related cancers of the oropharynx most commonly present with a new, painless level II (lymph nodes [LNs] at the upper jugular level) neck mass and an asymptomatic primary tumor. Patients with cancers of the larynx frequently present with hoarseness of voice, resulting in diagnosis at an early stage. If tumors are neglected, patients can present with dyspnea and airway obstruction prompting tracheostomy. In patients with tobacco-related HNSCC, the risk of a second tobacco-related primary tumor is significantly high, whether synchronous or metachronous, and can be localized at other sites in the HN region, or remotely in the esophagus or lungs.[3–10]

MR IMAGING TECHNIQUE
Routine MR Imaging Sequences

MR imaging offers better contrast resolution than computed tomography (CT) that helps to tumor margins from surrounding tissues. In addition, tumors appearing minimally enhancing on CT will be more evident on MR imaging because MR imaging is more sensitive to contrast enhancement. MR imaging is also more sensitive in the evaluation of perineural tumor spread, intracranial extension, and bone marrow infiltration. Conventional MR imaging sequences to assess HNSCC should include a T1 without fat suppression, T2 with and without fat suppression, and T1 postcontrast with fat suppression. These sequences are used to analyze certain characteristics of the primary tumor and possible nodal involvement.[6–9] Precontrast T1-weighted sequences should be performed without fat saturation for identification of the fat planes and delineation of normal anatomy. T2-weighted sequences should be acquired with fat suppression to increase the conspicuity of pathologic processes which often have increased T2 signal. The use of fat suppression on postcontrast T1-weighted sequence also maximizes the conspicuity of enhancement, because enhancing tissues may otherwise be the same signal intensity as surrounding fat. This technique is particularly important in the detection of perineural spread and for skull base involvement. Fat suppression for postcontrast T1 also increases the conspicuity of nodal necrosis and extranodal extension (ENE) of tumor which is currently added in the nodal staging for all tumors except nasopharyngeal carcinoma and HPV/p16 positive oropharyngeal tumors.[10–13] Some problems cannot be solved by anatomic sequences alone. Post-therapy changes such as inflammation and fibrosis show overlapping signal characteristics with recurrent or residual tumors. For LN assessment, the reactive LN that can be enlarged similar to nodal metastasis and normal-sized nodes can still contain tumors.[11–14]

Diffusion-Weighted Imaging
Routine diffusion-weighted imaging
Diffusion-weighted imaging (DWI) measures cellular density and cytoarchitecture by assessing water diffusivity. DWI is used in HN to differentiate SCC from lymphoma, diagnose LN metastasis, and differentiate recurrent neoplastic lesions from post-radiotherapy and chemotherapy changes. DWI is also able to detect changes in tumor prior size changes on anatomic sequences become visible, which can help to predict the early effect of treatment.[15–18]

Diffusion tensor imaging
Diffusion tensor imaging reflects micromovement of water molecules and can distinguish between different tissue compartments at the cellular level with different matrices. The most common metrics of diffusion tensor imaging used are mean diffusivity and fractional anisotropy (FA). Cellular tumors have a small extracellular space with low diffusivity and high anisotropy giving high FA values. Diffusion tensor imaging can be used in the HN to differentiate malignant from benign HN lesions, and can help prediction of recurrent HNSCC after treatment.[19,20]

Diffusion kurtosis imaging
The conventional DWI assess considers only water diffusion in one compartment which is the extracellular compartment. In diffusion kurtosis imaging, the interaction of water molecules with cell membranes is also considered. To estimate this motion, it is necessary to acquire b-values above 2000 mm^2/s. The main parameter derived from diffusion kurtosis imaging is the mean kurtosis (MK), which reflects the heterogeneity of the tissues. Aggressive lesions with higher mitotic index, presence of necrosis, and neoangiogenesis will show higher MK values than less aggressive lesions. However, in order to apply it, it is necessary to acquire multiple b-values and this means a longer examination time, with the consequent motion artifacts inherent to the HN region.[21]

Perfusion-Weighted Imaging

It provides a noninvasive assessment of microvascular characteristics of lesions. There are 3 main sequences of MR perfusion, contrast administration is used in 2 sequences: dynamic contrast-enhanced (DCE) and dynamic susceptibility contrast (DSC) techniques, in the third one, arterial spin labeling (ASL), no contrast administration is required, alternatively magnetically labeled arterial blood water is used as a tracer. DCE MR imaging and to a much lesser extent ASL are the perfusion techniques used to assess HN tumors.[8–13]

Dynamic contrast-enhanced MR imaging perfusion

It is the most commonly used technique, in which the passage of contrast bolus between the intravascular and extravascular compartments of the lesion is analyzed. An increase in the tissue signal is detected when the contrast reaches the extravascular space; the resulting signal intensity change over time creates the intensity-time curves. Data from this curve can be analyzed semiquantitatively or quantitatively. The semiquantitative method classifies the morphology of the signal intensity curve. The initial enhancement in the first 120 seconds is labeled as rapid, medium, or slow enhancement, and late enhancement beyond 120 seconds is described as persistent, plateau, or shout. In the quantitative method, additional tissue-specific parameters can be estimated including the transfer constant (Ktrans) which reflects the transfer rate of contrast from the plasma into the tissue extracellular space, the volume fraction of the extravascular extracellular space (ve), the volume fraction of plasma in tissue (vp), and the transfer rate from the extravascular extracellular space back to the plasma (kep).[12,22]

Dynamic susceptibility contrast MR imaging

DSC perfusion is based on the inhomogeneity of the magnetic field during the passage of a bolus of contrast through a capillary bed. Mean transit time, blood flow, and blood volume can be calculated. However, this technique is sensitive to motion artifacts because of the voluntary and involuntary movements in the HN region, which affects the reliability of the results. Also, blood products, calcifications, and air result in artificial signal loss.[23,24]

Arterial spin labeling

In ASL, blood flow can be calculated, which could reflect neovascularity within tumors. It is of particular clinical interest because of its relative speed, minimal postprocessing, and avoidance of gadolinium-based contrast agents. The main disadvantage of ASL is the low signal-to-noise ratio.[25–27]

MR Spectroscopy

Proton MR spectroscopy (MRS) is a noninvasive technique that can provide functional information through the evaluation of tissue metabolite concentrations. In HN lesions, the metabolites choline (Cho), creatine (Cr), lipid (Lip), and lactate (Lac) are often evaluated. Spectroscopy should be regarded as complementary to other functional MR imaging techniques in assessing HNSCC.[28]

Artificial Intelligence

Recently, advanced imaging analysis and processing is done with radiomics, deep learning with histogram analysis of quantitative parameters of MR imaging.[29–31]

ROLE OF IMAGING
Tumor Localization

The extent of mucosal involvement by the primary tumor is best assessed by endoscopic evaluation, whereas submucosal and deep extension is better documented at MR imaging. Tumors demonstrate isointense to hypointense signal on T1-weighted images (T1WIs) and hyperintense signal on T2-weighted images (T2WIs) compared to adjacent muscle (**Fig. 1**). Diffusion-weighted MR imaging can help to differentiate HNSCC from adjacent muscles as tumor shows lower apparent diffusion coefficient (ADC) values compared with benign tissue because of its high cellularity (**Fig. 2**). DCE may add benefits in discrimination between malignant

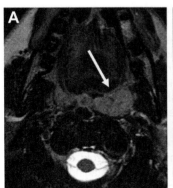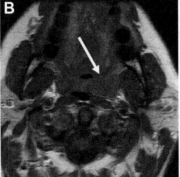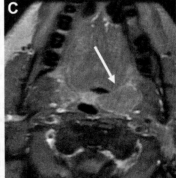

Fig. 1. MR imaging characteristics of squamous cell carcinoma. (*A*) Axial T2WI shows a left tonsillar carcinoma, which is a high signal. The lesion has T1 intermediate signal (*B*) and homogeneously enhances on fat-suppressed contrast-enhanced T1-weighted (T1W) sequences (*C*) (*arrows*).

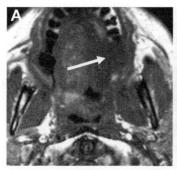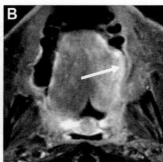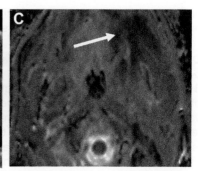

Fig. 2. DWI for identifying recurrent tumor. Noncontrast T1WI was obtained in a patient with a left retromolar trigone carcinoma that had been treated with combined chemotherapy and radiation therapy. (*A*) Axial noncontrast T1WIs show an intermediate signal involving the left retromolar trigone extending anteriorly to involve the posterior left maxillary alveolar ridge (*A*), which enhances following contrast (*B*). These imaging findings are indeterminant; however, the ADC maps show the area to have decreased signal (*C*), which was suspicious for recurrent tumor, and was confirmed with a biopsy (*arrows*).

lesions and adjacent normal tissues. The idea is based on that tumors with increased neoangiogenesis show earlier arrival of the contrast medium compared with normal tissue. Some studies showed that Ktrans, Kep, and Ve values are significantly higher in tumor areas than in the adjacent normal muscle. At MRS, the Cho/Cr ratio is found to be significantly elevated in cancer tissues in comparison with normal neck musculature due to increased cell membrane turnover in the cancer tissue.[7–12]

Locoregional Extension

Submucosal invasion

It is important to evaluate the full local extent of the primary tumor and detect submucosal and deep spread, perineural extension, bone and cartilage invasion, or intracranial involvement. Although there have been many changes in the updated eighth edition of the Cancer Staging Manual of the American Joint Committee on Cancer implemented in January 2018 (AJCC), it is necessary to ensure that all information that alters the tumor stage are included in the report. The location of the primary tumor can influence the selection of the initial imaging modality. MR imaging provides superior soft-tissue contrast is often the preferred imaging modality for evaluating the oral cavity, nasopharyngeal and oropharyngeal tumors. MR imaging can be affected by motion in the region of the larynx because of its relatively long scanning time. On MR imaging, the tumor usually appears hyperintense to muscle on T2WI and hypointense or isointense to muscle on T1WI (see **Fig. 1**).

The precontrast T1WI is particularly useful in differentiating tumor from surrounding fat. When evaluating the primary tumor (T), the specific criteria in the staging tables may require distinction by the size of the tumor or by specific invasion patterns.[32–34]

When measuring tumor size, the longest diameter is used. Conventional sequences can overestimate tumor size if inflammatory changes present. The use of DWI can help to better detect and demonstrate tumors because most squamous cell cancers are relatively hypercellular and can show diffusion restriction. The tumor typically shows an intermediate signal on T2WI and low ADC values at DWI, whereas peritumoral edema expresses a high signal on T2WI and high ADC values. Sometimes, delayed postcontrast T1 volumetric sequences (at least 5 min) may be used to demonstrate ish-out of tumor (which becomes darker) and progressive enhancement of surrounding inflammation (which becomes brighter).[31–35]

Tongue depth of invasion

In oral cavity tumors, of which tongue is the most common subsite, evaluation of the depth of invasion (DOI) is added as a critical determinant of T-staging. It can be measured on T1WIs by measuring the vertical distance between the deepest point of tumor infiltration and the simulated normal mucosal line. Many studies reported that MR imaging–determined DOI greater than 7.5 mm is significantly associated with the presence of neck LN metastasis, which added a nearly 3-fold risk of neck LN metastasis.[32–34,36] However, AJCC staging criteria emphasize that DOI is histologic measurement.

Thyroid and cricoid cartilage invasion

Accurate determination of thyroid cartilage invasion is essential for proper staging of laryngeal and hypopharyngeal cancers as they can upstage tumors to critical points where decision making for offered treatment is between chemoradiation and total laryngectomy. The first-line imaging for these

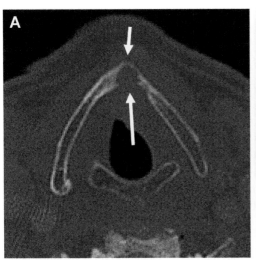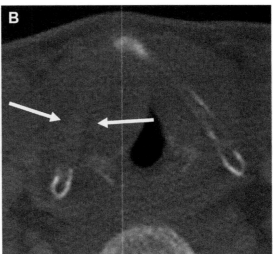

Fig. 3. CT of laryngeal cartilage invasion. (*A*) Axial CT was obtained through the thyroid cartilage reconstructed in bone algorithms in a patient with an SCCA of the anterior commissure. Cancer has eroded the inner cortex (*long arrow*) but the outer cortex is preserved (*short arrow*) indicating the stage of the tumor is T3. (*B*) Axial CT was obtained through the thyroid cartilage reconstructed in bone algorithms in a patient with an SCCA of the right true vocal cord. Cancer has eroded both the inner cortex (*long arrow*) and outer cortex (*short arrow*), indicating the stage of the tumor is T4.

tumor types is usually CT, which affords an excellent evaluation of these areas without swallowing artifacts in most cases. Tumor extending beyond the external margin of the cartilage ("extralaryngeal") is the most reliable feature of cartilage invasion. CT is able to pick up small defects of the cortical layer, while sclerosis is a nonspecific finding (**Fig. 3**). MR is superior in identifying intracartilaginous penetration: findings of infiltration are the copresence of low T1 (**Figs. 4** and **5**), intermediate T2 signals, and contrast-enhancement. Conversely, a high T2 signal is indicative of intracartilaginous edema, while the contribution of DWI is still not clear.[37,38]

Bone invasion

CT and MR are often used as complementary tools for preoperative planning. CT is more sensitive for demonstration of cortical erosion (**Fig. 6**). MR is better for early marrow invasion which appears as a defect in the low signal intensity of the bone cortex on T1WI and replacement of the high signal intensity marrow by low signal intensity tissue on T1WI with evident enhancement after contrast (**Fig. 7**). Marrow invasion of the mandible in oral cavity tumors will require surgical resection with a segmental mandibulectomy, rather than a marginal mandibulectomy for cortical erosion only. Marrow invasion will be evident on CT if the tumor is seen involving both sides of the mandible with extensive mandibular lytic destruction. When there is a subtle irregularity of the mandible and a critical surgical

decision must be made, as to whether there is marrow invasion, MR may be necessary.[39,40]

Prevertebral invasion

The prevertebral space can be invaded by carcinomas of the nasopharynx, oropharynx,

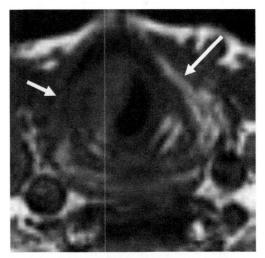

Fig. 4. MR imaging of cartilage invasion. Axial non-contrast T1W sequence was obtained through the thyroid cartilage in a patient with an SCCA of the right true vocal cord. Note the normal high T1W signal within the thyroid cartilage on the left side (*long arrow*) but replacement of the T1W (*short arrow*) adjacent to the tumor. The replacement of the normal T1W signal could be either due to tumoral invasion or peritumoral inflammation.

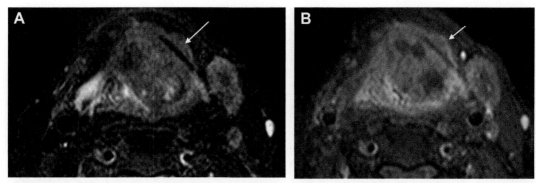

Fig. 5. MR imaging of cartilage invasion. Axial STIR and T1 postcontrast fat-saturated images (*A, B*) showing transglottic cancer obstructing the airway and transfixing the left thyroid cartilage (*white arrows*) with intermediate T2 signal and heterogeneous enhancement.

hypopharynx, or rarely larynx. The presence of obvious tumor fixation renders the tumor irresectable as tumor-free surgical margins cannot be achieved. In nasopharyngeal carcinoma, invasion to prevertebral muscles is currently clarified as T2 stage, yet associated with poor prognosis as the likelihood of locoregional recurrence and hematogenous metastases is increased. Several MR imaging signs may suggest the presence of prevertebral space invasion including obliteration of the retropharyngeal fat plane, ipsilateral muscle concavity, and T2 hyperintensity of the adjacent muscle (**Fig. 8**). However, these MR imaging findings are considered unreliable as they can be due to peritumoral edema, without actual muscle invasion. Still, accurate determination of neoplastic fixation to the prevertebral fascia is assessed most accurately intraoperatively during neck dissection

or with manual manipulation on endoscopy under general anesthesia. On the contrary, the absence of prevertebral space involvement can be clearly suggested on CT or MR imaging in cases where there is the preservation of the retropharyngeal fat plane.[34,41]

Esophageal invasion

Cervical esophageal invasion is reported in patients with hypopharyngeal cancer. MR imaging shows esophageal wall thickening, effacement of the adjacent fat plane, and T2 signal wall abnormality (**Figs. 9** and **10**). Circumferential mass more than 270° is a specific sign for esophageal invasion of HNSCC.[34,36–42]

Tracheal invasion

MR imaging is the modality of choice for the evaluation of tracheal invasion by thyroid cancer.

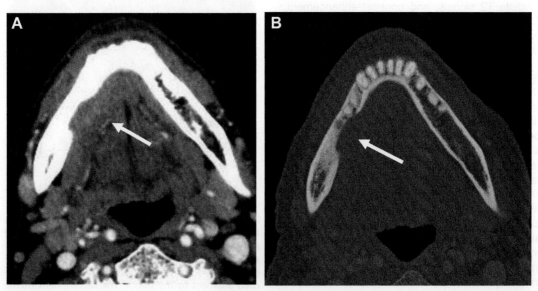

Fig. 6. CT findings of bone erosion. (*A*) Axial contrast-enhanced CT shows a right floor of mouth carcinoma (*arrow*). (*B*) Bone algorithm shows erosion of the adjacent lingual cortex (*arrow*).

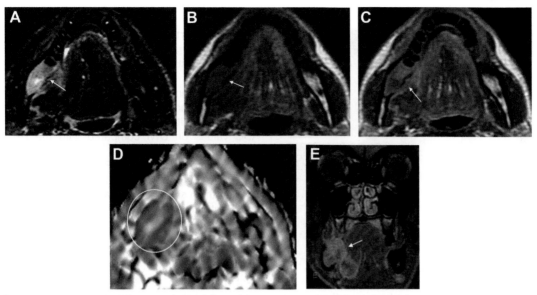

Fig. 7. Bone marrow invasion. Axial STIR (*A*), T1 (*B*), T1 postcontrast (*C*), and ADC map (*D*) of right retromolar trigone cancer showing hypointense mass invading the mandible with cortical erosions, expansion, and marrow replacement (*white arrows*). It shows a low ADC value of 0.9 in the ADC map (*circle*). T1 postcontrast fat-saturated coronal section (*E*) shows the heterogeneous enhancement of the tumor and infiltration of the mandible and floor of the mouth (*white arrow*).

Tracheal invasion is diagnosed by a combination of 3 criteria: tumor abutting circumference of the trachea for 180° or more, an intraluminal mass, or a soft-tissue signal within the cartilage (see **Figs. 9** and **10**). Invasion of the recurrent laryngeal nerve is predicted by the finding of effaced fatty tissue. The accuracy of these criteria is 90%.[43]

Cutaneous invasion
HNSCC may extend into the subcutaneous and cutaneous tissue. Imaging is important for surgical planning for the reconstruction of skin defects. Skin invasion at HNSCC is a bad prognostic sign. The presence of subcutaneous and cutaneous fat invasion appears as low signal intensity on T1WI and high signal on T2WI[44,45]

Perineural spread
It is critical to report this finding as, even if it does not change the tumor stage, it can significantly alter surgical and/or radiation planning. On CT scans, it can appear as a widening of the bony neural foramina at the skull base or at the mandibular or mental foramina of the mandible. MR imaging, with its higher contrast resolution and greater sensitivity to contrast enhancement, has been shown to be more sensitive on T1WIs, and there may be loss of normal fat padding around the nerve at the skull base. Characteristic findings of retrograde perineural are diffuse enhancement of an enlarged nerve (**Fig. 11**). On T2 and contrast-enhanced fat-saturated T1WIs, there is a thickening of the involved nerve. Muscle denervation subsequent to perineural tumor spread may also be evident and is much easier to detect on MR than on CT, due to early T2 hyperintensity and contrast enhancement of denervated muscles.[46,47]

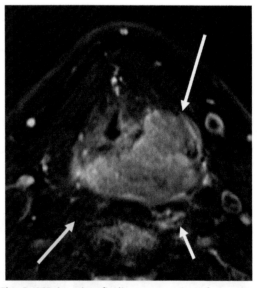

Fig. 8. MR imaging findings suggestive of prevertebral muscle involvement. Axial T2WI obtained in a patient with a large pyriform sinus carcinoma (*long white arrow*) shows increased T2 signal in the ipsilateral longus coli muscle (*short white arrow*), which is suspicious for muscle involvement. Compare this with the normal appearance of the contralateral longus coli muscle (*yellow arrow*).

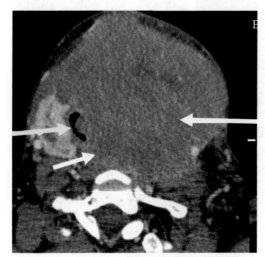

Fig. 9. Esophageal and tracheal invasion. Axial contrast-enhanced CT shows a large mass (*long white arrow*) extending medially to invade the trachea (*yellow arrow*) and extending posteriorly to involve the cervical esophagus (*short white arrow*).

Brachial plexus invasion

Brachial plexus invasion in HNSCC makes the tumor unresectable (**Fig. 12**). MR imaging shows high signal intensity on T2WI and enhancement along with brachial plexus or scalene muscles.[33,34]

Nodal Metastasis

Detection of nodal metastases in patients with HN cancer is important for treatment planning, the extent of radiation treatment field, or surgical neck dissection method. Morphologically, metastatic LNs should be rounded, with loss of the fatty hilum and more than 10 mm in short axis, focal necrosis may be present (**Fig. 13**). In addition to size and morphologic criteria, functional MR imaging techniques can add more data to suggest the presence of metastatic LNs, particularly in normal-sized nodes. There are multiple studies

that have reported significantly lower ADC in metastatic LNs (**Figs. 14** and **15**) than that of normal nodes. They suggested average ADC values of 1.02 to 1.38 × 10⁻³ mm²/s as a threshold value for differentiating malignant from benign LNs. It has been found that metastatic LNs associated with HPV-positive tumors tend to have lower ADC values on DWI compared with the HPV-negative LN metastasis.[6–10]

Few studies evaluated DCE-MR perfusion in the detection of metastatic LNs. Some studies showed that values of the Ktrans and Ve are found to be higher in metastatic LNs than in benign LNs. The Ktrans stands for the volume transfer constant, which is closely related to the perfusion and integrity of the endothelial cells. The Ve is a symbol of the extravascular extracellular volume fraction. Several studies on DCE MR imaging showed that the Ve is considered as an index of necrosis. Endothelial cells in tumor vessels are often pathologically immature, lacking in pericyte and smooth muscle coverage. Once an LN is invaded by tumor cells, new vessels with high permeability are generated. The increase in the number of new vessels can be detected as increased values of Ktrans of metastatic LNs corresponding to the histopathological changes. On the contrary, other studies showed that metastatic nodes have significantly lower Ktrans than the normal nodes. Such a low level of vascular-related parameters could be explained by necrosis, hypoxia, and elevated interstitial fluid pressure contributing to poor perfusion commonly observed in aggressive tumors.[48,49]

Extranodal extension

The new AJCC8 introduced the clinical ENE designation which is assessed on clinical examination (see **Fig. 13**). This finding should be looked for in all tumors except nasopharyngeal carcinoma and HPV/p16 positive oropharyngeal tumors. The presence of fixation of the nodal mass to adjacent

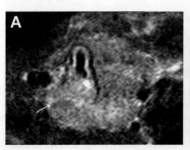 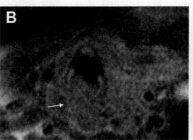 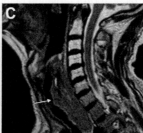

Fig. 10. Esophageal and tracheal invasion: Axial STIR (*A*), T1 postcontrast fat-saturated (*B*), and sagittal T2 (*C*) showing hypopharyngeal cancer invading the cervical esophagus, left thyroid lobe, and cervical trachea (*white arrows*). It shows a hypointense signal in T2 with heterogeneous enhancement.

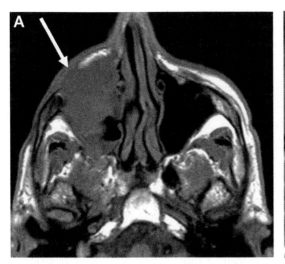
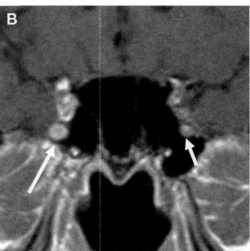

Fig. 11. MR imaging of perineural spread. (*A*) Axial noncontrast T1WI shows a large right maxillary sinus carcinoma (*arrow*). (*B*) Coronal contrast-enhanced T1WI shows diffuse enlargement and enhancement of the maxillary division of the trigeminal nerve (V2) indicative of retrograde perineural spread (*large arrow*). Compare this with the normal appearance of V2 on the contralateral site (*short arrow*).

structures such as skin or muscles or evidence of nerve dysfunction is suggesting the extranodal spread of the tumor, which upgrades the tumor to cN3b designation and grouping of stage IVB. Imaging may provide supportive evidence of this clinical ENE.[33,34]

On CT and MR imaging, different signs suggest the presence of ENE of the tumor. The most reliable imaging feature supporting the clinical diagnosis of ENE is the clear infiltration of perinodal tumor into adjacent fat or muscle. Other CT or MR imaging findings of ENE include indistinct nodal margins, irregular nodal capsular enhancement, and interruption in the nodal capsule. Several additional MR imaging signs have been reported such as the "vanishing border" sign where the fat space between node and adjacent tissues is obliterated on T1WIs, "flare" sign with high signal in interstitial tissues around and extending from the node on fat-suppressed T2WIs, and the "shaggy margin" sign where there is irregular or interrupted enhancement at the periphery of the nodes on axial gadolinium-enhanced T1WIs. Some studies indicated that ENE is more common in the presence of nodal necrosis and in nodes larger than 2 cm, while others find no correlation with nodal size.[50,51]

Distant Metastasis

The most common sites of distant metastasis in HNSCC are the lungs, followed by bone and liver. Variable factors increase the incidence of distant metastasis including advanced T-stage, poorly differentiated tumors, bilateral LN metastasis, and presence of ENE. Screening with integrated whole-body flouro deoxyglucose (FDG)-PET/CT including CT scan of the chest is currently the most valuable screening technique. Whole-body MR imaging (WB-MRI) has also become clinically feasible, with substantially reduced examination times. The use of whole-body diffusion-weighted MR imaging has even more advantages over standard anatomic WB-MRI sequences because of higher lesion-to-background contrast without the need for gadolinium contrast. Recently, images obtained with the PET-MR imaging system exhibited detailed resolution and greater image

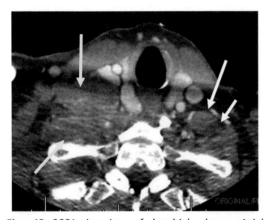

Fig. 12. SCCA invasion of brachial plexus. Axial contrast-enhanced CT shows normal appearance of the left anterior scalene (*long white arrow*) and supraclavicular brachial plexus (*small white arrow*). There is a large mass invading the right brachial plexus characterized by an invasion of the anterior scalene and supraclavicular brachial plexus (*yellow arrows*).

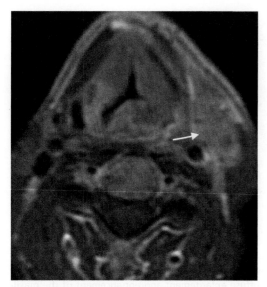

Fig. 13. Metastatic cervical lymph nodes. Axial T1 postcontrast image of a patient with SCC of the larynx showing left level II group metastatic lymph node (*white arrow*). It shows a globular shape, irregular outline, lost hilum, and invasion of left sternomastoid muscle; features of nodal metastases with ENE.

contrast in comparison to those from the PET/CT system, which may further improve detection of distant metastasis.[52,53]

Tumor, Node, Metastases Staging

Many changes have been added to the new AJCC8 for HNSCC. One of the significant changes is the staging of oropharyngeal tumors according to the HPV status. This change is based on the finding HPV-associated oropharyngeal SCC has a markedly better prognosis despite their

tendency to have early and extensive nodal metastasis. In the new classification, ipsilateral metastatic nodes are considered as N1, bilateral or contralateral nodes are to be designated as N2, and nodes that are larger than 6 cm are to be designated as N3. The prognostic table of the overall stage group is also changed. Stage I is determined by T1–2 and N0–1, stage II by T1–2 and N2 or T3 and N0–2, and stage III by T4 or N3, whereas stage IV is reserved for patients with metastatic disease. Accordingly, up to 80% of these tumors are classified as stage I. This is in contrast to p16−/non-HPV oropharyngeal SCC where most tumors are stage III or IV at presentation.[34,35]

Another important change regarding metastatic nodal SCCs is adding the pathologic and clinical criterion of ENE. This is applied in all HNSCCs except nasopharyngeal cancer and HPV-associated oropharyngeal cancer. Previously, pathologic diagnosis of ENE is found to be associated with poor prognosis for SCC, but it has not been part of the clinical or pathologic tables until AJCC8. Clinical ENE is suggested by the finding of fixation of the nodal mass to adjacent structures such as skin or muscles or evidence of nerve dysfunction suggesting nerve invasion. The designation of clinical ENE results in cN3b stage, which upstages tumors to stage group IVB. Details about the AJCC 8th classification will be discussed in the next article.[32–35]

Prognostic Parameters

Human papilloma virus
Oropharyngeal SCC has a different biology, and is associated with a better prognosis than HPV. In

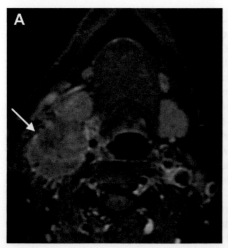
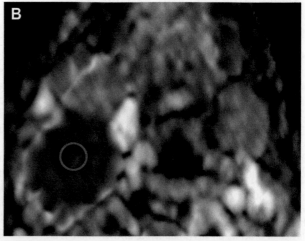

Fig. 14. Metastatic cervical lymph nodes. Axial T1WI (*A*) of a patient with metastatic SCC node shows irregular nodular periparotid lymph node (*white arrow*). In ADC map (*B*), it shows low signal intensity; ADC value 0.9×10^{-3} mm^2/s.

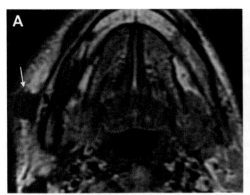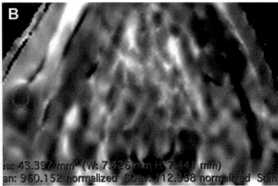

Fig. 15. Lymphomatous cervical LN. Axial T postcontrast fat-saturated image (*A*) showing large level II nodal mass with heterogeneous enhancement and invasion of the submandibular gland (*white arrow*) in a patient with nodal NHL. ADC map (*B*) showing a low signal intensity of the lymph node; ADC value 0.6×10^{-3} mm^2/s.

the AJCC8, the HPV-positive oropharyngeal SCC is staged separately from the HPV-negative type. DWI can offer a noninvasive imaging biomarker for HPV status of oropharyngeal SCC. Recent studies reported a lower mean ADC value in a primary lesion of HPV-positive oropharyngeal SCC compared with the HPV-negative tumors. HPV-negative oropharyngeal SCC showed higher ADC, reflecting histopathological features such as high stromal content, low cellularity, and micronecrosis. These prognostic characteristics likely contribute to the association of pretreatment high ADC values with poor outcomes in patients with HNSCC.[45,46]

Gross target volume

Tumor volume measured at MR imaging is referred to as gross target volume that correlates with local control and outcome for HNC and measure of the response to therapy. Tumor volume appears to be the strongest independent predictor of local failure after radiation therapy.[54]

Degree of differentiation

Differentiation of well-moderately differentiated HNSCC from poorly differentiated HNSCC is important for determining the prognosis and clinical outcome of patients. Some studies mentioned that poorly differentiated tumors may have lower ADC values than well/moderately tumors. Other authors, however, reported that ADC values could not distinguish between them. At histopathology, endothelial cells of poorly differentiated HNSCC are more immature, lacking in pericyte and smooth muscle coverage, these features can be highlighted at DCE. The increased permeability of these new vessels in poorly differentiated HNSCC results in increased values of Ktrans and Ve compared with well-differentiated HNSCC; corresponding to the histopathological changes.[5–25,26–59]

Treatment Planning

Detection of the best site for biopsy

Detection of the best biopsy site of the HN neoplasm is important for the best results. At routine MR imaging, biopsy is better taken from areas of lowest signal intensity at T2WIs and shows contrast enhancement and avoids areas of necrosis. An ADC map can differentiate viable from necrotic regions of malignancy. The viable regions of the tumor show restricted diffusion and necrotic regions display unrestricted diffusion. A biopsy is better when taken from the region of restricted diffusion with the lowest ADC value on the ADC map.[60]

Radiation therapy planning

Cross-sectional imaging has revolutionized radiation therapy planning and treatment effectiveness by allowing for conformational focus of radiation using 3-dimensional plans based on CT or MR imaging. The goal of radiation therapy is to control locoregional disease in the absence of distant metastatic disease. Here the value of adding FDG-PET to CT to detect unsuspected distant metastatic disease is a principal advantage of PET-CT in the evaluation of a patient under consideration for radiation therapy. To optimize conformational treatment plans, the radiation oncologist must know the precise delineation of the primary malignant mass and the extent of locoregional nodal disease (**Fig. 16**). Adding FDG-PET to the currently used CT imaging at simulation is becoming more widespread because of the improved delineation of tumor mass margins and assessment of locoregional tumor spread[60]

Differentiation from Lymphoma

SCC and lymphoma are the most common malignancies in the HN. Differentiation between these 2

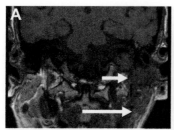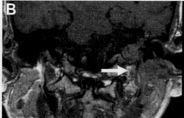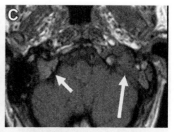

Fig. 16. Progressive SCCA due to inadequate treatment planning. Precontrast and postcontrast MR imaging were performed in a patient with an unknown primary tumor with extensive left-sided adenopathy which extended to the mastoid tip. The patient was treated with radiation therapy alone; however, the patient presented with progressive left neck pain. (C) Coronal noncontrast enhanced MR imaging shows a large low signal (A) enhancing mass (B) extending to the left skull base (*small arrow*) which has a higher signal compared with the adjacent parotid gland (*long arrow*). Axial images show diffuse replacement (*long arrow*) of the skull base compared to the contralateral side. These findings are consistent with a progressive tumor. These images were correlated with the treatment plan and the superior extent of the radiation did not include the mastoid tip with the superior extent of the field being between the long and short arrows on image A.

entities is crucial as management strategies differ completely. Both SCC and lymphoma arise from the same anatomic sites and show nearly similar imaging characteristics on conventional MR imaging sequences. On DWI, ADC is significantly lower in lymphoma (**Fig. 17**) than in SCC (**Fig. 18**) at primary or nodal sites, finding that is mostly attributed to higher cellularity in lymphoma. However, there is a greater possibility of overlap with the poorly differentiated SCCs, which tend to have a slightly lower ADC than their moderately or well-differentiated counterparts. Adding perfusion studies can help in the differentiation between these 2 pathologies. At DCE-MR, considering semiquantitative parameters derived from TIC, lymphoma shows longer TTP and lower enhancement peak than SCCs. Regarding quantitative assessment, several studies showed that lymphoma shows lower Ktrans and Ve values than

SCC, which means that lymphoma shows less vascular permeability and tight extravascular extracellular space when compared with SCC. This reflects the histopathologic nature of lymphoma where there is high cellular density, few microvessels, and the tumor cells often form a sleeve-like infiltration around the vessels.[61,62]

Prediction Response to Therapy

Many studies have investigated the application of pretreatment ADC value for the prediction of outcome in patients with HN SCC. Tumors that show necrosis due to tumor hypoxia and decreased vascularity and have higher ADC values are less responsive to chemotherapy and radiotherapy. DWI can be used as a pretreatment marker for tumor hypoxia. Many studies suggested that higher pretreatment ADC values are predictive of poor local control and treatment

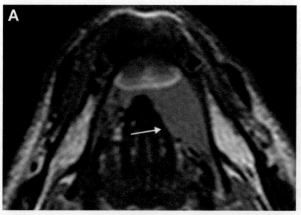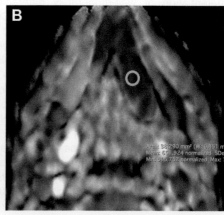

Fig. 17. Lingual lymphoma axial T2 and ADC map (A, B) showing left lingual lymphoma of intermediate signal intensity (*white arrow*) and ADC value 0.65×10^{-3} mm^2/s.

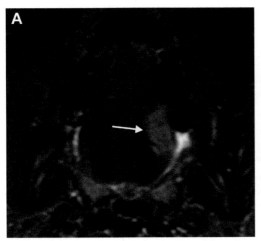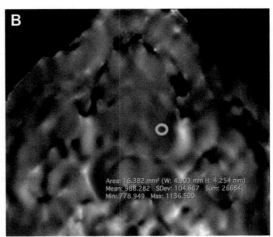

Fig. 18. Lingual SCC axial STIR and ADC map (*A, B*) showing left lingual SCC hyperintense to the muscle (*white arrow*) and ADC value 0.98×10^{-3} mm^2/s.

response. They found that an ADC greater than 1.15×10^{-3} mm^2/s in the primary tumor is associated with poor outcome after chemoradiation at 2-year follow-up.[7–12]

At DCE MR perfusion, low Ktrans value before the start of treatment, both in the primary tumor and the LN metastases, is associated with a worse prognosis, this could be explained as this lower permeability making it difficult for the chemotherapy agent to reach the cancer lesion. The role of DCE MR imaging metrics as predictors of response in HN cancers to conventional radiotherapy (CRT) and showed that HN cancer with higher pretreatment blood volume, and pretreatment Ktrans correlated with better response to CRT and disease-free survival. Tumors with higher blood flow and vascular permeability have better oxygenation with better access to CT and better response to RT.[22,34]

Intratreatment Assessment of Response to CRT

The efficacy of treatment is mainly evaluated by size changes of tumor and metastatic LNs before and after treatment. But actually, the size of the tumor will not change at the early stage, which makes it impossible to provide accurate information about the true response to treatment. As response adapted therapy becomes more widespread in cancer management, there will be greater interest in performing intratreatment scanning.[8–12]

DWI may help to closely monitor response in the early treatment phase and throughout treatment. Successful CRT results in rising in the ADC value in the first few weeks after the start of treatment. Some studies have shown that a smaller percentage of rising in the mean ADC value (<14–24%) in the first 3 weeks after the start of treatment is seen

in patients with disease failure compared to those with disease control. In addition, it has been observed that after the initial early ADC rise, a subsequent ADC fall predicts locoregional failure, which may be caused by the repopulation of cancer cells.[12–15]

At DCE MR imaging perfusion, successful chemoradiotherapy causes changes in the time-intensity curve. Initially, there is a decrease in the number of leaking vessels, which is reflected as a slower rise of the enhancement curve. With continued successful response to therapy, there is a regression of tumor angiogenic properties resulting in a decreased contrast peak and the development of fibrosis resulting in a gradual accumulation of contrast. So, the TIC will change from rapid rise and ish-out in the pretreatment state to a slow rise and ish-in in the post-treatment state. In patients with poor response to CRT, TIC showed a steep rise in the enhancement curve, which means a high initial contrast peak value and a short TTP. This could help in identifying patients at risk of local recurrence as candidates for dose escalation or salvage surgery.[22] Results showed that the values of Ktrans and Kep significantly decreased, whereas Ve significantly increased after treatment, compared with those before treatment. Differences are statistically significant. Some studies have shown that radiochemotherapy will induce the deformation and necrosis of capillary walls, consequently reducing blood perfusion of tumor tissues, reducing osmotic pressure of the blood vessel walls, and decreasing values of Ktrans and Kep after radiochemotherapy. Ve value increases maybe because the radiotherapy leads to osmotic pressure decreases of the tumor vessel walls, slows the flow rate of contrast agents, prolongs the

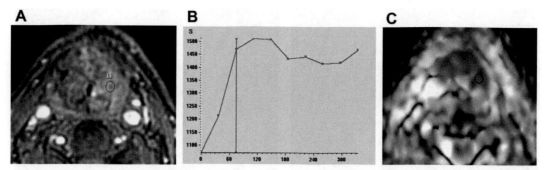

Fig. 19. Recurrent supraglottic SCC. Patient with left recurrent supraglottic SCC after management by chemoradiotherapy. DCE sequence and regenerated curve (*A, B*) show nodular enhancing left supraglottic mass with rapid enhancement followed by a gradual wash-out confirming its malignant nature. ADC map (*C*) showing hypointense signal of the lesion; ADC value 0.9 × 10⁻³ mm²/s.

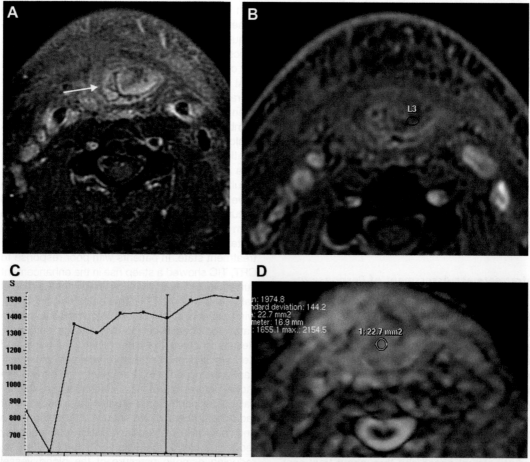

Fig. 20. Postradiation changes. Patient with laryngeal SCC managed by total laryngectomy and chemoradiotherapy. Axial T1 postcontrast fat-saturated image (*A*) showing diffuse thin linear enhancement of the mucosa of the reconstructed neopharynx and submucosal edema (*white arrow*). In the DCE sequence and regenerated curve (*B, C*), the curve shows rapid enhancement followed by a continuous regular rising curve representing benignity. ADC map (*D*) shows a high signal intensity of the reconstructed neopharynx ADC value 1.22 × 10⁻³ mm²/s representing postirradiation inflammation and edema.

residence time of contrast agents in the tissue vessels and outside the vascular, and eventually leads to an increase of Ve values.[8–13]

Recurrence Versus Postradiation Changes

The baseline scan is typically obtained at 8 to 10 weeks after chemoradiation, whereas postsurgical scans are often obtained around 10 to 12 weeks. The baseline cross-sectional scan serves as a "road map" of a deformed neck to increase sensitivity for early recurrent disease on the subsequent surveillance imaging. For this reason, it is ideal that the same cross-sectional modality chosen for baseline imaging, either CT or MR, is subsequently used for surveillance. Follow-up may be performed in 3 to 6 months intervals, depending on the initial tumor staging and histologic prognostic features and the ongoing clinical course and physical findings. At any follow-up imaging examination, the possibility of a second primary tumor must again be considered. Remember on every follow-up study to look for residual, recurrent, and new tumors.[8–13] Radiation with or without chemotherapy is associated with significant changes in the appearance of neck soft tissues. Radiation results in acute inflammation of all tissues in the radiation field with extensive edema. Over time this converts to fibrosis with atrophy and altered signal intensity and texture on

MR. Both acute and chronic expected radiation changes can be confusing on CT or MR, requiring careful evaluation and comparison with prior studies to detect early recurrences.[7–11]

On MR imaging, the recurrent tumors will have similar signal characteristics to the primary tumor, so it is important to review any preoperative imaging if available. A new nodule within the tumor bed or progressive thickening of the tissues deep to the flap is a concerning feature for recurrent disease. T2 sequences are useful to distinguish scar from a tumor, with scar tissue being of comparatively lower signal on T2. Several previous studies have reported that the imaging criteria for local tumor recurrence include an infiltrative mass, intermediate T1-weighted signal intensity, intermediate to high T2-weighted signal intensity, and enhancement. However, differentiating residual or recurrent tumor from scar using these imaging criteria is difficult because these findings could overlap with those for post-treatment edematous change, radiation-induced inflammation, or fibrosis. Quantitative analysis of diffusion MR imaging metrics can help distinguish between residual/recurrent malignant tissue and benign post-treatment changes. Prior studies suggested that residual HNSCC tends to have a lower average ADC compared with benign post-treatment changes (see **Fig. 2**). The suggested ADC thresholds in different studies for differentiating residual/recurrent (**Fig. 19**) malignant tissue

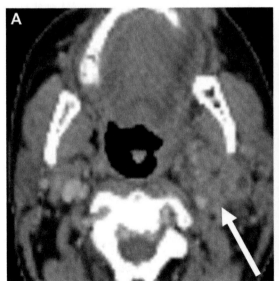 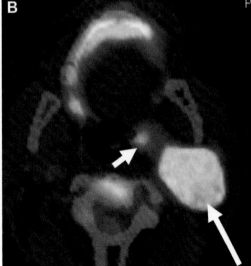

Fig. 21. Unknown primary detected with PET-CT. (*A*) Axial contrast-enhanced CT shows a large left level II nodal mass which was biopsy-proven SCC (*arrow*). No tumor was identified on direct endoscopy. The patient was thought to have an unknown primary and underwent PET-CT in an attempt to localize the tumor and help direct speculative biopsies. (*B*) PET-CT shows uptake in the large left nodal mass (*long arrow*) and focal uptake in the left tonsil (*small arrow*), which was suspicious for a left tonsillar carcinoma. The patient underwent a left tonsillectomy, which confirmed the diagnosis of a left tonsillar carcinoma, which was initially felt to be an unknown primary cancer eventually detected by PET-CT.

and benign post-treatment changes (**Fig. 20**) varied from 0.96 to 1.46×10^{-3} mm^2/s. These findings are likely reflective of the difference in cellularity of malignant tissue compared to fibrotic post-treatment changes. At DCE MR imaging, a rapid wash-in followed by a wash-out or plateau phase is indicative of tumor, while slowly progressive enhancements indicate benign post-treatment changes.[62–68]

Unknown Primary

An unknown primary tumor is defined as SCC detected from fine-needle aspiration of a nodal mass in the absence of a clinically evident primary source. More than 90% of unknown primary tumors are determined to be HPV-related OPSCC. As HPV-related tumors arise from the palatine tonsils and base of the tongue, it is essential to evaluate CT and MR scan for subtle asymmetry in the size and signal intensity to identify the primary lesion and direct surgeons to biopsy or tonsillectomy. PET-CT is often performed in the United States to help direct speculative biopsies and possibly identify the primary site in patients with metastatic LNs and negative endoscopy (**Fig. 21**). Determination of the true primary can markedly limit the radiation field used for therapy. High temporal resolution (ultrafast) DCE MR imaging has been found to improve the detection of clinically occult primary tumors in patients presenting with cervical SCC LN metastases. Qualitative reading of ultrafast-DCE images could depict early intensity changes and faster signal enhancement as indications for malignancy compared with normal tissue.[69]

SUMMARY

Routine and advanced MR imaging sequences are used for locoregional spread, nodal, and distant staging, aids treatment planning, predicts treatment response, differentiates recurrence for post-radiation changes, and monitor patients after chemoradiotherapy.

CLINICS CARE POINTS

- MRI helps asses soft tissue spread and provides better tumor characterization compared to MR.
- MRI is the study of choice for evaluating perineural spread.
- Advanced MRI techniques may be helpful to differentiate recurrent tumor from post-treatment changes.

REFERENCES

1. Chow LQM. Head and Neck Cancer. N Engl J Med 2020;382:60–72.
2. Argiris A, Karamouzis MV, Raben D, et al. Head and neck cancer. Lancet 2008;371:1695–709.
3. Pfister DG, Spencer S, Adelstein D, et al. Head and Neck Cancers, Version 2.2020, NCCN Clinical Practice Guidelines in Oncology. J Natl Compr Canc Netw 2020;18:873–98.
4. Lydiatt WM, Patel SG, O'Sullivan B, et al. Head and Neck cancers-major changes in the American Joint Committee on cancer eighth edition cancer staging manual. CA Cancer J Clin 2017;67:122–37.
5. Machiels JP, René Leemans C, Golusinski W, et al. Squamous cell carcinoma of the oral cavity, larynx, oropharynx and hypopharynx: EHNS-ESMO-ESTRO Clinical Practice Guidelines for diagnosis, treatment and follow-up. Ann Oncol 2020;31:1462–75.
6. Junn JC, Soderlund KA, Glastonbury CM. Imaging of Head and Neck Cancer With CT, MRI, and US. Semin Nucl Med 2021;51:3–12.
7. Glastonbury CM. Head and neck squamous cell cancer: approach to staging and surveillance. 2020. In: Hodler J, Kubik-Huch RA, von Schulthess GK, editors. Diseases of the brain, head and neck, spine 2020–2023.
8. Abdel Razek AA. Computed tomography and magnetic resonance imaging of lesions at masticator space. Jpn J Radiol 2014;32:123–37.
9. El Beltagi AH, Elsotouhy AH, Own AM, et al. Functional magnetic resonance imaging of head and neck cancer: Performance and potential. Neuroradiol J 2019;32:36–52.
10. Santos Armentia E, Martín Noguerol T, Suárez Vega V. Advanced magnetic resonance imaging techniques for tumors of the head and neck. Radiologia 2019;61:191–203.
11. Abdel Razek AA. Imaging of connective tissue diseases of the head and neck. Neuroradiol J 2016;29:222–30.
12. Juliano A, Moonis G. Computed Tomography Versus Magnetic Resonance in Head and Neck Cancer: When to Use What and Image Optimization Strategies. Magn Reson Imaging Clin N Am 2018;26:63–84.
13. Razek AA, Castillo M. Imaging appearance of granulomatous lesions of head and neck. Eur J Radiol 2010;76:52–60.
14. Seeburg DP, Baer AH, Aygun N. Imaging of Patients with Head and Neck Cancer: From Staging to Surveillance. Oral Maxillofac Surg Clin North Am 2018; 30:421–33.
15. Abdel Razek AA. Assessment of solid lesions of the temporal fossa with diffusion-weighted magnetic resonance imaging. Int J Oral Maxillofac Surg 2015;44:1081–5.

16. Thoeny HC, De Keyzer F, King AD. Diffusion-weighted MR imaging in the head and neck. Radiology 2012;263:19–32.

17. Abdel Razek AA, Nada N. Role of diffusion-weighted MRI in differentiation of masticator space malignancy from infection. Dentomaxillofac Radiol 2013; 42:20120183.

18. Abdel Razek A, Mossad A, Ghonim M. Role of diffusion-weighted MR imaging in assessing malignant versus benign skull-base lesions. Radiol Med 2011;116:125–32.

19. Abdel Razek AAK. Routine and Advanced Diffusion Imaging Modules of the Salivary Glands. Neuroimaging Clin N Am 2018;28:245–54.

20. Khalek Abdel Razek AA. Characterization of salivary gland tumours with diffusion tensor imaging. Dentomaxillofac Radiol 2018;47:20170343.

21. Ma G, Xu XQ, Hu H, et al. Utility of Readout-Segmented Echo-Planar Imaging-Based Diffusion Kurtosis Imaging for Differentiating Malignant from Benign Masses in Head and Neck Region. Korean J Radiol 2018;19:443–51.

22. Kabadi SJ, Fatterpekar GM, Anzai Y, et al. Dynamic Contrast-Enhanced MR Imaging in Head and Neck Cancer. Magn Reson Imaging Clin N Am 2018;26: 135–49.

23. Razek AA, Elsorogy LG, Soliman NY, et al. Dynamic susceptibility contrast perfusion MR imaging in distinguishing malignant from benign head and neck tumors: a pilot study. Eur J Radiol 2011;77:73–9.

24. Abdel Razek AA, Samir S, Ashmalla GA. Characterization of Parotid Tumors With Dynamic Susceptibility Contrast Perfusion-Weighted Magnetic Resonance Imaging and Diffusion-Weighted MR Imaging. J Comput Assist Tomogr 2017;41:131–6.

25. Abdel Razek AAK, Talaat M, El-Serougy L, et al. Clinical Applications of Arterial Spin Labeling in Brain Tumors. J Comput Assist Tomogr 2019;43:525–32.

26. Abdel Razek AAK, Nada N. Arterial spin labeling perfusion-weighted MR imaging: correlation of tumor blood flow with pathological degree of tumor differentiation, clinical stage and nodal metastasis of head and neck squamous cell carcinoma. Eur Arch Otorhinolaryngol 2018;275:1301–7.

27. Razek AAKA. Multi-parametric MR imaging using pseudo-continuous arterial-spin labeling and diffusion-weighted MR imaging in differentiating subtypes of parotid tumors. Magn Reson Imaging 2019;63:55–9.

28. Abdel Razek AA, Poptani H. MR spectroscopy of head and neck cancer. Eur J Radiol 2013;82:982–9.

29. Abdel Razek AAK. Editorial for "Preliminary Assessment of Intravoxel Incoherent Motion Diffusion-Weighted MRI (IVIM-DWI) Metrics in Alzheimer's Disease. J Magn Reson Imaging 2020;52:1827–8.

30. Razek AAKA. Editorial for "Preoperative MRI-Based Radiomic Machine-Learning Nomogram May Accurately Distinguish Between Benign and Malignant Soft Tissue Lesions: A Two-Center Study. J Magn Reson Imaging 2020;52:883–4.

31. Abdel Razek AAK, Gadelhak BN, El Zahabey IA, et al. Diffusion-weighted imaging with histogram analysis of the apparent diffusion coefficient maps in the diagnosis of parotid tumours. Int J Oral Maxillofac Surg 2021. https://doi.org/10.1016/j.ijom.2021.03.019.

32. Glastonbury CM. Critical Changes in the Staging of Head and Neck Cancer. Radiol Imaging Cancer 2020;2:e190022.

33. Glastonbury CM, Mukherji SK, O'Sullivan B, et al. Setting the Stage for 2018: How the Changes in the American Joint Committee on Cancer/Union for International Cancer Control Cancer Staging Manual Eighth Edition Impact Radiologists. AJNR Am J Neuroradiol 2017;38:2231–7.

34. Yousem D, Gad K, Tufano R. Resectability Issues with Head and Neck Cancer. AJNR Am J Neuroradiol 2006;27:2024–36.

35. Lydiatt W, O'Sullivan B, Patel S. Major Changes in Head and Neck Staging for 2018. Am Soc Clin Oncol Educ Book 2018;38:505–14.

36. Huopainen P, Jouhi L, Hagstrom J, et al. MRI correlates to histopathological data in oral tongue squamous cell carcinoma diagnostics. Acta Odontol Scand 2021;79:161–6.

37. Cho SJ, Lee JH, Suh CH, et al. Comparison of diagnostic performance between CT and MRI for detection of cartilage invasion for primary tumor staging in patients with laryngo-hypopharyngeal cancer: a systematic review and meta-analysis. Eur Radiol 2020;30:3803–12.

38. Kuno H, Sakamaki K, Fujii S, et al. Comparison of MR Imaging and Dual-Energy CT for the Evaluation of Cartilage Invasion by Laryngeal and Hypopharyngeal Squamous Cell Carcinoma. AJNR Am J Neuroradiol 2018;39:524–31.

39. Ogawa T, Kojima I, Wakamori S, et al. Clinical utility of apparent diffusion coefficient and diffusion-weighted magnetic resonance imaging for resectability assessment of head and neck tumors with skull base invasion. Head Neck 2020;42:2896–904.

40. Lee YC, Jung AR, Kwon OE, et al. Comparison of Computed Tomography, Magnetic Resonance Imaging, and Positron Emission Tomography and Computed Tomography for the Evaluation Bone Invasion in Upper and Lower Gingival Cancers. J Oral Maxillofac Surg 2019;77:875.e1-9.

41. Meerwein CM, Pizzuto DA, Vital D, et al. Use of MRI and FDG-PET/CT to predict fixation of advanced hypopharyngeal squamous cell carcinoma to prevertebral space. Head Neck 2019;41:503–10.

42. Tian D, Huang H, Yang YS, et al. Depth of Invasion into the Circular and Longitudinal Muscle Layers in T2 Esophageal Squamous Cell Carcinoma Does Not Affect Prognosis or Lymph Node Metastasis: A

Multicenter Retrospective Study. World J Surg 2020; 44:171–8.

43. Wang JC, Takashima S, Takayama F, et al. Tracheal invasion by thyroid carcinoma: prediction using MR imaging. AJR Am J Roentgenol 2001;177:929–36.

44. Spector ME, Gallagher KK, McHugh JB, et al. Correlation of radiographic and pathologic findings of dermal lymphatic invasion in head and neck squamous cell carcinoma. AJNR Am J Neuroradiol 2012;33:462–4.

45. Nemec SF, Linecker A, Czerny C, et al. Detection of cutaneous invasion by malignant head and neck tumors with MDCT. Eur J Radiol 2008;68:335–9.

46. Agarwal M, Wangaryattawanich P, Rath TJ. Perineural Tumor Spread in Head and Neck Malignancies. Semin Roentgenol 2019;54:258–75.

47. Dankbaar JW, Pameijer FA, Hendrikse J, et al. Easily detected signs of perineural tumour spread in head and neck cancer. Insights Imaging 2018;9:1089–95.

48. Abdel Razek AA, Gaballa G. Role of perfusion magnetic resonance imaging in cervical lymphadenopathy. J Comput Assist Tomogr 2011;35:21–5.

49. Razek AAKA, Helmy E. Multi-parametric arterial spin labeling and diffusion-weighted imaging in differentiation of metastatic from reactive lymph nodes in head and neck squamous cell carcinoma. Eur Arch Otorhinolaryngol 2021;278:2529–35.

50. Pons Y, Ukkola-Pons E, Clément P, et al. Relevance of 5 different imaging signs in the evaluation of carotid artery invasion by cervical lymphadenopathy in head and neck squamous cell carcinoma. Oral Surg Oral Med Oral Pathol Oral Radiol Endod 2010;109:775–8.

51. Yousem DM, Hatabu H, Hurst RW, et al. Carotid artery invasion by head and neck masses: prediction with MR imaging. Radiology 1995;195:715–20.

52. Razek AA, Tawfik A, Rahman MA, et al. Whole-body diffusion-weighted imaging with background body signal suppression in the detection of osseous and extra-osseous metastases. Pol J Radiol 2019;84: e453–8.

53. Razek AAKA, Shamaa S, Lattif MA, et al. Interobserver agreement of whole-body computed tomography in staging and response assessment in lymphoma: the lugano classification. Pol J Radiol 2017;82:441–7.

54. Razek AA, Nada N. Correlation of choline/creatine and apparent diffusion coefficient values with the prognostic parameters of head and neck squamous cell carcinoma. NMR Biomed 2016;29:483–589.

55. Javadi S, Menias CO, Karbasian N, et al. HIV-related Malignancies and Mimics: Imaging Findings and Management. Radiographics 2018;38:2051–68.

56. Payabvash S, Chan A, Jabehdar, et al. Quantitative diffusion magnetic resonance imaging for prediction of human papillomavirus status in head and neck squamous-cell carcinoma: A systematic review and meta-analysis. Neuroradiol J 2019;32(4):232–40.

57. Abdel Razek AA, Kamal E. Nasopharyngeal carcinoma: correlation of apparent diffusion coefficient value with prognostic parameters. Radiol Med 2013;118:534–9.

58. Abdel Razek AA, Elkhamary S, Al-Mesfer S, et al. Correlation of apparent diffusion coefficient at 3T with prognostic parameters of retinoblastoma. AJNR Am J Neuroradiol 2012;33:944–8.

59. Abdel Razek AAK, Elkhamary SM, Nada N. Correlation of apparent diffusion coefficient with histopathological parameters of salivary gland cancer. Int J Oral Maxillofac Surg 2019;48:995–1000.

60. Razek AA. Diffusion-weighted magnetic resonance imaging of head and neck. J Comput Assist Tomogr 2010;34:808–15.

61. Bae S, Choi YS, Sohn B, et al. Squamous Cell Carcinoma and Lymphoma of the Oropharynx: Differentiation Using a Radiomics Approach. Yonsei Med J 2020;61:895–900.

62. Eissa L, Abdel Razek AAK, Helmy E. Arterial spin labeling and diffusion-weighted MR imaging: Utility in differentiating idiopathic orbital inflammatory pseudotumor from orbital lymphoma. Clin Imaging 2021;71:63–8.

63. Chung SR, Choi YJ, Suh CH, et al. Diffusion-weighted Magnetic Resonance Imaging for Predicting Response to Chemoradiation Therapy for Head and Neck Squamous Cell Carcinoma: A Systematic Review. Korean J Radiol 2019;20:649–61.

64. Abdel Razek AAK, Abdelaziz TT. Neck Imaging Reporting and Data System: What Does Radiologist Want to Know? J Comput Assist Tomogr 2020;44: 527–32.

65. Abdelaziz TT, Abdel Razk AAK, Ashour MMM, et al. Interreader reproducibility of the Neck Imaging Reporting and Data system (NI-RADS) lexicon for the detection of residual/recurrent disease in treated head and neck squamous cell carcinoma (HNSCC). Cancer Imaging 2020;20:61.

66. Abdel Razek AAK. Arterial spin labelling and diffusion-weighted magnetic resonance imaging in differentiation of recurrent head and neck cancer from post-radiation changes. J Laryngol Otol 2018; 132:923–8.

67. Abdel Razek AA, Gaballa G, Ashamalla G, et al. Dynamic Susceptibility Contrast Perfusion-Weighted Magnetic Resonance Imaging and Diffusion-Weighted Magnetic Resonance Imaging in Differentiating Recurrent Head and Neck Cancer From Postradiation Changes. J Comput Assist Tomogr 2015;39:849–54.

68. Razek AAKA. Diffusion tensor imaging in differentiation of residual head and neck squamous cell carcinoma from post-radiation changes. Magn Reson Imaging 2018;54:84–9.

69. Donta TS, Smoker WR. Head and neck cancer: carcinoma of unknown primary. Top Magn Reson Imaging 2007;18:281–92.

MR Imaging of Nasopharyngeal Carcinoma

Ann D. King, MBChB, FRCR, MD

KEYWORDS

- Nasopharyngeal carcinoma • MR imaging • Staging • Screening • Structured report

KEY POINTS

- Most nasopharyngeal carcinomas arise in endemic regions and are a radiosensitive undifferentiated carcinoma with a strong genetic basis and close association with the Epstein-Barr virus.
- MR imaging can detect early cancers that cannot be detected by endoscopy, including those identified by plasma Epstein-Barr virus–related marker screening.
- Primary and nodal MR staging is aided by a structured report and forms the cornerstone for radiation field planning and determining the need for chemotherapy.
- Distant metastases most commonly present after treatment.

INTRODUCTION

Nasopharyngeal carcinoma (NPC) is prevalent in distinct geographic regions, including southern China, Southeast Asia, North Africa, Greenland, and Alaska, and most commonly affects middle-aged men. Unlike most squamous cell carcinomas of the head and neck, those that develop in the nasopharynx of patients from endemic and certain nonendemic regions are mostly of the nonkeratinizing undifferentiated subtype. Several etiologic factors have been implicated in undifferentiated NPC,[1] the most predominant of which is the Epstein-Barr virus (EBV). NPC also has a strong genetic basis; nearly 12% of patients have a first-degree relative with NPC,[2] and the risk of NPC remains even after emigration.

NPC has a propensity for local invasion and for spreading to lymph nodes in the neck and at distant sites. Early-stage NPCs can be asymptomatic or can cause nonspecific symptoms such as nasal stuffiness, epistaxis, and hearing loss due to middle ear effusion from eustachian tube obstruction. Therefore, patients often present at a later stage with symptoms such as neurologic deficits or a lump in the neck. Distant metastases are uncommon at presentation (approximately 8% of patients),[3] and most are detectable only after treatment. Undifferentiated NPC is sensitive to radiotherapy. Intensity-modulated radiotherapy is used for locoregional disease, and chemotherapy is added for advanced cancers.

For several decades, MR imaging has been the technique of choice for staging of NPC in the head and neck.[4–8] MR imaging maps the sites and boundaries of the primary tumor and nodal metastases when planning for radiation therapy, and it also provides indicators of the need for chemotherapy. It remains the cornerstone of treatment planning because of its advantages over 18F-fluorodeoxyglucose positron emission tomography (PET)/computed tomography (CT) in mapping the extent of the primary tumor.[9,10] MR images are fused with those from the planning CT scan for three-dimensional radiation planning.[11] An advanced stage, especially N3 nodal disease, and high plasma EBV DNA levels are

Department of Imaging and Interventional Radiology, The Chinese University of Hong Kong, Prince of Wales Hospital, 30–32 Ngan Shing Street, Shatin, New Territories, Hong Kong SAR, China
E-mail address: king2015@cuhk.edu.hk

Magn Reson Imaging Clin N Am 30 (2022) 19–33
https://doi.org/10.1016/j.mric.2021.06.015
1064-9689/22/© 2021 The Author. Published by Elsevier Inc. This is an open access article under the CC BY-NC-ND license (http://creativecommons.org/licenses/by-nc-nd/4.0/).

often considered in NPC endemic regions to select patients at risk of distant metastases who would benefit from a whole-body PET/CT scan. Whole-body MR imaging and, more recently, PET-MR imaging are promising techniques with some advantages over PET-CT scanning.[12–14]

After treatment, MR imaging is used to detect and map residual or recurrent locoregional disease (which tends to have the same signal intensity as the original tumor) and to identify long-term radiation-induced complications.[15] PET-CT scanning has greater value in the posttreatment setting for the detection of locoregional recurrence and distant metastases; the latter are now the major cause of death from this disease. However, posttreatment imaging is beyond the scope of this article, which instead focuses on the use of MR imaging at the initial diagnosis for detection or early cancer, staging, and management and briefly covers differential diagnoses.

NORMAL ANATOMY

The nasopharynx lies behind the nasal cavity and just below and in front of the sloping skull base. It comprises a roof, lateral and posterior walls, and a floor formed by the soft palate. **Fig. 1** shows an MR image of the anatomy of the nasopharynx in a patient with early NPC. In brief, the lining of the nasopharynx comprises mucosa and submucosa and contains abundant lymphoid tissue, with focal accumulation in the center of the roof and the upper posterior wall of the site of the adenoids. The pharyngeal recess, also known as the fossa of Rosenmüller, is a posterolateral outpouching from each side of the nasopharynx that lies posterior to the eustachian tube and its expanded distal cartilaginous portion, known as the torus tubarius. The nasopharynx is bounded by fascia, which is best appreciated as a thin line on MR images along the lateral aspect of the nasopharynx and curving around the deep aspect of the pharyngeal recess. The levator veli palatini muscle and the eustachian tube enter the nasopharynx through a gap in the fascia. Lateral to the fascia is the tensor palatini muscle, the parapharyngeal fat space that contains the pterygoid venous plexus and the mandibular branch (V3) of the trigeminal nerve, and the medial and lateral pterygoid muscles. The retropharyngeal region contains the prevertebral muscles, Batson's venous plexus, lymph nodes, and lymphatic channels. The internal carotid artery lies posterolateral to the nasopharynx near the deep aspect of the pharyngeal recess. The anatomy of the skull base and other closely related structures is discussed in the section on Staging.

IMAGING PROTOCOLS

MR imaging is performed with a head and neck coil on a 1.5-T or 3.0-T MR imaging system. The optimal choice of sequences and planes is compromised by the scanning time. **Table 1** shows a suggested protocol. Two-dimensional sequences should be obtained with a slice thickness of 3 or 4 mm, with the scan coverage separated into upper and lower regions. It is suggested that at least one T1-weighted postcontrast sequence should be a spin-echo sequence without fat saturation and that diffusion-weighted imaging (DWI) should include a high b-value (ie, at least 800). The addition of a three-dimensional T1-weighted fat saturation after contrast gradient echo scan in the coronal plane allows for volumetric scanning with thin contiguous slices (0.8 mm with 0.4-mm overlap) and multiplanar reconstruction (0.4 mm).

IMAGING FINDINGS
Early Detection

NPC is one of the few cancers for which a blood test exists that can successfully screen for early-stage disease. Plasma EBV DNA screening for NPC was recently shown to successfully detect early-stage cancers in asymptomatic patients[16];

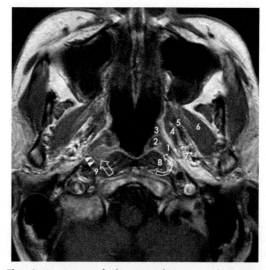

Fig. 1. Anatomy of the nasopharynx and primary stage T1 focal NPC. Axial T1-weighted postcontrast MR image shows a small focal cancer confined to the right pharyngeal recess (*open straight arrow*) and normal anatomy; pharyngeal recess on the left (*open curved arrow*), levator palatini muscle (1), torus tubarius (2), eustachian tube orifice (3), tensor palatini muscle (4), medial pterygoid muscle (5), lateral pterygoid muscle (6), parapharyngeal fat space (7), prevertebral muscles (8), internal carotid artery (9), and fascia (*arrow heads*).

Table 1
MR imaging protocol for nasopharyngeal carcinoma

Region	Sequences and Planes	[a]Coverage	Plane Tilt
Two-dimensional sequences			
Head/upper neck	Axial T2WFS, DWI, T1W before and after contrast	Above the skull base (level of superior orbital rim/inferior frontal sinuses) to lower margin of mandible or C3.	Perpendicular to posterior nasopharyngeal wall
	Sagittal T1W	Include medial half of maxillary sinus on each side.	Parallel to midline
	Coronal T2W and T1W after contrast	Mid portion of the hard palate to posterior spinal canal	Parallel to posterior nasopharyngeal wall
Neck	Axial T1W after contrast (±T2WFS)	Several sections above the lower margin of the mandible or C3 (overlap with the head/upper neck) to several sections below the suprasternal notch	Perpendicular to cervical spine
Three-dimensional sequences			
Nasopharynx and whole neck	Coronal volumetric T1WFS after contrast with reconstruction into coronal, axial, and sagittal planes	Mid portion of hard palate to posterior spinal canal	Parallel to posterior nasopharyngeal wall

Abbreviations: DWI, diffusion-weighted imaging; FS, Fat saturation; W, weighted.
[a] Coverage may need to be extended for the most advanced cases.

70% of NPCs were stage I or II carcinomas (compared with 21% from the literature data).[16] However, small cancers may be hidden from the endoscopic view in the pharyngeal recess (see **Fig. 1**), the corner of the roof, or the submucosa. Detection via endoscopy is also hampered by coexisting benign hyperplasia. Prospective studies on the performance of endoscopic examination and MR imaging have shown that MR imaging is highly sensitive[17] and that 11% of all NPCs in symptomatic patients were detected only by MR imaging,[17,18] and this figure increased to between 17% and 35% in asymptomatic patients screened for the disease, a high proportion of whom had early-stage cancer.[19,20] MR imaging can also detect early NPCs as long as 3 years before they are visible on endoscopy.[18,19]

Primary tumors tend to be nonnecrotic, homogeneous, or mildly heterogeneous, and the signal characteristics, that is, intermittent T2 signal intensity, low signal on the apparent diffusion coefficient (ADC) map (restricted diffusion), and moderate contrast enhancement on non–fat-saturated images, although early cancers may show less contrast enhancement,[21] are similar to those of other carcinomas (**Fig. 2**). Detection of NPC is straightforward when the tumor invades beyond the nasopharynx or when early-stage tumors form a focal mass on one side of the nasopharynx (see **Fig. 1**), but it is more challenging when an early-stage tumor forms a focal mass in the midline of the roof or spreads in a diffuse manner to involve both sides of the nasopharynx (see **Fig. 2**). In these cases, early-stage NPC must be differentiated from benign hyperplasia, which also causes enlargement of the adenoid and/or diffuse thickening of the nasopharyngeal walls.[21–24] NPC and benign hyperplasia may also coexist. Detection of NPC in these cases relies heavily on asymmetry in the thickness or signal intensity when comparing the right and left halves of the nasopharynx (see **Fig. 2A**), excluding

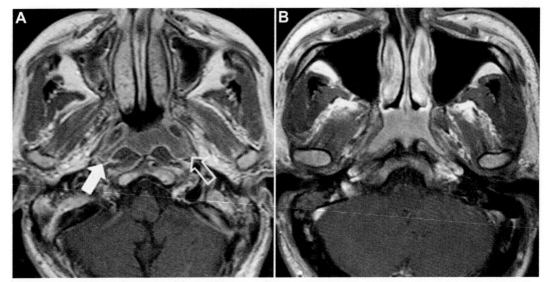

Fig. 2. Stage T1 NPC causing (*A*) diffuse asymmetrical thickening with low enhancement along the nasopharyngeal walls that is greater on the left (*open straight arrow*) than on the right (*solid straight arrow*) and (*B*) a central roof mass with moderate enhancement at the site of the adenoid without the normal adenoidal stripped pattern.

asymmetry caused by cysts. In addition, alternating septa of enhancement and columns of lower enhancement, which give adenoidal hyperplasia a stripped appearance, is lost in NPC (see **Fig. 2**B). Tumors that arise in the corner of the roof adjacent to benign hyperplasia in the adenoid may also displace the normal adenoidal striped pattern toward the opposite side. A four-grade system for MR imaging detection of NPC was first proposed in 2011[17] and was recently updated in 2020 to a five-grade system to achieve a sensitivity of 98% and a specificity of 90% for NPC detection.[25]

An MR imaging grading system was recently evaluated for use with a non–contrast-enhanced scan,[25] and studies on DWI[26] and automatic discrimination using artificial intelligence[27,28] have shown promise for expanding the role of MR imaging in EBV-related marker screening programs.

Staging

All sites of local invasion and sites of nodal metastases should be indicated in the MR imaging report for radiation field planning, and the stage also indicates when additional chemotherapy is required. The use of a structured report based on tumor, node, and metastasis staging[29] ensures that all relevant structures in the head and neck are scrutinized systematically and presented clearly and concisely to facilitate the transfer of information to the referring radiotherapist and oncologist. These sites are illustrated in the following

paragraphs, and a basic template for evaluation is shown in **Box 1**.

Local staging

The primary tumor size is only a weak predictor of outcome[30] and is not a criterion for NPC staging, but the size should be indicated on the report (using at least two dimensions; a single dimension does not reflect the volume of NPCs with irregular shapes[31]).

Stage T1 (nasopharynx, nasal cavity, and oropharynx) NPCs confined to the nasopharynx tend to form a focal mass in the pharyngeal recess or roof, but they may also be diffuse and involve both sides of the nasopharynx and fill the nasopharyngeal cavity (**Figs. 1** and **2B**).[21] Superficial spread outside the nasopharynx is included in stage T1; spread into the nasal cavity along the nasal septum and/or lateral walls is common but is often limited to the posterior aspect. NPC tends to spread in a superior direction rather than an inferior direction, so superficial spread to the oropharynx is usually accompanied by deep spread elsewhere.[5]

Stage T2 (parapharynx and retropharynx) Deep invasion of the soft tissues that lie lateral and posterior to the nasopharynx involves the parapharynx, retropharynx, and carotid sheath (**Fig. 3**). The parapharyngeal fat space may be compressed by tumor confined within the nasopharynx (TI) instead of being invaded (T2). In either scenario, middle ear or mastoid effusion is common.

Box 1
Suggested template for staging nasopharyngeal carcinoma

Primary Tumor

- (*T1*) Nasopharyngeal carcinoma measuring (X × X cm) and predominantly arising from (left/right side). Nasal cavity and oropharynx
- (*T2*) Parapharyngeal, retropharyngeal, and carotid sheath
- (*T3*) Skull base bones (*clivus, right and left pterygoid processes, right and left petrous apices and body of the sphenoid*); foramina (*rotundum, ovale, and lacerum*); canals (*vidian, pterygopalatine, and hypoglossal*); fissures (*pterygomaxillary, orbital [inferior and superior] and petroclival*); pterygopalatine fossa; large tumors, jugular foramen, optic canal, infraorbital canal, sphenoid wings, and occipital condyles. Upper cervical spine, sphenoid, ethmoid, and maxillary sinus
- (*T4*) Cavernous sinus, cranial nerves (especially V3, V2, infraorbital, auriculotemporal, and 12th), middle and posterior cranial fossa dura orbit, infratemporal fossa, parotid gland, and hypopharynx

Nodal Metastases

- General description for staging. Unilateral/bilateral (*N1/N2*); size of the largest node/conglomeration of nodes (*>6 cm N3*); groups below the level of the cricoid cartilage (*N3*). Necrosis and extranodal tumor spread
- Sites of metastatic nodes (right and left sides). retropharyngeal; parotid/periparotid; submental (level IA); submandibular (level IB); upper, middle, and lower internal jugular chain (levels II, III, IV); posterior triangle (levels VA, VB); and paratracheal (level VI). Mediastinal and axillary (if partially covered on the scan)

Distant metastases (M1) and second primary tumors

- Lung apices and bones

Additional findings

- Middle ear/mastoid effusion
- Mucosal inflammatory changes in the paranasal sinuses
- Other findings

Conclusion

- Nasopharyngeal carcinoma with unilateral/bilateral cervical nodal metastases (Head and neck scan stage *T_N_M_* according to the 8th edition of AJCC)

Spread to the prevertebral muscles in the retropharynx can be subtle or bulky providing the main route of inferior spread.

Stage T3 (skull base, paranasal sinuses, and cervical spine) Skull base invasion is common (approximately 65%)[5,32] and may be the only site of invasion outside the nasopharynx (**Figs. 4–7**). The skull base should be assessed systematically at the most common sites of invasion, which comprise six bony sites (*clivus, right and left pterygoid processes, right and left petrous apices, and body of the sphenoid, especially the floor of the sphenoid sinus*); three foramina (*rotundum, ovale, and lacerum*); three canals (*vidian, pterygopalatine, and hypoglossal*); three fissures (*pterygomaxillary, orbital, and petroclival*); and one fossa (*pterygopalatine fossa*). Tumor in the pterygopalatine fossa spreads in many sites, including the nasal cavity (via the sphenopalatine foramen), middle cranial fossa (via foramen rotundum), orbit (via the inferior orbital fissure), infratemporal fossa (via the pterygomaxillary fissure), and oropharynx (via the pterygopalatine canal). Larger tumors invade beyond these sites such as to the jugular foramen, optic canal, infraorbital canal, wings of the sphenoid, occipital condyles, and upper cervical spine. The roof of the nasopharynx forms the floor of the sphenoid sinus, so the sphenoid sinus frequently undergoes invasion by NPC, whereas invasion of the ethmoid sinus and maxillary sinus is less frequent.

Stage T4 (brain, cranial nerves, orbits, parotid gland, infratemporal fossa, and hypopharynx) Intracranial invasion most commonly involves the cavernous sinus and dura of the middle and posterior cranial fossa (see **Figs. 5** and **6**). Spread into the cavernous sinus may occur through the foramina, along the internal carotid artery, or directly through the bone. The cranial nerves are frequently surrounded and may be invaded by tumor in the parapharyngeal region, skull base foramina, cavernous sinus and orbital fissures, especially the mandibular nerve (foramen ovale and parapharyngeal region), the maxillary nerve (foramen rotundum), and the hypoglossal nerve (hypoglossal canal). Perineural spread distal to the main tumor bulk is less common, but it is important to scrutinize distal pathways such as the auriculotemporal nerve in the parotid gland (via the mandibular nerve) and the infraorbital nerve in the floor of the orbit (via the maxillary nerve) which lie outside the standard radiation field. Muscle denervation in the tongue or in the muscles of mastication provides clues regarding

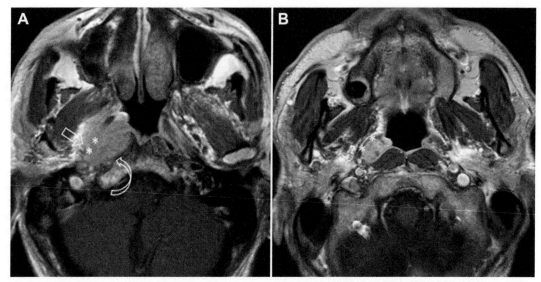

Fig. 3. Primary stage T2 NPC. Axial T1-weighted postcontrast MR image shows a case of (*A*) NPC in the right pharyngeal recess with early invasion through the levator palatini muscle (*) into the parapharynx (*open straight arrow*) and into the retropharynx (*open curved arrow*) compared with (*B*) stage T1 NPC causing a focal mass in the right pharyngeal recess that is confined to the nasopharynx and displaces and thins the levator palatini muscle (*).

cranial nerve involvement. Invasion of the infra-temporal fossa (defined for NPC staging purposes as anterior to the anterior margin of the lateral pterygoid muscle) is usually via the pterygomaxillary fissure or through the lateral pterygoid muscle. The parotid gland, orbit, and hypopharynx are further indicators of the most advanced patterns of local disease.

Nodal staging

Nodal metastases occur in approximately 80% of patients,[33] but even though small early T-stage tumors can have extensive nodal metastases, they are not necessarily present in late T-stage tumors (**Fig. 8**). Diagnosis of a metastatic NPC node by MR imaging relies on criteria similar to those used for other carcinomas of the head and neck,

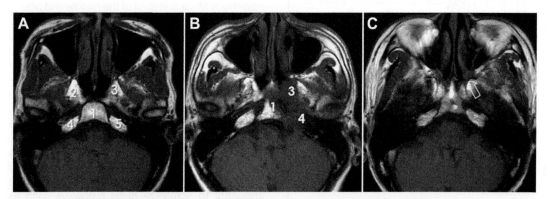

Fig. 4. Primary stage T3 NPC with invasion into skull base bones. Axial T1-weighted MR images of the skull base superior to the roof of the nasopharynx show (*A*) a normal skull base with high T1 signal intensity of the fatty bone marrow in five of the six bones invaded commonly by NPC: clivus (1), right pterygoid process (2), left pterygoid process (3), right petrous apex (4), and left petrous apex (5); (*B*) invasion into the clivus (1), left pterygoid process (3), and left petrous apex (4); and (*C*) subtle invasion of the pterygoid process and left pterygopalatine fossa (*open straight arrow*) with early invasion on the right side as well. The floor and walls of the sphenoid sinus are best assessed in the coronal plane (not shown).

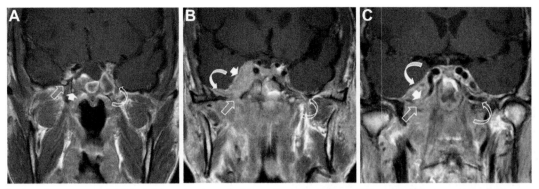

Fig. 5. Primary stage T3 NPC with invasion into skull base foramina. Coronal T1-weighted postcontrast MR images show the foramina invaded commonly by NPC (*open straight arrows*) and normal foramina on the opposite side (*open curved arrows*). From anterior to posterior: (*A*) foramen rotundum, which contains the maxillary nerve, the vidian canal is also invaded (*solid straight arrow*); (*B*) foramen ovale, which contains the mandibular nerve and invasion of cavernous sinus (*solid straight arrow*) and dura of the middle cranial fossa (*solid curved arrow*); (*C*) foramen lacerum just below the horizontal portion of the internal carotid artery, the artery is encased (*solid straight arrow*) and intracranial invasion into the cavernous sinus (*solid curved arrow*).

such as size, necrosis, and extracapsular extension.

Nodes are frequently bilateral and may show necrosis and extranodal spread. The first groups of metastatic spread are either the lateral retropharyngeal or the upper internal jugular chain (level II), especially those that lie posterior to the vein (IIA and IIB).[6,7,34,35] The lateral retropharyngeal nodes are located between the internal carotid artery and the anterolateral margin of the prevertebral muscle and extend from approximately the level of the lateral recess of the nasopharynx to the third cervical vertebra.[6] The minimum axial dimension for retropharyngeal nodes is controversial, and 5 mm and 6 mm have both been advocated.[6,36] The nodes that lie immediately deep to the lateral margin of the recess are separated from the primary tumor by a thin line of fascia that is best appreciated on an MR image,[9] but the fascia may be disrupted or totally lost if direct spread occurs between the two sites. The medial retropharyngeal nodes lie in the midline anterior to the prevertebral muscles. Discrete nodes at this site are rarely seen, but it is likely that spread along the abundant lymphatic channels in this region contributes to the extensive retropharyngeal pattern of inferior spread seen in some patients. Orderly spread down the neck occurs along the internal jugular chain and/or spinal accessory chain in the posterior triangle to the lower neck and the

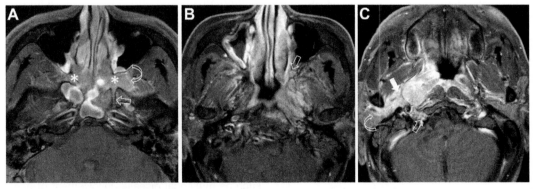

Fig. 6. Primary stage T3 NPC with invasion into skull base canals. Axial T1-weighted postcontrast MR images with fat saturation show the canals invaded commonly by NPC (*straight open arrows*). From superior to inferior: (*A*) vidian canal (connects the pterygopalatine fossa (***) and foramen lacerum), tumor is also spreading from the pterygopalatine fossa (***) to the infratemporal fossa via the pterygomaxillary fissure (*open curved arrow*); (*B*) pterygopalatine canal (connects the pterygopalatine fossa and palate); and (*C*) hypoglossal canal. Note also extensive parapharyngeal invasion (*solid straight arrow*) and perineural spread into the parotid gland along the auriculotemporal nerve (*open curved arrow*).

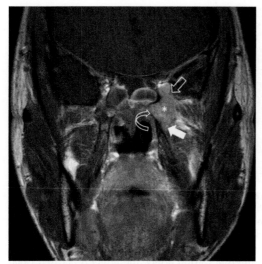

Fig. 7. Primary stage T3 NPC with invasion into skull base pterygopalatine fossa/fissures. Coronal T1-weighted postcontrast MR images show tumor in the pterygopalatine fossa (*) with spread into the inferior orbital fissure (*open straight arrow*) to the orbit; the sphenopalatine foramen (*open curved arrow*) to the nasal cavity; pterygopalatine canal to the palate (*solid straight arrow*). Tumor in the pterygopalatine also spreads along the pterygomaxillary fissure to the infratemporal fossa (**Fig. 6**A), vidian canal to the foramen lacerum (see **Fig. 6**A), and foramen rotundum to the middle cranial fossa (not shown).

supraclavicular fossa. Involvement of the parotid/periparotid, submandibular, and submental nodes is less common.[6]

Nodal staging differs from that of other head and neck cancers. It is based on (1) laterality, unilateral or bilateral disease (N1 or N2, respectively, except for bilateral retropharyngeal nodes, which are staged as N1); (2) size, any node larger than 6 cm (N3); and (3) involvement of nodes in the lower neck below the level of the cricoid cartilage (N3). The best method for measuring the maximum size for staging purposes is controversial, but a recent study showed that the maximum measurement of matted or contiguous nodes may be the best predictor of outcome.[37] The nodal volume[38-40] and extracapsular extension[41,42] also show promise for prediction of the outcome.

Staging of distant metastases

Identification of distant metastases on the head and neck staging MR scan is uncommon, but they may sometimes be found in the lung apices, while bony metastases in the cervical spine are rare.

Functional MR Imaging Markers for the Prediction of Response

Several promising pretreatment and intratreatment functional MR imaging markers are available for the prediction of short-term and long-term treatment response, including markers from DWI,[43-46] dynamic contrast-enhanced MR imaging (DCE-MR imaging),[47-49] and amide proton transfer imaging (APT imaging).[50,51] High pretreatment ADC from DWI or pure diffusion coefficient (D) from intravoxel incoherent motion is an indicator of poor treatment response[44-46] (**Fig. 9**). These results are in keeping with those from other head and neck cancers where high ADC/D is associated with histologic findings seen in resistant tumors, such as low cell density and high stromal content. In the early intratreatment period, the ADC rises as cell death and blood supply increase. Similar to other head and neck cancers, NPC with a higher rise in ADC indicates a better response based on short-term outcomes.[43]

There are only limited DCE data. Two studies found poor long-term response in tumors with a large extracellular extravascular volume, as indicated by a high Ve,[47,49] while another found poor short-term response in tumors with a low Ktrans.[48]

APT imaging is a fairly new chemical exchange-saturation transfer MRI technique that has recently been applied to NPC. Preliminary results show high pretreatment APT values or a rise in APT in the early-intratreatment period may be an indicator of poor response.[50,51] Parametric imaging has the potential to provide more comprehensive treatment prediction, for example, diffusion may have predictive advantages for NPC locoregional resistance and APT for distant metastases.[46,50]

Diagnostic Criteria and Differential Diagnosis

Other malignant and nonmalignant diseases produce abnormalities centered in the nasopharynx with or without spread to adjacent structures. The MR imaging appearance of NPC may overlap with that of these other processes, so diagnosis requires biopsy and histologic examination in most cases. The most common differential diagnosis for NPC is non-Hodgkin's lymphoma (**Fig. 10**). Lymphoma is commonly exophytic, but it may be invasive and mimic early- or late-stage NPC. The diagnosis of lymphoma relies on clues such as multifocal disease, involvement of unexpected nodal groups,[52,53] and differences in functional MR imaging parameters. Notably, the ADC and Ktrans of lymphoma are lower than those of undifferentiated NPC.[54-56] Other tumors that originate in the nasopharynx include adenoid cystic carcinoma, sarcoma and radiation-induced

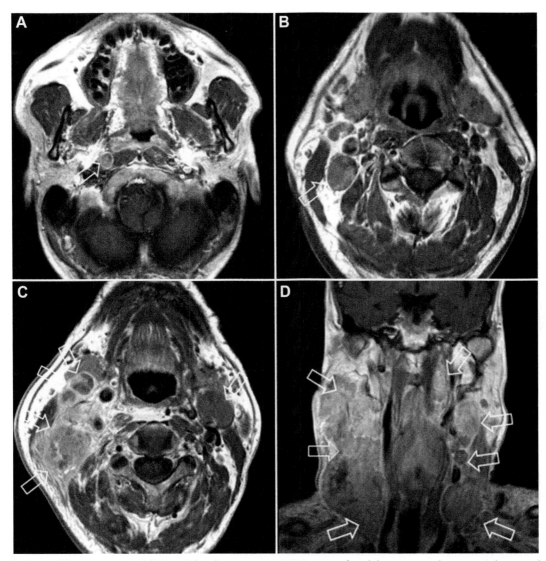

Fig. 8. Nodal metastases. Axial T1-weighted postcontrast MR images of nodal metastases (*open straight arrows*). (*A*) Lateral retropharyngeal nodes and (*B*) upper internal jugular nodes (level II), including those posterior to the internal jugular vein (level IIA/B), are both common groups for the first echelons of nodal spread, and (*C*) bilateral nodes, extranodal spread, and necrosis are common. (Bilateral nodal metastases increase the stage from N1 to N2, except for bilateral retropharyngeal nodes, which are still classified as N1.) Coronal T1-weighted postcontrast image shows (*D*) orderly spread down the neck with bilateral nodal metastases and the most advanced nodal stage comprising bulky matted nodes larger than 6 cm in maximum dimension (N3) and involvement of groups in the lower neck (N3).

sarcoma, plasmacytoma, melanoma, and (rarely) pleomorphic adenoma. Inflammatory and infectious disease processes include skull base osteomyelitis,[57] nasopharyngeal tuberculosis, sarcoid granulomatosis with polyangiitis, and amyloid and IgG4-related disease.[58] Discussion of these pathologies is beyond the scope of this article, but diseases other than NPC should be suspected when the nasopharyngeal abnormality is very heterogeneous or necrotic or when the scan shows calcification (amyloid or sarcoma), high T2 signal intensity (sarcoma and infection), low T2 signal intensity (IgG4-related disease), high signal intensity on the ADC map (infection, inflammation, pleomorphic adenoma), marked contrast enhancement (granulomatous polyps, infection, vascular tumors), multifocal disease, or prominent perineural spread (adenoid cystic carcinoma).

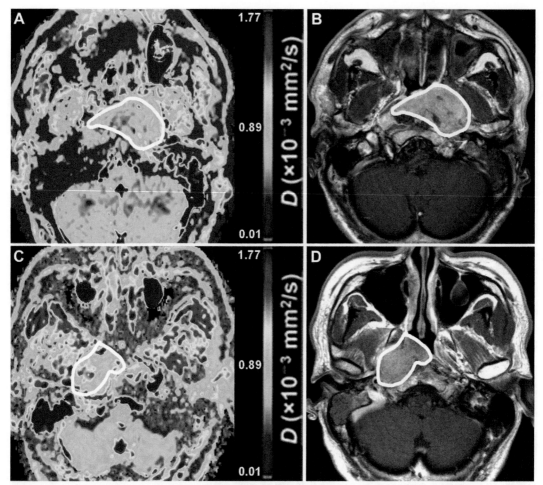

Fig. 9. The pretreatment pure diffusion maps derived from intravoxel incoherent motion diffusion weighted imaging and contrast-enhanced MR images of a primary nasopharyngeal carcinoma in two patients with NPC; one without relapse (*A, B*) in whom the pure diffusion coefficient was 0.62×10^{-3} mm^2/s and one with relapse (*C, D*) in whom the pure diffusion coefficient was higher at 0.81×10^{-3} mm^2/s.

PEARLS, PITFALLS, AND VARIANTS
Detection

- The pharyngeal recess and lateral aspect of the roof are common sites of early NPC and require scrutiny in the axial and coronal planes, respectively, to ensure that no small tumors are missed.
- The contrast-enhanced striped appearance of adenoidal hyperplasia is best appreciated on a scan dedicated to the nasopharynx.
- Benign hyperplasia is common in the general population and may be mildly asymmetrical on an MR image, so the MR grading systems should be applied only to patients in whom NPC is suspected.

Staging

T1 and T2 staging

- Tumor sites within the nasopharynx do not influence staging or radiation planning.
- The C1/2 junction is a useful landmark for demarcating the junction of the nasopharynx and oropharynx and can overcome difficulties with the use of the soft palate.

T3 staging

- For skull base invasion, it is helpful to begin by assessing the five of the six major bones on the axial T1-weighted image immediately above the level of the nasopharynx (see

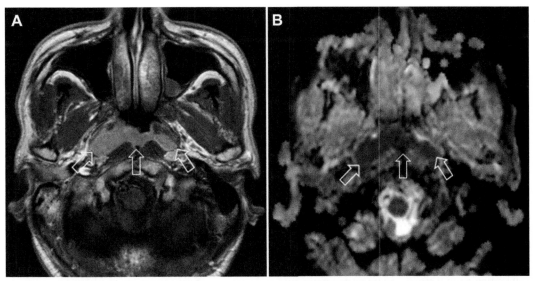

Fig. 10. Non-Hodgkin's lymphoma (*open straight arrows*). (*A*) Nasopharyngeal lymphoma is indistinguishable from NPC on this axial T1-weighted postcontrast MR image, although (*B*) very low signal intensity on the apparent diffusion coefficient map is a clue to the diagnosis. Diagnosis requires biopsy, but other features on MR images of the head and neck that suggest lymphoma include multisite involvement or nodes outside the expected pathway of metastatic spread for NPC (such as parotid/periparotid, submandibular, and external jugular chain nodes).

Fig. 4) for any loss of high T1 signal intensity of fatty bone marrow. One must also verify that signal loss in the pterygoid processes or petrous apices is not due to fluid in aerated bone.

- Assessment of all skull base bones, foramina, canals, fissures, and pterygopalatine fossae requires multiple sequences and planes. In addition to the axial plane, the coronal plane is valuable for assessment of the body of the sphenoid (including the sphenoid sinus floor), foramina, vidian canals, and orbital fissures, and the sagittal plane is valuable for assessment of the clivus.
- Skull base invasion may be of small volume and easily missed, so one must check for sites of anterior spread into the medial aspect of the pterygoid processes or pterygopalatine fossa and for spread into the floor of the sphenoid sinus and clivus. The presence of tumor in the pterygopalatine fossa requires systematic scrutiny of all connecting sites, including subtle superior spread to the inferior orbital fissure.
- Red marrow hyperplasia or edema may cause heterogeneous or generalized loss of the fatty bone marrow signal, especially in the clivus. To identify tumor invasion, one must look for a signal intensity similar to that of tumor on

all sequences that are in direct continuity with the primary tumor in the nasopharynx.
- Sites of bony sclerosis adjacent to the tumor should be included in the report because they are usually covered in the radiation field.
- Even large areas of bone invasion will be overlooked on the postcontrast T1-weighted MR image without fat saturation.

T4 staging

- Compared with local invasion, the emissary veins in the hypoglossal nerve canal and inferior petrosal sinus and basilar plexus posterior to the clivus show more marked contrast enhancement.
- Denervation in the pterygoid muscles adjacent to the tumor is characterized by less diffusion restriction and preservation of muscle striations.

N staging

- The minimum axial diameter is used to identify a metastatic node, but the maximum diameter is used to designate the nodal stage.
- The difficulty in defining the supraclavicular fossa boundary has been overcome by using the lower border of the cricoid cartilage as the landmark to define N3 disease.

- A nodule in the parotid gland has a high chance of being a benign salivary gland tumor than a metastatic node.
- Superior cervical sympathetic ganglia occur in a location similar to that of metastatic retropharyngeal nodes. The ganglia, however, are usually bilateral and more fusiform in shape, show greater contrast enhancement and less restriction of diffusion, and contain a small T2 hypointense spot. These ganglia also tend to have a more posterolateral location, and the minimum axial dimension is usually smaller than that of a metastatic node.[59]

WHAT THE REFERRING PHYSICIAN NEEDS TO KNOW
Detection

- In a patient in whom NPC is suspected and who has normal results on an endoscopic examination or an indeterminate submucosal bulge or enlarged adenoid, the detection of a small cancer on an MR image guides the site and depth of biopsy (which is especially important for tumors in the pharyngeal recess near the internal carotid artery). Small suspected tumors in the pharyngeal recess may require biopsy under navigation and general anesthesia or close surveillance via MR imaging.
- Normal MR imaging reassures the physician that the patient does not have NPC and that sampling biopsies are not required.

Staging

- The MR imaging report should indicate all sites of local tumor invasion and nodal metastases for radiation planning. Special note should be made when the NPC (1) approaches or invades the orbit, neurologic structures (ie, the cavernous sinus, temporal lobes, brain stem, cervical cord, or brachial plexus), or salivary glands (which are normally spared from the radiation field to reduce xerostomia) or (2) spreads to sites distal to the main tumor bulk (ie, perineural spread especially along the infraorbital and auriculotemporal nerves).
- Indications for the addition of chemotherapy may vary between centers, but in general, advanced local disease (T3/T4, and in some institutions, bulky T2) or nodal disease (N2/3) is an indication for concurrent chemoradiation. Neoadjuvant chemotherapy is also used to shrink the tumor before concurrent chemoradiation when a bulky primary or nodal metastasis lies close to neurologic structures,

when extensive perineural spread is found, or when the oropharynx is involved (to reduce the severity of radiation-induced mucositis).
- Advanced-stage disease (especially N3) is a marker for distant metastases and an indication for PET/CT scanning at centers where it is not routinely performed. The detection of distant metastases may lead to a change in the treatment of primary and nodal disease from curative to palliative.

SUMMARY

MR imaging plays a major role in the imaging of head and neck NPC because of its ability to detect and depict the boundaries of the primary tumor site and regional nodal metastases. The staging report is critical for staging and for planning radiation or chemoradiation therapy. A structured approach ensures that all sites that influence management in this complex region are covered in the report. New morphologic and function parameters for MR imaging show promise for improving outcome prediction. MR imaging also plays a new role in the detection of early-stage cancers that cannot be detected via endoscopy, and this role is likely to expand in regions in which NPC is endemic as the use of NPC screening programs becomes more widespread. Distant metastases tend to present after treatment, but PET-MR imaging shows promise for whole-body evaluation of patients in whom distant metastases are detected at the initial presentation.

ACKNOWLEDGMENTS

The author would like to acknowledge Dr Qi-Yong Ai from the Department of Imaging and Interventional Radiology, The Chinese University of Hong Kong, for literature search, content editing, and image preparation.

DISCLOSURE

The author declares no conflicts of interest.

REFERENCES

1. Tsao SW, Yip YL, Tsang CM, et al. Etiological factors of nasopharyngeal carcinoma. Oral Oncol 2014;50: 330–8.
2. Ouyang PY, Su Z, Mao YP, et al. Prognostic impact of family history in southern Chinese patients with undifferentiated nasopharyngeal carcinoma. Br J Cancer 2013;109:788–94.
3. Chua MLK, Ong SC, Wee JTS, et al. Comparison of 4 modalities for distant metastasis staging in

endemic nasopharyngeal carcinoma. Head Neck 2009;31:346–54.

4. Ng SH, Chang TC, Ko SF, et al. Nasopharyngeal carcinoma: MRI and CT assessment. Neuroradiology 1997;39:741–6.

5. King AD, Lam WWM, Leung SF, et al. MRI of local disease in nasopharyngeal carcinoma: Tumour extent vs tumour stage. Br J Radiol 1999;72:734–41.

6. King AD, Ahuja AT, Leung SF, et al. Neck node metastases from nasopharyngeal carcinoma: MR imaging of patterns of disease. Head Neck 2000;22:275–81.

7. Ng S-H, Chang JT-C, Chan S-C, et al. Nodal metastases of nasopharyngeal carcinoma: patterns of disease on MRI and FDG PET. Eur J Nucl Med Mol Imaging 2004;31:1073–80.

8. Abdel Khalek Abdel Razek A, King A. MRI and CT of nasopharyngeal carcinoma. AJR Am J Roentgenol 2012;198:11–8.

9. King AD, Ma BB, Yau YY, et al. The impact of 18F-FDG PET/CT on assessment of nasopharyngeal carcinoma at diagnosis. Br J Radiol 2008;81:291–8.

10. Chen W, Li J, Hong L, et al. Comparison of MRI , CT and 18F-FDG PET/CT in the diagnosis of local and metastatic of nasopharyngeal carcinomas : an updated meta analysis of clinical studies. Am J Transl Res 2016;8:4532–47.

11. Emami B, Sethi A, Petruzzelli GJ. Influence of MRI on target volume delineation and IMRT planning in nasopharyngeal carcinoma. Int J Radiat Oncol Biol Phys 2003;57:481–8.

12. Ng SH, Chan SC, Yen TC, et al. Pretreatment evaluation of distant-site status in patients with nasopharyngeal carcinoma: accuracy of whole-body MRI at 3-Tesla and FDG-PET-CT. Eur Radiol 2009;19:2965–76.

13. Ng S-H, Chan S-C, Yen T-C, et al. Comprehensive imaging of residual/recurrent nasopharyngeal carcinoma using whole-body MRI at 3 T compared with FDG-PET-CT. Eur Radiol 2010;20:2229–40.

14. Chan SC, Yeh CH, Yen TC, et al. Clinical utility of simultaneous whole-body 18F-FDG PET/MRI as a single-step imaging modality in the staging of primary nasopharyngeal carcinoma. Eur J Nucl Med Mol Imaging 2018;45:1297–308.

15. King AD, Ahuja AT, Yeung DK, et al. Delayed complications of radiotherapy treatment for nasopharyngeal carcinoma: imaging findings. Clin Radiol 2007;62:195–203.

16. Chan KCA, Woo JKS, King A, et al. Analysis of plasma epstein–barr virus DNA to screen for nasopharyngeal cancer. N Engl J Med 2017;377:513–22.

17. King AD, Vlantis AC, Bhatia KSS, et al. Primary nasopharyngeal carcinoma: diagnostic accuracy of MR imaging versus that of endoscopy and endoscopic biopsy. Radiology 2011;258:531–7.

18. King AD, Vlantis AC, Yuen TWC, et al. Detection of nasopharyngeal carcinoma by MR imaging: diagnostic accuracy of MRI compared with endoscopy and endoscopic biopsy based on long-term follow-up. Am J Neuroradiol 2015;36:2380–5.

19. King AD, Woo JKS, Ai QY, et al. Complementary roles of MRI and endoscopic examination in the early detection of nasopharyngeal carcinoma. Ann Oncol 2019;30:977–82.

20. Liu Z, Li H, Yu K, et al. Comparison of new magnetic resonance imaging grading system to conventional endoscopy for the early detection of nasopharyngeal carcinoma. Cancer 2021. https://doi.org/10.1002/cncr.33552.

21. King AD, Wong LYS, Law BKH, et al. MR imaging criteria for the detection of nasopharyngeal carcinoma: discrimination of early-stage primary tumors from benign hyperplasia. Am J Neuroradiol 2018;39:515–23.

22. Bhatia KSS, King AD, Vlantis AC, et al. Nasopharyngeal mucosa and adenoids: appearance at MR imaging. Radiology 2012;263:437–43.

23. Wang M-L, Wei X-E, Yu M-M, et al. Value of contrast-enhanced MRI in the differentiation between nasopharyngeal lymphoid hyperplasia and T1 stage nasopharyngeal carcinoma. Radiol Med 2017;122(10):743–51.

24. Surov A, Ryl I, Bartel-Friedrich S, et al. MRI of nasopharyngeal adenoid hypertrophy. Neuroradiol J 2016;29:408–12.

25. King AD, Woo JKS, Ai Q-Y, et al. Early detection of cancer: evaluation of MR imaging grading systems in patients with suspected nasopharyngeal carcinoma. Am J Neuroradiol 2020;41:515–20.

26. Ai QY, King AD, Chan JSM, et al. Distinguishing early-stage nasopharyngeal carcinoma from benign hyperplasia using intravoxel incoherent motion diffusion-weighted MRI. Eur Radiol 2019;29:5627–34.

27. Ke L, Deng Y, Xia W, et al. Development of a self-constrained 3D DenseNet model in automatic detection and segmentation of nasopharyngeal carcinoma using magnetic resonance images. Oral Oncol 2020;110:104862.

28. Wong LM, King AD, Ai Q-YH, et al. Convolutional neural network for discriminating nasopharyngeal carcinoma and benign hyperplasia on MRI. Eur Radiol 2021;31(6):3856–63.

29. Amin MB, Edge SB, Greene FL, et al, editors. AJCC cancer staging manual. 8th ed. New York (NY): Springer; 2017.

30. Feng M, Wang W, Fan Z, et al. Tumor volume is an independent prognostic indicator of local control in nasopharyngeal carcinoma patients treated with intensity-modulated radiotherapy. Radiat Oncol 2013;8:208.

31. King AD, Zee B, Yuen EHY, et al. Nasopharyngeal cancers: which method should be used to measure these irregularly shaped tumors on cross-sectional imaging? Int J Radiat Oncol Biol Phys 2007;69: 148–54.

32. Li YZ, Cai PQ, Xie CM, et al. Nasopharyngeal cancer: impact of skull base invasion on patients prognosis and its potential implications on TNM staging. Eur J Radiol 2013;82:e107–11.

33. Au KH, Ngan RKC, Ng AWY, et al. Treatment outcomes of nasopharyngeal carcinoma in modern era after intensity modulated radiotherapy (IMRT) in Hong Kong: a report of 3328 patients (HKNPCSG 1301 study). Oral Oncol 2018;77:16–21.

34. Liu L-Z, Zhang G-Y, Xie C-M, et al. Magnetic resonance imaging of retropharyngeal lymph node metastasis in nasopharyngeal carcinoma: patterns of spread. Int J Radiat Oncol Biol Phys 2006;66: 721–30.

35. Wang XS, Hu CS, Ying HM, et al. Patterns of retropharyngeal node metastasis in nasopharyngeal carcinoma. Int J Radiat Oncol Biol Phys 2009;73: 194–201.

36. Zhang G, Liu L, Wei W, et al. Radiologic criteria of retropharyngeal lymph node metastasis in nasopharyngeal carcinoma treated with radiation therapy. Radiology 2010;255:605–12.

37. Ai QY, King AD, Mo FKF, et al. Staging nodal metastases in nasopharyngeal carcinoma: which method should be used to measure nodal dimension on MRI? Clin Radiol 2018;73:640–6.

38. Chen FP, Zhou GQ, Qi ZY, et al. Prognostic value of cervical nodal tumor volume in nasopharyngeal carcinoma: analysis of 1230 patients with positive cervical nodal metastasis. PLoS One 2017;12:1–13.

39. Ai Q-Y, King AD, Mo FKF, et al. Prediction of distant metastases from nasopharyngeal carcinoma: improved diagnostic performance of MRI using nodal volume in N1 and N2 stage disease. Oral Oncol 2017;69:74–9.

40. Yuan H, Ai QY, Kwong DLW, et al. Cervical nodal volume for prognostication and risk stratification of patients with nasopharyngeal carcinoma, and implications on the TNM-staging system. Sci Rep 2017;7:10387.

41. Mao YP, Liang SB, Liu LZ, et al. The N staging system in nasopharyngeal carcinoma with radiation therapy oncology group guidelines for lymph node levels based on magnetic resonance imaging. Clin Cancer Res 2008;14:7497–503.

42. Ai Q-Y, King AD, Poon DMC, et al. Extranodal extension is a criterion for poor outcome in patients with metastatic nodes from cancer of the nasopharynx. Oral Oncol 2019;88:124–30.

43. Hong J, Yao Y, Zhang Y, et al. Value of magnetic resonance diffusion-weighted imaging for the prediction of radiosensitivity in nasopharyngeal carcinoma. Otolaryngol Neck Surg 2013;149: 707–13.

44. Zhang Y, Liu X, Zhang Y, et al. Prognostic value of the primary lesion apparent diffusion coefficient (ADC) in nasopharyngeal carcinoma: a retrospective study of 541 cases. Sci Rep 2015;5:12242.

45. Tu N, Zhong Y, Wang X, et al. Treatment response prediction of nasopharyngeal carcinoma based on histogram analysis of diffusional kurtosis imaging. Am J Neuroradiol 2019;40:326–33.

46. Qamar S, King AD, Ai QYH, et al. Pre-treatment intravoxel incoherent motion diffusion-weighted imaging predicts treatment outcome in nasopharyngeal carcinoma. Eur J Radiol 2020;129:109127.

47. Qin Y, Yu X, Hou J, et al. Prognostic value of the pre-treatment primary lesion quantitative dynamic contrast-enhanced magnetic resonance imaging for nasopharyngeal carcinoma. Acad Radiol 2019; 26:1473–82.

48. Zheng D, Yue Q, Ren W, et al. Early responses assessment of neoadjuvant chemotherapy in nasopharyngeal carcinoma by serial dynamic contrast-enhanced MR imaging. Magn Reson Imaging 2017;35:125–31.

49. Chan S-C, Yeh C-H, Chang JT-C, et al. Combing MRI perfusion and 18F-FDG PET/CT metabolic biomarkers helps predict survival in advanced nasopharyngeal carcinoma: a prospective multimodal imaging study. Cancers (Basel) 2021;13:1550.

50. Qamar S, King AD, Ai QYH, et al. Pre-treatment amide proton transfer imaging predicts treatment outcome in nasopharyngeal carcinoma. Eur Radiol 2020;30:6339–47.

51. Qamar S, King AD, Ai QY, et al. Amide proton transfer MRI detects early changes in nasopharyngeal carcinoma: providing a potential imaging marker for treatment response. Eur Arch Otorhinolaryngol 2019;276:505–12.

52. King AD, Lei KIK, Richards PS, et al. Non-Hodgkin's lymphoma of the nasopharynx: CT and MR imaging. Clin Radiol 2003;58:621–5.

53. Liu XW, Xie CM, Mo YX, et al. Magnetic resonance imaging features of nasopharyngeal carcinoma and nasopharyngeal non-Hodgkin's lymphoma: are there differences? Eur J Radiol 2012;81: 1146–54.

54. Fong D, Bhatia KSS, Yeung D, et al. Diagnostic accuracy of diffusion-weighted MR imaging for nasopharyngeal carcinoma, head and neck lymphoma and squamous cell carcinoma at the primary site. Oral Oncol 2010;46:603–6.

55. Song C, Cheng P, Cheng J, et al. Differential diagnosis of nasopharyngeal carcinoma and nasopharyngeal lymphoma based on DCE-MRI and RESOLVE-DWI. Eur Radiol 2020;30:110–8.

56. Lee FK, King AD, Ma BB-Y, et al. Dynamic contrast enhancement magnetic resonance imaging (DCE-MRI) for differential diagnosis in head and neck cancers. Eur J Radiol 2012;81:784–8.

57. Goh JPN, Karandikar A, Loke SC, et al. Skull base osteomyelitis secondary to malignant otitis externa mimicking advanced nasopharyngeal cancer: MR imaging features at initial presentation. Am J Otolaryngol 2017;38:466–71.

58. Liu J, Zhang B, Sun H, et al. Immunoglobulin G4-related disease in the skull base mimicking nasopharyngeal carcinoma. J Craniofac Surg 2015;26: e144–5.

59. Yokota H, Mukai H, Hattori S, et al. MR imaging of the superior cervical ganglion and inferior ganglion of the vagus nerve: structures that can mimic pathologic retropharyngeal lymph nodes. Am J Neuroradiol 2018;39:170–6.

MR imaging of Oral Cavity and Oropharyngeal Cancer

Ahmed Abdel Khalek Abdel Razek, MD[a,†], Manar Mansour, MD[a], Elsharawy Kamal, MD[b], Suresh K. Mukherji, MD, MBA, FACR[c,*]

KEYWORDS

- Oral cavity cancer • OPC • MR imaging

KEY POINTS

- Understanding the anatomy is essential of evaluating patients with oropharynx SCCA.
- MRI is superior to CT for providing soft tissue detail of oropharynx SCCA.
- MRI helps identify locoregional spread, define tumor extent and identify lymph node metastases.

INTRODUCTION

Oral cavity cancer (OCC) represents approximately 1.4% of all new malignancies and oropharyngeal cancer (OPC) is the most common head and neck cancer diagnosed in the Western world. Squamous cell carcinoma (SCC) comprises 90% of all oral malignancies. The average age of diagnosis is 60 years, with a male-to-female ratio of 2.2:1.[1] Smoking tobacco and alcohol consumption are the traditional risk factors for developing OCC and OPC. However, in the past decade and a half, the oncogenic human papillomavirus (HPV) has emerged as a recognized causative agent for OPC. Infection with high-risk HPV (HR-HPV) types (ie, HPV16 and HPV18) explains 17% to 56% of OPCs in developed countries and, to a lesser extent (13%), OPCs in less developed countries. HPV-driven OPC and tobacco-related OPC differ in the underlying molecular and genetic profiles, socioeconomic demographics, and response to treatment. HPV-related OPC tends to occur in younger patients and has a significantly better response. Less studied risk factors for OCC include poor oral hygiene, ill-fitting dentures, and the subsequent development of oral sores in which mechanical irritation could result in dysplasia and potentially carcinoma.[2,3]

ANATOMY
Oral Cavity

The oral cavity is the most ventral portion of the aerodigestive tract; it is bounded by the lips anteriorly and separated from the oropharynx posteriorly by a ring of structures consisting of the circumvallate papillae inferiorly, the soft palate superiorly, and the anterior tonsillar pillars on both sides. The oral cavity can be divided into 2 parts, namely, the oral vestibule and oral cavity proper by the upper and lower alveolus forming the lateral margins of the oral cavity proper and medial margins of the vestibule. The vestibule is bounded laterally by the buccal mucosa, which reflects superiorly and inferiorly over the maxilla and mandible, respectively, forming the upper and lower gingivobuccal sulcus and it continues over the gingiva as gingival mucosa. Posteriorly it leads to the retromolar trigone. The anatomic subdivisions of the oral cavity are the lips, the floor of the mouth (FOM), the oral tongue (ie, the anterior two-thirds of the tongue), the buccal mucosa, the upper and lower gingivae, the hard palate, and the retromolar trigone.[4–6]

Oropharynx

The oropharynx is the part of the pharynx that is posterior to the oral cavity, between the

[a] Faculty of Medicine, Department of Diagnostic Radiology, Mansoura University, Elgomhoria Street, Mansoura 35512, Egypt; [b] Faculty of Medicine, Department of Otorhinolaryngology Head and Neck Surgery, Mansoura University, Elgomhoria Street, Mansoura 35512, Egypt; [c] Marian University, Head and Neck Radiology, ProScan Imaging, Carmel, IN, USA
[†] Deceased
* Corresponding author.
E-mail address: sureshmukherji@hotmil.com

Magn Reson Imaging Clin N Am 30 (2022) 35–51
https://doi.org/10.1016/j.mric.2021.07.002

mri.theclinics.com

nasopharynx and the hypopharynx. The anterior border of the oropharynx is the plane formed by the circumvallate papillae, anterior tonsillar pillars, and soft palate. Its posterior border is the posterior pharyngeal wall. The oropharynx is bordered superiorly by the level of the elevated soft palate and inferiorly by the valleculae. The anatomic subdivisions of the oropharynx are divided into the base of the tongue, including the glossoepiglottic and pharyngeoepiglottic folds, the palatine tonsils (including the tonsillar fossa), the anterior and posterior tonsillar pillars, the ventral soft palate (including the uvula), and the lateral and posterior oropharyngeal walls.[6]

MR IMAGING TECHNIQUE

The role of imaging in OCC/OPC is for tumor staging and surveillance. Imaging options include panoramic radiography, CT scan, MR imaging, and PET scan. Using these tools, radiologists contribute information regarding the characteristics of the primary tumor, lymphatic spread, and distant metastasis.[7] In malignancies that have a higher incidence of early bone involvement such as gingivobuccal sulcus and retromolar trigone carcinoma, it usually begins cortical and has a direct impact on surgical planning. Multidetector CT scans have a very high specificity (87%–90%) for the detection the minor cortical bone erosions.[8]

MR imaging is preferred over CT scanning in the evaluation of OCC/OPC because it provides superior soft tissue contrast to depict the detailed anatomy and accurately delineate the borders and extent of infiltration of tumor (Fig. 1). It is optimum in the evaluation of perineural tumor spread and bone marrow invasion, which are important factors in treatment planning. Although MR imaging has

the advantage of decreased metallic artifacts from dental amalgam, which often hampers evaluation of the primary carcinoma with a CT scan. Extensive dental hardware may produce susceptibility artifacts in MR images that can obscure the primary tumor. This can be minimized by avoidance of gradient echo, the use of lower field strength magnets, a decrease in echo train length and echo time, and increase in bandwidth.[9,10]

Routine MR Imaging

MR imaging should be performed with a dedicated neck coil and should include small field of view (FOV) images (14–18 cm) with thin sections (3–4 mm) dedicated to the oral cavity and large FOV (20 cm) images of the entire neck to evaluate for nodal metastases. Small FOV images should include thin section axial, sagittal, and coronal T1-weighted images; thin section axial, sagittal, and coronal postcontrast T1-weighted images with or without fat suppression (fat suppression is recommended to make enhancing lesions more conspicuous); and a coronal T2-weighted fat-saturated or short T1 inversion recovery (STIR) sequence is required. Large FOV images should include axial T2 with fat saturation or STIR sequence for entire neck, sagittal T1 precontrast, and axial postcontrast T1 images.[11] Because the structures within the oral cavity abut one another when imaged with the mouth closed, placement of a rolled 2 × 2–inch gauze adjacent to the tumor just before the MR examination has been shown to effectively separate the mucosal surfaces and significantly improve tumor delineation, particularly for the evaluation of small mucosal tumors and tumors in certain locations, such as the gingiva and buccal mucosa.[12]

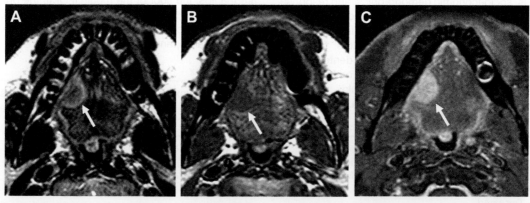

Fig. 1. SCC of the oral tongue. (A) Axial T2-weighted images shows a lateralized high signal mass (arrow) involving the right lateral oral tongue extending to involve the floor of mouth. Axial noncontrast T1-weighted image (B) show the mass to be intermediate signal (arrows) and homogeneous enhances (arrow) on the postcontrast fat-suppressed images (C).

Diffusion-Weighted Imaging

Diffusion-weighted imaging (DWI) evaluates the relative diffusivity of water protons through tissues, which can be affected by changes in tissue organization at the cellular level leading to alteration in the MR signal. The average extent of molecular motion that is affected by cellular organization and integrity (apparent diffusion coefficient [ADC]) can be measured. Restricted diffusion is manifested as a hyperintense signal on the diffusion-weighted image and signal drop out on the corresponding ADC map. Because of their highly cellular nature, head and neck SCCs have been shown to demonstrate restricted diffusion, with ADC values of less than 0.9 to 1.3 mm^2/s in the primary site and in metastatic lymph nodes (LNs). DWI also has higher sensitivity and specificity for detecting LN metastases than conventional MR imaging and CT scans. DWI is particularly useful in the post-treatment setting owing to its ability to distinguish tumor recurrence from inflammatory changes. Recurrent tumor demonstrates decreased ADC, reflecting the high cellularity compared with post-treatment change, which demonstrates normal to elevated ADC. DWI helps to predict and monitor tumor response to chemoradiation. Low ADC values on the baseline pretreatment scan have been correlated with a better response to treatment. A high degree of ADC increase from the baseline scan compared with scans obtained in the early treatment phase also predicts better treatment response. DWI in the oral cavity may be degraded by susceptibility artifacts from dental amalgam; parallel imaging can decrease susceptibility artifacts.[13,14]

Diffusion Tensor Imaging

Diffusion tensor imaging provides information on the degree of alignment of cellular structures, as well as their structural integrity (fractional anisotropy). In some studies, diffusion tensor imaging derived metrics (mean diffusivity and fractional anisotropy) are proved to be reliable and reproducible parameters that can help in the differentiation of residual head and neck SCC from postradiation changes. Recently, DWI techniques have entered the head and neck cancer clinic, in which images are acquired with multiple b-values, yielding techniques such as intravoxel incoherent imaging or diffusion kurtosis imaging, techniques that aim to provide information that extends diffusion of water, such as perfusion (for intravoxel incoherent imaging) or non-Gaussian diffusion behavior (for diffusion kurtosis imaging).[15,16]

Perfusion-Weighted Imaging

Dynamic perfusion MR imaging gives an idea about the delivery of the blood to tissue and reflect the degree of angiogenesis of the tissues by 2 approaches: either by application of exogenous contrast agents in dynamic susceptibility contrast-enhanced and dynamic contrast-enhanced MR perfusion or endogenous contrast agent, namely, magnetically labeled arterial blood water in arterial spin labeling MR perfusion (**Fig. 2**). It distinguishes between malignant and benign tumors using perfusion

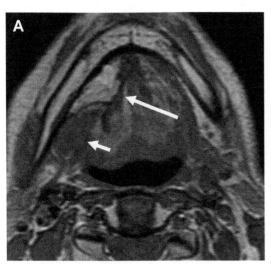 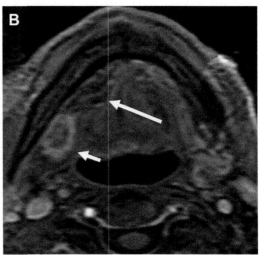

Fig. 2. Recurrent tumor detected with dynamic contrast-enhanced sequences. (*A*) Axial noncontrast enhanced T1-weighted images shows postoperative changes following primary resection with reconstruction with a forearm flap (*long arrow*). There is a focal soft tissue mass posterior to the free flap (*short arrow*). (*B*) Axial postcontrast dynamic contrast-enhanced images shows diffuse enhancement of the recurrent tumor (*short arrow*) with suppression of the forearm free flap (*long arrow*).

parameters, including blood flow, blood volume, permeability, and mean transit time, with increased perfusion values reflecting the increased degree of angiogenesis of malignant lesions. It also can distinguish tumor recurrence from a postsurgical change in the treated neck, with recurrent tumor having elevated blood flow and volume relative to post-treatment change. Perfusion MR may have a role in predicting treatment response, with tumors of greater vascularity showing greater response to chemoradiation therapy. In the oral cavity, susceptibility artifacts from dental amalgam and the soft tissue–air interfaces often limit the use of perfusion imaging using the dynamic susceptibility contrast-enhanced technique.[16,17]

MR Spectroscopy

MR spectroscopy detects the presence of specific metabolites in areas of interest. Studies have shown head and neck malignancies to have elevated choline/creatine ratios compared with normal tissues and benign tumors head and neck. However, MR spectroscopy is difficult to perform in the head and neck and is often severely degraded by patient motion and susceptibility artifacts, in addition to contamination of the spectra by a dominant fat peak.[18]

Radiomics

Recent advances in image processing and segmentation have led to a specialized field called radiomics, which is the high-throughput extraction of large amounts of quantitative features and their subsequent analysis and correlation with clinical features. Radiomics and deep learning not only complement and facilitate but will probably also accelerate advancement toward precision cancer medicine. The imaging biomarkers extracted by deep learning and radiomics have been found to significantly correlate with the phenotype of the tumor and will likely impact the field of head and neck SCC management in the following areas: tumor segmentation and pathologic classification; risk stratification, as prognostic and/or predictive biomarker(s); and monitoring of alteration in normal tissue as sequelae of radiotherapy dose deposition.[8]

ROLE OF MR IMAGING
Tumor Localization

Tumors seem to be isointense to hypointense signal to muscle on noncontrast T1-weighted images and can be distinguished accurately from the muscles by variable fat content within the muscles and interspersed fat in between. Disruption of the fat planes is a good indicator for invasion. Tumors demonstrate hyperintense signal on T2-weighted images and enhance on postgadolinium T1-weighted images. Although the conspicuity of lesions is greater with T2-weighted and contrast-enhanced images, the extent of a tumor may be overestimated in T2-weighted images, because of the similar signal characteristics of surrounding edema and inflammation.[9,12]

Locoregional Extension

Depth of invasion
Depth of invasion (DOI) is measured as the histologic tumor infiltration below the basement membrane, which is equivalent to the endophytic component. In the eighth edition T classification, the DOI incorporates the relationship of tumor infiltration with the outcome; it replaces the criterion of the invasion of the deep extrinsic muscles of the tongue at the previous seventh edition. Several studies have reported that DOI of oral tongue carcinoma of more than 4 mm is a strong predictor of cervical LN involvement and local tumor recurrence and implicate elective neck dissection, whereas a DOI of more than 10 mm is a poor prognostic marker so adjuvant treatment is considered.[8,19]

Accurate assessment of the DOI is challenging on imaging and it is important to understand that the tumor thickness measured on imaging is not equivalent to the DOI. Exophytic and ulcerative tumors can create inconsistencies in the histopathological determination of thickness. An exophytic tumor may seem to be thick, but may have minimal invasion and exposure to the underlying lymphovascular networks. Although an ulcerative lesion may have been in contact with deep lymphovascular channels, a measure of thickness would not show this factor. However, there is evidence of prognostic equivalence of these 2 parameters and, hence, imaging can play a vital role in assigning the T category for staging. CT scans and MR imaging may have limited utility in assessing DOI and ultrasound examination has been reported to be a more accurate method for assessing DOI.[8,19]

Tumor thickness
Tumor thickness is an important component of tumor staging and strongly correlates with the presence of nodal metastases, risk of local recurrence, and overall survival. MR imaging has higher sensitivity and specificity compared with CT scans and PET/CT scans for the evaluation of tumor depth and muscle invasion.[20]

Bone involvement
Bone involvement upstages the tumor to at least a T4a; hence, accurate preoperative determination

of bone involvement is essential in staging and treatment planning. A CT scan better demonstrates small cortical bony erosions, whereas MR imaging is superior in the detection of bone marrow invasion (**Fig. 3**). It appears as a low signal intensity replacing the high signal of the medullary fat in nonenhanced T1-weighted images and hyperintense signal on fat-suppressed T2-weighted images and enhancement on fat-suppressed postcontrast images. Replacement of the hypointense signal of the bony cortex on T1- and T2-weighted images with the signal intensity of the tumor is a strong indicator for cortical invasion. MR imaging has higher sensitivity than a CT scan in evaluating bone involvement, but it has a lower specificity, with false-positive cases attributed to the inflammatory change from dental infections or procedures and to chemical shift artifact from bone marrow fat on a T1-weighted MR image.[21,22]

Determining the presence and extent of bone invasion is critical to determine the planned osteotomy sites. Segmental mandibulectomy involves the removal of a section of the mandible is required for bone marrow invasion. Marginal mandibulectomy, however, involves the removal of only the cortex and a portion of the marrow with mandibular continuity. This procedure is used for minor cortical erosion and tumors in close proximity to the mandible. However, obtaining a 1-cm margin often leaves a thin residual mandible that is prone to fracture, which is particularly problematic in edentulous patients with mandibular atrophy; this subset of patients often requires a segmental mandibulectomy, even with minimal osseous invasion.[21]

Perineural spread

MR imaging is better at detecting perineural tumor spread, most commonly associated with SCCs and adenoid cystic carcinomas. The most commonly involved nerves with OCC and OPC are branches of the maxillary (V2) and mandibular (V3) divisions of the trigeminal nerve. Hard palate tumors can spread along the greater palatine nerve (branch of V2) to the pterygopalatine fossa. Tumors invading the mandible and specifically the mandibular canal can spread along the inferior alveolar nerve (branch of V3). Findings of perineural tumor spread include enlargement of the nerves with abnormal enhancement on postcontrast T1-weighted images and obliteration of the hyperintense fat signal in the skull base foramina and pterygopalatine fossa on precontrast T1-weighted images. Perineural tumor spread can be antegrade or retrograde, and therefore the entire course of the nerve should be evaluated, with attention to the pterygopalatine fossa, cavernous sinus, and Meckel's cave (**Fig. 4**). Findings of secondary muscle denervation of the masticator space musculature may also be evident.[11]

Nodal Metastasis

Nodal spread

Neck nodal metastasis has a direct impact on treatment and outcomes. A systematic search for abnormal nodes is performed particularly in the expected sites of drainage. Gingivobuccal and

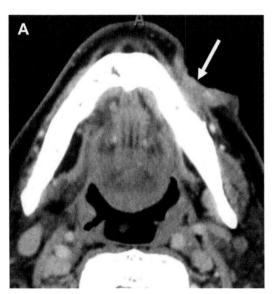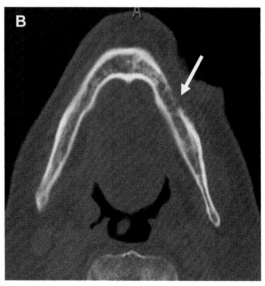

Fig. 3. Buccal cancer with bone erosion. (*A*) Axial contrast-enhanced CT scan reconstructed in soft tissue algorithms shows an aggressive soft tissue mass involving the left gingivobuccal sulcus (*arrow*). (*B*) Bone algorithm shows erosion of the buccal cortex upstaging the tumor to T4b (*arrow*).

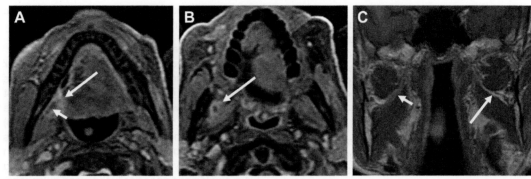

Fig. 4. Retrograde perineural spread along the lingual nerve. (*A*) Axial dynamic contrast-enhanced image obtained in the same patient illustrated in **Fig. 2** shows an area of enhancement (*long arrow*) surrounding a focal nonenhancing area (*short arrow*). This patient presented with unexplained right neuropathic pain. (*B*) Axial dynamic contrast-enhanced images at the level of the ramus of the mandible show the "target-like" enhancing pattern with a peripheral enhancement surrounding an area of nonenhancement (*arrow*). These findings were suspicious for retrograde perineural spread along the lingual nerve. (*C*) Coronal contrast-enhanced T1-weighted images shows linear enhancement involving the expected course of the right lingual nerve (*small arrow*) coursing between the lateral and medial pterygoid muscles. Compare this enhancement ("evil gray") with the normal appearance of the fat on the contralateral side (*long arrow*). These findings confirmed the presence of retrograde perineural spread along the right lingual nerve.

retromolar trigone malignancies drain at levels IB and II, and oral tongue malignancies drain at levels I, II, and III. However, skip metastasis is also known with an incidence ranging from 6% to 10% to level III and IV. Contralateral adenopathy is also seen in tongue malignancies as a result of disease crossing over the midline. Occult nodal micrometastases in which there is no clinical or imaging evidence of LN involvement, are common for oral cavity carcinomas; therefore, an ipsilateral selective neck dissection is performed for almost all oral cavity carcinomas, except those arising from the lips.[23,24]

Imaging helps to detect nodal metastasis in the absence of suspicious lymphadenopathy on clinical examination. The morphologic loss of fatty hilum, a rounded appearance, necrosis, and cystic changes are indicators of nodal metastasis. Nodal necrosis is the most reliable indicator, with a specificity between 95% and 100%, even for sub-centimeter nodes. Imaging helps to measure the nodal burden and identify adverse features such as extranodal extension (ENE) and carotid artery encasement (>270°), which are associated with poorer outcomes.[25,26]

Extranodal extension

In addition to the number, size, and laterality of the involved regional LNs, ENE has been added to the N stage category. ENE is considered as a second major change in the American Joint Committee on Cancer (AJCC) eighth edition. Two separate clinical and pathologic nodal staging has been introduced. Radiologic imaging and clinical examination are current methods of assessment of clinical ENE, which are less accurate than

pathologic examination. Radiologic examination lacks sensitivity and specificity in the detection of early or minor ENE. Therefore, imaging used only in gross ENE which could be classified as either macroscopic or clinical ENE.[8,19]

Imaging features such as perinodal fat stranding and infiltration into the adjacent fat or muscle have high specificity for predicting ENE. Indirect imaging signs of ENE, especially in a high level II node include denervation atrophy or signs of dysfunction of muscles innervated by the upper cranial nerves IX to XII[27] (**Fig. 5**).

Distant Metastasis

Patients with a risk for distant metastasis will be assessed through imaging the chest and the liver. However, as PET scans become more available, this modality is used frequently to assess for distant disease.[19]

TNM Staging

The recently published eighth edition of the AJCC manual has introduced some changes from the prior seventh edition, which has implications on the management and outcomes of OCC/OPC[8,19,28]: **Boxes 1–3** shows update eighth edition of AJCC of OCC/OPC.

Changes in eighth Edition of the American Joint Committee on Cancer for Oral Cavity Cancer

1. *DOI* in determining the T stage of primary tumors and replaces the item of extrinsic tongue muscle invasion.

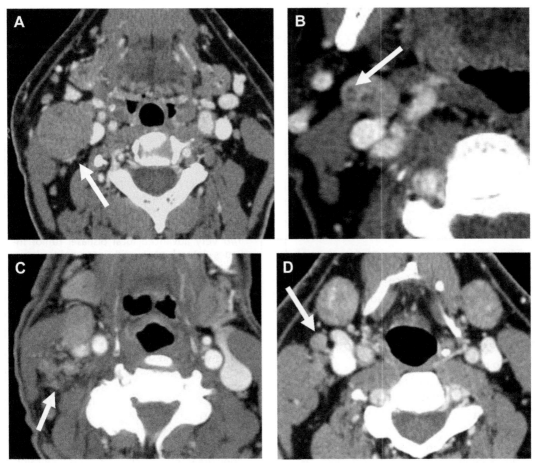

Fig. 5. Diagnostic criteria for detecting metastatic LNs. Axial images show the following criteria can be used to detect lymph metastases (*arrows*). (*A*) Size, (*B*) internal low attenuation, (*C*) extracapsular penetration, and (*D*) clumping of LNs in the ipsilateral primary echelon lymphatic drainage.

2. *ENE* in nodal staging: histologically, ENE is defined as an extension of metastatic carcinoma through the fibrous capsule of the node and spilling out to the adjacent connective tissue, regardless of the presence of stromal reaction. The clinically positive ENE is classified as the involvement of the skin overlying the nodes or soft tissue invasion around LNs with deep fixation/tethering or clinical signs of nerve invasion.
3. *Removed of T0 stage* carcinoma of unknown primary in head and neck has new chapter in the eighth edition staging system.
4. *Removal of cutaneous malignancies of dry vermilion* that moved to a new chapter in cutaneous malignancies of head and neck.[19]

Changes in eighth Edition of the American Joint Committee on Cancer for Oropharyngeal Cancer

The eighth edition of the AJCC TNM staging system introduced significant changes to the classification of OPC. It made major changes to OPC staging according to HPV status. In the eighth edition, HPV positivity is determined by p16 testing of tumor tissue. The main differences from seventh edition with regard to OPC are as follows:

1. *T-staging of OPC*: Tis (in situ) is not included in p16-positive OPC, T0 category is only used in p16-positive metastatic LNs; the primary tumor is presumed to be OPC, stages T4a and T4b are now unified in a single category (T4) in p16-positive OPC.
2. *N-staging of OPC*: N-staging for p16-positive OPC is N1: ipsilateral LNs (1 or multiple) not larger than 6 cm are characterized. N2: bilateral or contralateral nodes not larger than 6 cm. No subcategories are included in the N2 stage. N3: nodes larger than 6 cm. For p16-negative OPC, N3 is divided into 2 subcategories: N3a if the nodes are larger than 6 cm but without ENE and stage N3b if there are any signs of ENE.[29,30]

Box 1
TN staging of OCC

T Staging

T1 Tumor 2 cm or less in greatest dimension and 5 mm or less depth invasion

T2 Tumor 2 cm or less in greatest dimension and more than 5 mm but no more than 10 mm DOI or tumor more than 2 cm but not more than 4 cm in greatest dimension and DOI no more than 10 mm

T3 Tumor more than 4 cm in greatest dimension or any tumor with a DOI more than 10 mm

T4 T4a (*lip*) Tumor invades through cortical bone, inferior alveolar nerve, FOM, or skin

T4a (*oral cavity*) Tumor invades through cortical bone of the mandible or maxillary sinus or invades skin of face

T4b Tumor invades masticator space, pterygoid plates, or skull base or encases internal carotid artery

N Staging

N0 No regional LN metastasis

N1 Metastasis in single ipsilateral LN less than 3 cm and ENE negative

N2 Metastasis in a single ipsilateral or contralateral node

N2a Metastasis in a single ipsilateral or contralateral node 3 to 6 cm and ENE negative

N2b Metastasis in multiple ipsilateral nodes less than 6 cm and ENE negative

N2c Metastasis in contralateral or bilateral nodes less than 6 cm and ENE negative

N3a Metastasis in a single node greater than 6 cm and ENE negative

N3b Metastasis in a single ipsilateral, multiple ipsilateral, contralateral, or bilateral nodes of any size and ENE+

Box 2
TN staging of p16-negative OPC

T Staging

T1 Tumor 2 cm or smaller in greatest dimension

T2 Tumor greater than 2 cm but 4 cm or smaller in greatest dimension

T3 Tumor greater than 4 cm in greatest dimension or extension to lingual surface of epiglottis

T4a Moderately advanced local disease: tumor invades larynx, extrinsic muscles of tongue, medial pterygoid, hard palate, or mandible

T4b Very advanced local disease: tumor invades lateral pterygoid, pterygoid plates, lateral nasopharynx, or skull base or encases the carotid artery

N Staging

Nx Regional LNs cannot be assessed

N0 No regional LN metastasis

N1 Metastasis in single ipsilateral LN 3 cm or smaller in greatest dimension and ENE negative

N2a Metastasis in single ipsilateral LN more than 3 cm but 6 cm or less in greatest dimension and ENE negative

N2b Metastasis in multiple ipsilateral LNs, none greater than 6 cm in greatest dimension and ENE negative

N2c Metastasis in bilateral or contralateral LN(s), none more than 6 cm in greatest dimension and ENE negative

N3a Metastasis in LN more than 6 cm in greatest dimension and ENE negative

N3b Metastasis in any node(s) with clinically overt ENE (clinical ENE)

SPECIFIC SITE FEATURES

Patterns of tumor spread and treatment approaches depending on the site of origin in the oral cavity and oropharynx. The general routes of spread of OCC/OPC are the same for all subsites: direct extension over mucosal surfaces, muscle, and bone; lymphatic drainage pathways; and extension along neurovascular bundles. However, the particular subsite of involvement of the oral cavity and oropharynx may dictate the routine assessment of certain anatomic structures. The relevant imaging anatomy and the patterns of spread for each primary subsite carcinoma are discussed.[1–5]

Oral Tongue Cancer

The oral tongue is the main content of the oral cavity proper; it is composed of intrinsic and extrinsic muscles and is divided into equal halves by midline fatty lingual septum. The intrinsic muscles include the superior and inferior longitudinal, transverse, and vertical muscles. The extrinsic muscles include the genioglossus, hyoglossus, styloglossus, and palatoglossus muscles. The genioglossus muscle is the largest. It originates from the

---

Box 3
TN staging of p16-positivve OPC

T Staging

T0 No primary tumor identified

T1 Tumor 2 cm or smaller in greatest dimension

T2 Tumor more than 2 cm but 4 cm or less in greatest dimension

T3 Tumor more than 4 cm in greatest dimension or extension to lingual surface of epiglottis

T4 Moderately advanced local disease: tumor invades larynx, extrinsic tongue muscles, medial pterygoid, hard palate, or mandible or beyond

N Staging

Nx Regional LNs cannot be assessed

N0 No regional LN metastasis

N1 One or more ipsilateral LNs, none more than 6 cm

N2 Contralateral or bilateral LNs, none more than 6 cm

N3 LN(s) >more than 6 cm

---

superior genial tubercle in the midline mandible and fans out in the tongue superiorly interdigitating with the intrinsic muscles. The hyoglossus muscles are depicted in the coronal and axial planes as thin rectangular muscles parallel and medial to the mylohyoid muscles and lateral to the genioglossus muscles. Because the neurovascular bundles are closely related to the hyoglossus muscles, involvement of the hyoglossus muscle by tumor is a strong marker for neurovascular invasion.[9,31]

The oral tongue is the most frequently involved site in the oral cavity, accounting for approximately 33% of oral cavity carcinomas. Contrast-enhanced MR imaging is the preferred imaging modality for the evaluation of tongue carcinomas. The muscular anatomy is best appreciated on precontrast T1-weighted imaging. The tumor is represented as intermediate to higher signal on T2-weighted and STIR images.[32]

The following features must be assessed on cross-sectional imaging: size of tumor and DOI, extension across the midline, extension into adjacent structures, neurovascular bundle involvement, mandibular involvement, and radiologic nodal metastasis.[25] The DOI can be measured on coronal contrast-enhanced T1-weighted images, because its measurement on T2-weighted/STIR images may lead to overestimation owing to perilesional edema.[33] Tumors may extend posteriorly into the base of the tongue and glossotonsillar sulcus, inferiorly to the FOM, laterally to the gingiva and mandible, and medially to the lingual septum and contralateral tongue. From the floor of mouth, a tumor may invade the mandible or inferiorly extend through the mylohyoid sling into the submandibular space. Infiltration of the hyoglossus muscle with tumors indicates neurovascular bundle involvement. Bone involvement is less frequent than gingivobuccal sulcus and retromolar trigone malignancies. It predominantly occurs if the disease extends to FOM, which can be either midline or lateral.[34]

Surgical treatments range from transoral wide excision for small (T1 or T2) lesions to partial, subtotal, or total glossectomy, with or without resection of the base of the tongue. Disease extension posteriorly into the tonsil, lateral pharyngeal wall, and posteroinferiorly to the valleculae, pre-epiglottic space, and hyoid bone are relative contraindications for primary surgical management. Disease involving or in close proximity to the hyoid bone (5 mm) leads to high morbidity from the functional sequelae of removal of the hyoid bone. Invasion across the midline and involvement of the contralateral neurovascular bundle are contraindications to partial glossectomy and require a subtotal or total glossectomy.[35] Bilateral elective neck dissections are indicated in tumors that cross the midline and in tumors where the 1-cm surgical margin crosses the midline. If there is associated ENE, adjuvant treatment is indicated, whereas if there is more than 270° carotid artery encasement either primary nonsurgical treatment or induction chemotherapy followed by reassessment for resectability are indicated (**Fig. 6**). Midthird mandibulectomy with appropriate reconstruction is required for midline involvement of the mandible.[36,37]

Floor of the Mouth Cancer

The mylohyoid muscle forms a muscular U-shaped sling of FOM. It originates from the mandibular mylohyoid line on both sides and inserts into the midline fibrous raphe that extends from the mandibular symphysis to the hyoid bone. It separates the submandibular space located inferiorly and lateral from the sublingual space being superomedial. Both spaces are connecting together along the posterior margin of the myelohoid muscle.[9]

FOM cancer accounts for 18% of OCC, with most originating anteriorly at the midline (**Fig. 7**). These tumors are particularly difficult to evaluate on clinical examination, and surgeons rely heavily on imaging for surgical planning. Tumors of the

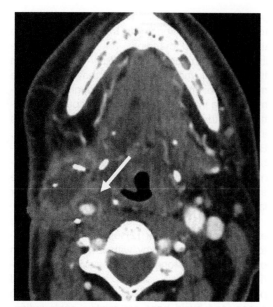

Fig. 6. Carotid encasement. Axial contrast-enhanced CT scan shows recurrent tumor involving the right neck encasing the carotid artery.

FOM may extend superiorly into the ventral oral tongue, inferiorly through the mylohyoid muscle into the submandibular space, anteriorly and laterally into the bordering mandible, and posteriorly into the base of the tongue. Carcinomas arising from the anterior FOM can obstruct the Wharton ducts, and ductal dilatation, and glandular enlargement. The sublingual glands are more likely to be directly invaded by tumor or be secondarily obstructed. Involvement of the midline is common and important to determine preoperatively, because it necessitates bilateral nodal dissections. Neurovascular spread is much more common in carcinoma of the FOM, so close inspection of the neurovascular bundle is mandatory. Osseous and nodal involvement should be ruled out.[6,11]

Retromolar Trigone Cancer

The retromolar trigone is a triangular-shaped mucosal fold with its base behind the last mandibular molar, extending superiorly with an apex behind the last maxillary molar. The mucosa blends medially with the anterior tonsillar pillar and laterally with the buccal mucosa. Deep to the mucosa of the retromolar trigone lies the pterygomandibular raphe, which is a fibrous band extending from the mylohyoid line on the lingual aspect of the mandible inferiorly to the pterygoid hamulus of the medial pterygoid plate superiorly. It also connects to the buccinators muscle anteriorly and the superior constrictor muscle of the pharynx posteriorly. The pterygomandibular raphe has been implicated in the route of tumor spread from the retromolar trigone (**Fig. 8**).[38,39]

Retromolar trigone carcinoma accounts for 7% to 12% of oral cavity carcinomas. This site is also the second most common site of minor salivary gland tumors. Imaging evaluation of the retromolar trigone is critical because the extent of SCC

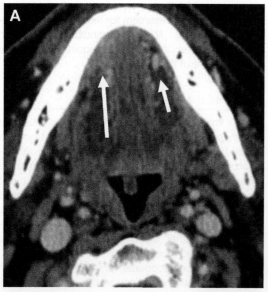
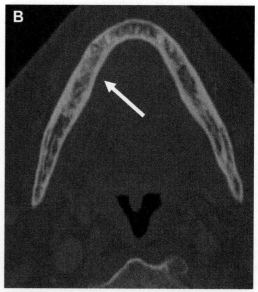

Fig. 7. FOM SCCA. (*A*) Axial contrast-enhanced CT scan shows a soft tissues mass involving the anterior right FOM (*long arrow*). Compare the tumoral involvement with the normal fat on the left side (*small arrow*). (*B*) Bone algorithms shows no evidence of cortical erosion (*arrow*).

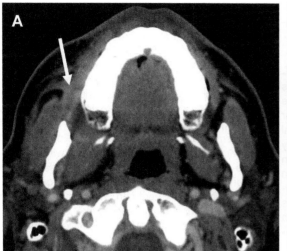
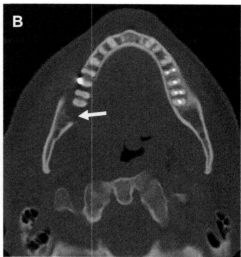

Fig. 8. Retromolar trigone carcinoma (CT scan). (*A*) Axial contrast-enhanced CT scan reconstructed in soft tissue algorithms shows a soft tissue mass involving the right retromolar trigone (*arrow*). (*B*) Bone algorithms shows clinically occult erosion of the anterior mandibular cortex (*arrow*).

involvement of this subsite cannot be determined clinically. Evaluation of SCC involvement of the retromolar trigone should include assessment of submucosal spread, including involvement of the muscles of mastication; osseous involvement; neurovascular extension; and cervical lymphatic spread.[40] The retromolar trigone may be primary or may result from a regional extension. The clinical significance of the retromolar trigone is that it provides easy access to numerous routes of spread. SCC originating from the retromolar trigone may spread anteriorly along the buccal mucosa and gingiva, posteriorly to the adjacent anterior tonsillar pillar and soft palate, and posterolaterally to the masticator space. The pterygomandibular raphe provides access for these tumors to invade the buccinator muscle and buccal space, pterygoid plates and musculature, posterior mandible and maxilla, and the skull base. Perineural tumor spread may occur along

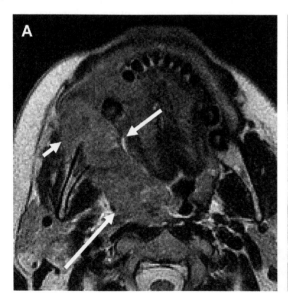
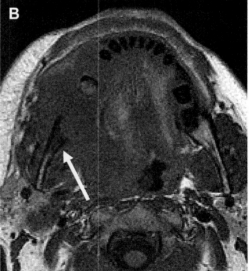

Fig. 9. Retromolar trigone carcinoma (MR imaging). (*A*) Axial T2-weighted image shows a large right retromolar trigone carcinoma centered in the right pterygomandibular raphe (*medium arrow*). The mass extends anteriorly to the buccinator muscle (*small arrow*) and posteriorly to involve the superior constrictor muscle (*large arrow*). (*B*) Axial noncontrast T1-weighted images shows invasion of the right mandibular marrow (*arrow*).

the inferior alveolar nerve (branch of V3) because of the proximity of the nerve to the retromolar trigone[39,40] (**Fig. 9**).

Buccal and Gingival Cancer

The buccal mucosa covers the cheeks and lips and is continuous with the buccal aspect of the gingiva of the maxillary and mandibular alveolar ridge, as well as the retromolar trigone. Buccal SCC accounts for a large percentage of oral cavity carcinomas in Asia and are much more common in men than in women, likely related to the common practice of chewing betel quid by men in this region. Buccal cancer frequently demonstrates aggressive behavior and is associated with a high rate of treatment failure with poor locoregional control. The superficial spread of these lesions is best assessed clinically, but their detection at imaging can be improved by having the patient perform special maneuvers during image acquisition, such as puffing the cheeks outward during a CT scan or the placement of gauze during an MR imaging evaluation of these tumors. The gauze separates the buccal mucosa from the adjacent gingiva and enables better tumor delineation.[6]

Evaluation of the buccal or gingival mucosal lesion should address the extent of submucosal spread, osseous involvement, involvement of the retromolar trigone and pterygomandibular raphe, and cervical lymphatic spread. Submucosal invasion of the underlying buccinator muscle is common, with potential further spread into the buccal and masticator spaces. Invasion of the Stensen (parotid) duct may occur, which pierces the buccinator muscle at the level of the second maxillary molar. A tumor may also spread craniocaudally to the gingivobuccal sulci and the maxilla and mandible. Although skin involvement is better evaluated with clinical examination, the extent of subcutaneous invasion especially above the zygoma is better assessed on imaging. An assessment of spread along the masticator space/infratemporal fossa can only be discerned with imaging and is critical for management planning. As per eighth AJCC, the involvement of masticator space is T4b and unresectable. However, Liao and colleagues[41] suggested that there is a subset of infratemporal fossa involvement (low infratemporal fossa) that is, potentially resectable, with acceptable outcomes. High infratemporal fossa disease when treated with surgery had dismal outcomes. Early bone involvement can only be assessed with imaging. Perineural spread in the gingivobuccal carcinoma is less than 10% and predominantly occurs along the mandibular division of the trigeminal nerve. LN drainage is most commonly to the submental, submandibular, and periparotid LNs. Buccal mucosal carcinomas are associated with a high rate of recurrence even in the setting of negative margins. Therefore, postoperative radiotherapy is commonly indicated for these cancers[41] (see **Fig. 3**).

Hard Palate Cancer

SCCs arising from the hard palate are rare and often represent an extension from an adjacent gingival lesion. The palate is the most common site of origin for minor salivary gland neoplasms because it contains the highest concentration of minor salivary glands in the aerodigestive tract. Adenoid cystic carcinoma is the most frequently observed minor salivary gland malignancy, followed by mucoepidermoid carcinoma and adenocarcinoma. Minor salivary gland tumors are more likely to be submucosal in locations with early bone invasion. The bone invasion has been shown to be more radioresistant with a high risk of

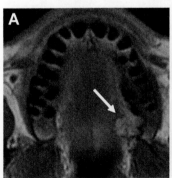 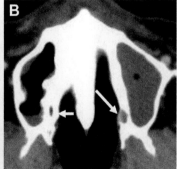 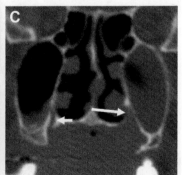

Fig. 10. Hard palate SCCA. (*A*) Axial contrast-enhanced MR imaging performed shows an enhancing mass involving the left side of the hard palate. (*B*) Axial and coronal CT scans show enlargement of the left greater palatine foramen (*long arrow*) compared with the normal appearance of the contralateral greater palatine foramen (*small arrow*), indicative of retrograde perineural spread along the greater palatine foramen.

osteoradionecrosis. Hard palate carcinoma may extend laterally to invade the maxillary alveolar ridge or superiorly to involve the nasal cavity and maxillary sinuses. Perineural tumors spread along the greater palatine nerve (branch of V2) to the pterygopalatine fossa particularly adenoid cystic carcinomas. Careful attention must be paid to the pterygopalatine canal and fossa, along with other sites of retrograde and antegrade spread, including the foramen rotundum, cavernous sinuses, and Meckel's cave[42] (**Fig. 10**).

Lip Cancer

Ultraviolet radiation is the major risk factor for lip carcinoma. Lip lesions are easily assessed with direct visualization, and only infiltrative tumors with uncertain margins require imaging. SCC of the lip tends to arise from the vermilion border and spread by lateral extension to the skin or by deep extension to the orbicularis oris muscle. Even so, early stage lesions are often difficult to differentiate from the normal orbicularis oris muscle. The key features that should be sought in the presence of an SCC of the lip include osseous invasion and lymphatic involvement. Sagittal plane images are particularly useful in the evaluation of lip carcinomas. Osseous involvement usually occurs along the buccal surface of the maxillary or mandibular alveolar ridge. Osseous infiltration creates the opportunity for the perineural invasion along the inferior alveolar nerves, which makes locoregional control particularly difficult. The risk for LN metastases is low for lip carcinomas, particularly with low-grade lesions. Elective LN dissections are thus not performed routinely. LN metastases are most frequently seen at levels IA and IB, followed by level II. Unlike tumors arising from other sites in the oral cavity, carcinomas arising from the lips are radiosensitive and have similar success rates in patients treated with surgery and those treated with radiation therapy.[6,9,11]

Base of Tongue Cancer

The base of the tongue extends from the circumvallate papillae anteriorly to the valleculae inferiorly. The base of tongue cancers is difficult to diagnosis with imaging when small because the base of the tongue consists of dense musculature and lacks the fat planes that provide a contrasting background, in addition to the great variability in the size of the lingual tonsils. Therefore, direct inspection by referring physicians is vital before imaging particularly for small mucosal lesions.[6] SCCs of the base of the tongue tend to be poorly differentiated and aggressive, with a survival rate of only 20%. Although SCCs in this subsite often manifest with dysphagia, odynophagia, or the sensation of a mass, many cases are clinically silent and manifest by a neck mass that corresponds with the nodal disease.[43]

Tumors arising in the tongue base spread anteriorly into the root of the tongue and extrinsic tongue muscles, and into the sublingual space and neurovascular bundle of the oral cavity, although it can extend inferiorly to the vallecula and potentially the pre-epiglottic fat. A lateral extension is potentially into the lateral wall, pterygomandibular raphe, and mandible. Posteriorly, a tumor can invade the parapharyngeal fat and carotid space. Tumors can extend superiorly along the tonsillar pillars. There is a high rate of nodal involvement by SCCs of the dorsum of the tongue owing to the rich lymphatic network with significant cross-drainage. The primary lymphatic drainage is to level II, III, and IV LNs[6,43] (**Fig. 11**).

Early stage SCC of the base of the tongue is treated initially with surgical excision or radiation therapy. As much as one-half of the base of the tongue may be resected with acceptable functional outcomes. Posterior and inferior extension of SCCs of the tongue base is particularly important because the involvement of the larynx or the pre-epiglottic fat precludes the surgical option of partial glossectomy and supraglottic laryngectomy may be included. Advanced stage SCCs of the base of the tongue require treatment with a combination of chemotherapy, radiation therapy, and surgical resection.[44]

Tonsillar Cancer

Tonsillar subsites include the anterior and posterior tonsillar pillars, which overlie the palatoglossus and palatopharyngeus muscles, respectively, and the palatine tonsils. Most SCCs of the tonsil originate in the anterior tonsillar pillar. These tumors tend to spread superiorly along the palatoglossus muscle to the soft palate. The tumor may spread to the masticator space (pterygoid muscles), nasopharynx, and the skull base. Inferior extension to the base of the tongue can occur, although anteriorly and laterally it can travel along the pharyngeal constrictor muscles and pterygomandibular raphe to the oral cavity at the retromolar trigone and into the buccinator muscle. The tumor also may extend posteriorly to the retropharyngeal or carotid space or to the pharyngoepiglottic fold to the top of the pyriform sinus. Osseous involvement in tonsillar SCCs occurs primarily along the pterygoid plates and the maxilla. Lymphatic involvement is common, occurring in nearly one-half of cases of tonsillar SCC to level I, II, and III LNs[45] (**Fig. 12**).

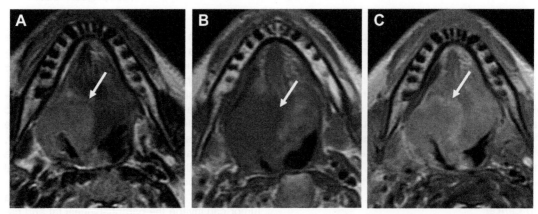

Fig. 11. Tongue base SCCA. (*A*) Axial T2-weighted image shows a large aggressive mass (*arrow*) involving the right tongue base extending into the right glossotonsillar sulcus. Axial precontrast (*A*) and postcontrast (*C*) enhanced T1-weighted images shows the mass to have intermediate T1-weighted signal (*B*) and homogeneously enhance with contrast (*C*) (*arrow*).

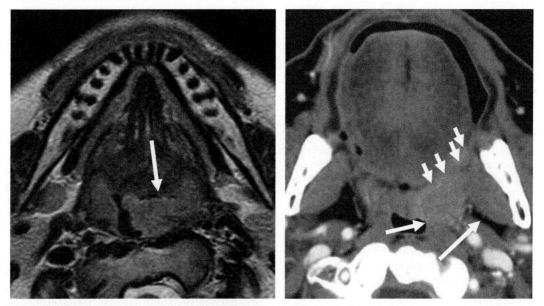

Fig. 12. Tonsil SCCA. (*A*) Axial T2-weighted image shows and exophytic left tonsillar carcinoma arising from the palatine (faucil) tonsil. (*B*) Axial contrast-enhanced CT scan shows a left tonsillar carcinoma (*medium arrow*) in a different patient. This cancer extends deeply to involve the parapharyngeal space (*long arrow*) and extends anteriorly to involve the pterygomandibular raphe and buccinator muscle (*small arrows*).

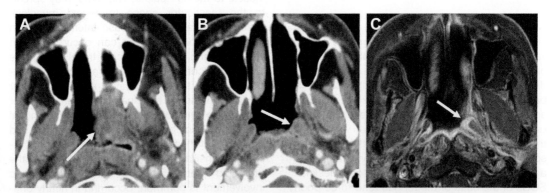

Fig. 13. Soft palate cancer involving the nasopharynx:. (*A*) Axial contrast-enhanced CT shows a large mass involving the left half of the soft palate (*arrow*). (*B*) Axial contrast-enhanced CT performed through the nasopharynx suggests enlargement of the left torus tubarius (*arrow*). (*C*) Axial fat-suppressed contrast-enhanced MR confirms enlargement of the left torus tubarius and enhancing tumor extending along the surface of the torus. These findings indicated superior spread of tumor to the nasopharynx, which was clinically occult.

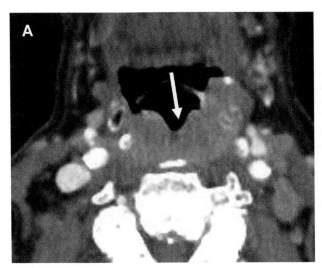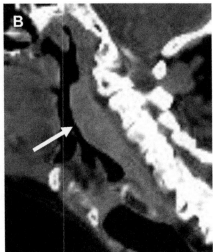

Fig. 14. Posterior pharyngeal wall SCCA. Axial (*A*) contrast-enhanced CT scan with sagittal (*B*) reconstructions shows the characteristic appearance of a posterior pharyngeal wall carcinoma (*arrow*).

Soft Palate Cancer

Soft palate tumors are commonly found on the ventral surface and are generally small at the time of diagnosis. These tumors are often well-differentiated and have the best prognosis of the OPCs. A local extension can occur anteriorly onto the hard palate; laterally into palatine muscles and the parapharyngeal space, and from there to skull base and nasopharynx, and inferiorly onto the tonsillar pillars. Perineural extension of disease can occur along the palatine nerves and to the pterygopalatine fossa and cavernous sinus. Lymphatic drainage from the soft palate is to levels II and III as well as the retropharyngeal nodes[1–5] (**Fig 13**).

Posterior Pharyngeal Wall Cancer

Posterior pharyngeal wall tumors are often large at the time of diagnosis and can spread superiorly to the nasopharynx, laterally into the parapharyngeal space, inferiorly into the hypopharynx, and anteriorly into the tonsil. If the tumor has deep extension, it invades the prevertebral musculature (longus colli and capitus). Recognition of prevertebral muscle invasion is important, as this finding renders the patient unresectable. Many of these tumors extend past midline. Lymphatic drainage of the posterior pharyngeal wall includes bilateral jugular chain LNs and the retropharyngeal LNs[45,46] (**Fig. 14**).

SUMMARY

Routine MR imaging is the preferable imaging modality of diagnosis and staging of OCC/OPC. It has an important role in the fulfillment of the new changes in the eighth edition AJCC staging system of the OCC/OPC. MR imaging helps identify locoregional spread, delineate true tumor extent, and determine LN metastases.

CLINICS CARE POINTS

- The role of imaging is to describe tumor size and sprea which assists with staging.
- Imaging helps accurately TMN staging.
- Imaging findings can suggest extranodal extension (ENE), however, ENE is a clinical diagnosis in the new 8th edition of the AJCC staging manual.

REFERENCES

1. Prisman E, Miles BA, Genden EM. Oral malignancies: etiology, distribution, and treatment considerations. In: Greenberg A, Schmelzeisen R, editors. Craniomaxillofacial reconstructive and corrective bone surgery. New York, NY: Springer; 2019.
2. Varghese J, Kirsch C. Magnetic resonance imaging of the oral cavity and oropharynx. Top Magn Reson Imaging 2021;30:79–83.
3. Parvathaneni U, Lavertu P, Gibson MK, et al. Advances in diagnosis and multidisciplinary management of oropharyngeal squamous cell carcinoma: state of the art. Radiographics 2019;39:2055–68.
4. Standring S. Gray's anatomy, the anatomical basis of clinical practice. 40th edition. Philadelphia: Churchill Livingstone Elsevier; 2011.

5. Loevner LA, Hoang JK. Extramucosal spaces of the head and neck. In: Diseases of the brain, head and neck, spine 2016-2019. Cham: Springer; 2016. p. 169–76.

6. Trotta BM, Pease CS, Rasamny JJ, et al. Oral cavity and oropharyngeal squamous cell cancer: key imaging findings for staging and treatment planning. Radiographics 2011;31:339–54.

7. Aulino JM, Strother MK, Shipman JL. Imaging of oral cavity squamous cell carcinoma. Oral Maxillofac Surg Clin North Am 2006;18:445–63.

8. Mahajan A, Ahuja A, Sable N, et al. Imaging in oral cancers: a comprehensive overview of imaging findings for staging and treatment planning. Oral Oncol 2020;04:104658.

9. Hagiwara M, Nusbaum A, Schmidt BL. MR assessment of oral cavity carcinomas. Magn Reson Imaging Clin 2012;20:473–94.

10. Lee MJ, Kim S, Lee SA, et al. Overcoming artifacts from metallic orthopedic implants at high-field strength MR imaging and multi-detector CT. Radiographics 2007;27:791–803.

11. Forghani R, Smoker WRK, Curtin HD. Pathology of the oral region. In: Som PM, Curtin HD, editors. Head and neck imaging, vol. 2, 5th edition. St Louis (MO): Elsevier; 2011. p. 1643–748.

12. Dillon JK, Glastonbury CM, Jabeen F, et al. Gauze padding: a simple technique to delineate small oral cavity tumors. AJNR Am J Neuroradiol 2011; 32:934–7.

13. Srinivasan A, Mohan S, Mukherji SK. Biologic imaging of head and neck cancer: the present and the future. AJNR Am J Neuroradiol 2012;33:586–94.

14. Vandecaveye V, Dirix P, De Keyzer F, et al. Diffusion weighted magnetic resonance imaging early after chemoradiotherapy to monitor treatment response in head-and-neck squamous cell carcinoma. Int J Radiat Oncol Biol Phys 2012;82:1098–107.

15. Abdel Razek AAK. Diffusion tensor imaging in differentiation of residual head and neck squamous cell carcinoma from post-radiation changes. Magn Reson Imaging 2018;54:84–9.

16. Jansen JF, Parra C, Lu Y, et al. Evaluation of head and neck tumors with functional MR imaging. Magn Reson Imaging Clin 2016;24:123–33.

17. Razek AA, Elsorogy LG, Soliman NY, et al. Dynamic susceptibility contrast perfusion MR imaging in distinguishing malignant from benign head and neck tumors: a pilot study. Eur J Radiol 2011;77:73–9.

18. Razek AA, Poptani H. MR spectrsocopy of head and neck cancer. Eur J Radiol 2013;82:982–9.

19. Hay A, Shah J. Staging of oral cancer. Textbook of oral cancer. Cham: Springer; 2020. p. 55–67.

20. Park JO, Jung SL, Joo YH, et al. Diagnostic accuracy of magnetic resonance imaging (MRI) in the assessment of tumor invasion depth in oral/oropharyngeal cancer. Oral Oncol 2011;47:381–6.

21. Vidiri A, Guerrisi A, Pellini R, et al. Multi-detector row computed tomography (MDCT) and magnetic resonance imaging (MRI) in the evaluation of the mandibular invasion by squamous cell carcinomas (SCC) of the oral cavity. Correlation with pathological data. J Exp Clin Cancer Res 2010;29:73.

22. Imaizumi A, Yoshino N, Yamada I, et al. A potential pitfall of MR imaging for assessing mandibular invasion of squamous cell carcinoma in the oral cavity. AJNR Am J Neuroradiol 2006;27:114–22.

23. Schmidt BL. Principles of oral cavity management. In: Andersson L, Kahnberg K, Pogrel MA, editors. Oral and maxillofacial surgery. West Sussex (United-Kingdom): John Wiley & Sons; 2010. p. 705–34.

24. Tsang RK, Chung JC, To VS, et al. Efficacy of salvage neck dissection for isolated nodal recurrences in early carcinoma of oral tongue with watchful waiting management of initial N0 neck. Head Neck 2011;33:1482–5.

25. Mahajan A, Peter P, Arya S. Should 18F FDG PET/CT really be indicated in routine clinical practice for detecting contralateral neck node metastasis in head and necks squamous cell carcinoma? Radiology 2016;280:651–2.

26. Kelly HR, Curtin HD. Squamous cell carcinoma of the head and neck—imaging evaluation of regional lymph nodes and implications for management. Semin Ultrasound CT MR 2017;38:466–78.

27. Kimura Y, Sumi M, Sakihama N, et al. MR imaging criteria for the prediction of extranodal spread of metastatic cancer in the neck. Am J Neuroradiol 2008;29:1355–9.

28. Liu J, Ebrahimi A, Low TH, et al. Predictive value of the 8th edition American Joint Commission Cancer (AJCC) nodal staging system for patients with cutaneous squamous cell carcinoma of the head and neck. J Surg Oncol 2018;117:765–72.

29. Machczyński P, Majchrzak E, Niewinski P, et al. A review of the 8th edition of the AJCC staging system for oropharyngeal cancer according to HPV status. Eur Arch Otorhinolaryngol 2020;277: 2407–12.

30. Baba A, Hashimoto K, Kayama R, et al. Radiological approach for the newly incorporated T staging factor, depth of invasion (DOI), of the oral tongue cancer in the 8th edition of American Joint Committee on Cancer (AJCC) staging manual: assessment of the necessity for elective neck dissection. JAP J Radiol 2020;38:821–32.

31. Amin MB, American Joint Committee on Cancer. AJCC cancer staging manual. 8th edition. Chicago: American Joint Committee on Cancer: Springer; 2017.

32. Weber AL, Romo L, Hashmi S. Malignant tumors of the oral cavity and oropharynx: clinical, pathologic, and radiologic evaluation. Neuroimaging Clin 2003; 13:443–64.

33. Murakami R, Shiraishi S, Yoshida R, et al. Reliability of MRI-derived depth of invasion of oral tongue cancer. Acad Radiol 2019;26:e180–6.

34. Chandler K, Vance C, Budnick S, et al. Muscle invasion in oral tongue squamous cell carcinoma as a predictor of nodal status and local recurrence: just as effective as depth of invasion? Head Neck Pathol 2011;5:359–63.

35. Piazza C, Grammatica A, Montalto N, et al. Compartmental surgery for oral tongue and floor of the mouth cancer: oncologic outcomes. Head Neck 2019;41: 110–5.

36. Baik SH, Seo JW, Kim JH, et al. Prognostic value of cervical nodal necrosis observed in preoperative CT and MRI of patients with tongue squamous cell carcinoma and cervical node metastases: a retrospective study. Am J Roentgenol 2019;30:1–7.

37. Gou L, Yang W, Qiao X, et al. Marginal or segmental mandibulectomy: treatment modality selection for oral cancer: a systematic review and meta-analysis. Int J Oral Maxillofac Surg 2018;47:1.

38. Mazziotti S, Pandolfo I, D'Angelo T, et al. Diagnostic approach to retromolar trigone cancer by multiplanar computed tomography reconstructions. Can Assoc Radiol J 2014;65:335–44.

39. Crecco M, Vidiri A, Angelone ML, et al. Retromolar trigone tumors: evaluation by magnetic resonance imaging and correlation with pathological data. Eur J Radiol 1999;32:182–8.

40. Stambuk HE, Karimi S, Lee N, et al. Oral cavity and oropharynx tumors. Radiol Clin North Am 2007;45: 1–20.

41. Liao CT, Ng SH, Chang JT, et al. T4b oral cavity cancer below the mandibular notch is resectable with a favorable outcome. Oral Oncol 2007;43:570–9.

42. Chijiwa H, Sakamoto K, Umeno H, et al. Minor salivary gland carcinomas of oral cavity and oropharynx. J Laryngol Otol 2009;123:52–7.

43. Corey A. Pitfalls in the staging of cancer of the oropharyngeal squamous cell carcinoma. Neuroimaging Clin 2013;23:47–66.

44. Sessions DG, Lenox J, Spector GJ, et al. Analysis of treatment results for base of tongue cancer. Laryngoscope 2003;113:1252–61.

45. Wesolowski JR, Mukherhi S. Pathology of the pharynx. In: Som PM, Curtin HD, editors. Head and neck imaging. 5th edition. St. Louis: Elsevier; 2011. p. 1749–810.

46. Cohan DM, Popat S, Kaplan SE, et al. Oropharyngeal cancer: current understanding and management. Curr Opin Otolaryngol Head Neck Surg 2009;17:88–94.

MR Imaging of Laryngeal and Hypopharyngeal Cancer

Minerva Becker, MD[a],*, Yann Monnier, MD, PhD[b], Claudio de Vito, MD, PhD[c]

KEYWORDS

• MR imaging • Diffusion-weighted imaging • Larynx and hypopharynx • Head and neck cancer

KEY POINTS

• State-of-the-art MR imaging of the larynx and hypopharynx with high-resolution morphologic and DWI sequences has an increased precision for tumor delineation than CT, thereby facilitating tailored treatment with the ultimate goal to improve patient care.

• Current diagnostic MR imaging criteria combining DWI features with distinct signal intensity patterns on morphologic sequences allow improved discrimination between tumor, peritumoral inflammation, and fibrosis.

• Multiparametric MR imaging is particularly useful for the assessment of paraglottic space invasion, for the characterization of laryngeal cartilage abnormalities, and for the detection of extralaryngeal tumor spread, all of which can be misinterpreted on CT scans.

• DWI MR imaging has a higher diagnostic performance than CT for the detection and precise depiction of post-treatment residual and recurrent disease in the larynx and hypopharynx.

INTRODUCTION

Laryngeal cancer represents about 1% to 2% of cancers worldwide and, although the incidence is decreasing in some countries, the global incidence is increasing.[1] The highest incidence is seen in Europe followed by the Americas, whereas the ratio between death and incidence is highest in Africa.[1] The worldwide incidence of hypopharyngeal cancer is about 0.5% to 1% with a well-documented increasing incidence in women in several countries.[2,3] Over 95% of laryngeal and hypopharyngeal cancers are squamous cell carcinomas (SCCs) caused mainly by tobacco and alcohol consumption and, in contrast to oropharyngeal cancer, infection with the human papillomavirus does not play an important role.[4]

During the past 20 years, the work-up of patients with suspected cancer of the larynx and hypopharynx has been primarily done with endoscopic biopsy for the assessment of mucosal abnormalities and with multislice computed tomography (CT) for the detection of submucosal tumor spread, the complementarity of both diagnostic tools requiring a close, multidisciplinary cooperation.[5–7] This combined information allows tumors to be classified according to AJCC/UICC guidelines[8,9] and therapeutic decisions to be made. However, MR imaging is increasingly regarded in many institutions as the method of choice not only for precise localization of laryngeal and hypopharyngeal cancer but also for accurate assessment of key anatomic subsites. Advantages of MR imaging in comparison to CT include a

[a] Diagnostic Department, Division of Radiology, Unit of Head and Neck and Maxillo-facial Radiology, Geneva University Hospitals, University of Geneva, Rue Gabrielle-Perret-Gentil 4, Geneva 14, Geneva 1211, Switzerland; [b] Department of Clinical Neurosciences, Clinic of Otorhinolaryngology, Head and Neck Surgery, Unit of Cervicofacial Surgery, Geneva University Hospitals, Rue Gabrielle-Perret-Gentil 4, Geneva 14, Geneva 1211, Switzerland; [c] Diagnostic Department, Division of Clinical Pathology, Geneva University Hospitals, Rue Gabrielle-Perret-Gentil 4, Geneva 14, Geneva 1211, Switzerland
* Corresponding author.
E-mail address: Minerva.Becker@hcuge.ch

Magn Reson Imaging Clin N Am 30 (2022) 53–72
https://doi.org/10.1016/j.mric.2021.08.002

superior soft-tissue contrast enabling the detection of subtle soft-tissue abnormalities, an increased discrimination capability between tumor and peritumoral inflammatory changes, improved assessment of laryngeal cartilage abnormalities, improved tumor delineation for highly focused radiotherapy and transoral laser microsurgery, and a higher diagnostic performance for the detection and precise depiction of post-treatment residual or recurrent disease.[7,10–19] However, some relative drawbacks of MR imaging in comparison to CT persist, including a longer acquisition time and motion artifacts requiring improved patient cooperation, a lower spatial resolution, and technical challenges related to air-tissue interfaces affecting image quality of diffusion-weighted imaging (DWI) sequences.

This review discusses the current state-of-the-art MR imaging examination protocols for oncologic imaging of the larynx and hypopharynx, key anatomic areas, and characteristic imaging features of laryngeal and hypopharyngeal tumors focusing on clinically relevant information in SCC and it equally addresses potential pitfalls of image interpretation. Correlation with endoscopic and histopathologic features is provided to highlight key concepts and imaging pearls.

IMAGING TECHNIQUE AND PROTOCOLS

One of the key issues when imaging laryngeal and hypopharyngeal cancer is spatial resolution, which is crucial for accurate tumor evaluation. For routine MR imaging, most authors advocate the use of either 1.5T or 3T scanners, the latter providing a higher signal-to-noise ratio, which is preferable if thinner slices are used for imaging. The coils routinely used to image laryngeal and hypopharyngeal cancers include dedicated head and neck phased array coils (groups of overlapping coils linked to a common output), parallel imaging array coils (groups of coils with a high level of decoupling optimized for artifact-free parallel imaging performance), or local circular receive surface coils placed around the larynx.[11–13,20–23] Local circular surface coils can be used alone or they can be combined with head coils. They have a small field of view and an increased signal-to-noise ratio for tissues adjacent to the loop, hence, slice thickness and in-plane resolution can be substantially improved. Nevertheless, the area covered is restricted allowing imaging of the larynx/hypopharynx only. In addition, the placement of loop surface coils around the larynx can be challenging and requires precise positioning by an experienced technician. Incorrect coil positioning can result in a reduced signal to noise, limited

penetration depth, signal void in the anterior larynx, or fold-back artifacts.[24] As the circular surface coils need to be positioned relatively tightly on the patient's neck, the uncomfortable position can further lead to motion artifacts during image acquisition. In contrast, phased array head/neck coils and the latest generation parallel imaging array coils are rather straightforward to use in clinical routine. The area covered is large and evaluation of the primary tumor and lymph nodes in the neck is possible within a reasonable time. Therefore, in most institutions, phased array or parallel imaging array coils are used for routine MR imaging scanning of laryngeal and hypopharyngeal cancers. At the authors' institution, we use parallel imaging array coils which combine 64 or 20 channel head coils (for 3T and 1.5T, respectively) with flexible superficial coils placed on the anterior neck.

According to the literature, a slice thickness of 3 to 4 mm is recommended for MR imaging of the larynx/hypopharynx as a compromise between a decreased signal-to-noise ratio due to thinner slices (in particular at 1.5T) and an increased acquisition time necessary to cover the required anatomic area. The recommended in-plane resolution is in the range of 0.4×0.4 mm to 0.8×0.8 mm,[7,11] whereas local circular surface coils placed around the larynx may achieve an in-plane resolution as high as 0.2×0.5 mm.[12,23]

Although MR imaging protocols are subject to rapid technical evolutions, at the authors' institution routine MR imaging protocols for the larynx and hypopharynx include coronal short tau inversion recovery (STIR) followed by axial DWI, T2, and precontrast and postcontrast T1, as well as additional acquisitions in the coronal and/or sagittal plane. DWI is routinely performed with a single shot echoplanar imaging (SS-EPI) sequence with 2 b values (b = 0 and b = 1000) and with apparent diffusion coefficient (ADC) maps generated automatically by the MR imaging software. The imaging protocols from the authors' institution are shown in **Table 1**. Tips and tricks to optimize image quality include the following:

- The comfortably immobilized patient should be instructed to breathe regularly and not too deep and, whenever possible, with an open mouth during image acquisition (as swallowing is not possible with an open mouth)
- The patient should clear the throat between sequences (to avoid coughing during image acquisition)
- Axial images should be strictly parallel to the plane of the true vocal cords (based on sagittal and coronal localizers)

Table 1
Summary of the MR imaging protocol for laryngeal and hypopharyngeal cancer at the authors' institution

Series Number	Sequence Type	Plane	Slice Thickness	Phase Encoding
Series 1	Survey/localizer	Axial, coronal, sagittal		
Series 2	T2 STIR	Coronal	3 mm	Caudal-cranial
Series 3	DWI SS-EPI 2b values (0 and 1000)	Axial	3 mm	Anteroposterior
Series 4	T2 TSE/FSE	Axial	3 mm	Anteroposterior
Series 5	T1 TSE/FSE	Axial	3 mm	Anteroposterior
Series 6[a]	Perfusion T1 cartography (vibe T1 map)	Axial	3 mm	Anteroposterior
Injection: iv. Contrast				
Series 7[a]	Perfusion T1 dynamic vibe	Axial	3 mm	Anteroposterior
Series 8	T1 TSE/FSE	Axial	3 mm	Anteroposterior
Series 9	T1 TSE/FSE with fat saturation	Axial	3 mm	Anteroposterior
Series 10[b]	T1 Dixon	Coronal/sagittal	3 mm	Caudal-cranial

Routinely, a subtraction series (subtracting series 5 from series 8) is obtained by postprocessing to evaluate the enhancement patterns more precisely.
[a] Series 6 and 7 are routinely performed in the post-treatment setting, otherwise optional.
[b] Depending on tumor localization and findings on previous images, either coronal or sagittal or both coronal and sagittal imaging planes are acquired.

- The smallest possible field of view should be chosen (dependent on neck morphotype, 16 × 18 cm – 18 × 20 cm) and an acquisition matrix of 350 to 512 × 450 to 512 should be used
- The phase encoding gradient should be either in the anteroposterior direction (axial and sagittal plane) or in the caudal-cranial direction (coronal plane) to move flow artifacts (especially after iv. contrast) away from the larynx and hypopharynx
- Meticulous shimming for DWI sequences is a must

KEY ANATOMIC CONSIDERATIONS AND IMPLICATIONS FOR PATTERNS OF SUBMUCOSAL TUMOR SPREAD

Accurate radiological assessment of submucosal tumor spread plays a key role in the T classification of laryngeal and hypopharyngeal cancers and in treatment planning, especially for transoral laser excision, open partial laryngectomy, and highly focused radiotherapy. Although knowledge of the anatomy of the larynx and hypopharynx is essential for the correct interpretation of MR imaging scans, a detailed review of the pertinent anatomy

is beyond the scope of this article. Nevertheless, to understand what the referring physician needs to know and to deliver actionable information to the patient care team, the clinically relevant anatomy of the paraglottic space, pre-epiglottic space, and laryngeal cartilages will be reviewed.

Paraglottic Space

The paraglottic space plays an important role in the T classification of laryngeal cancers because if it is invaded, SCC is classified as T3 according to the AJCC/UICC guidelines.[8,9] Whether neoplastic involvement of the paraglottic space influences the outcome after radiotherapy is still a matter of debate.[25–27] However, invasion of the posterior paraglottic space and of the thyrocricoarytenoid space (TCAS, see below) is associated with a poorer outcome in terms of overall survival, disease-free survival, and locoregional control after radiotherapy and open partial laryngectomy.[28,29] Furthermore, if the posterior paraglottic space is invaded, transoral laser surgery is contraindicated.[12,23,30]

The paired and symmetric paraglottic space found in the supraglottic and glottic region (**Fig. 1**) mainly contains adipose tissue, loose

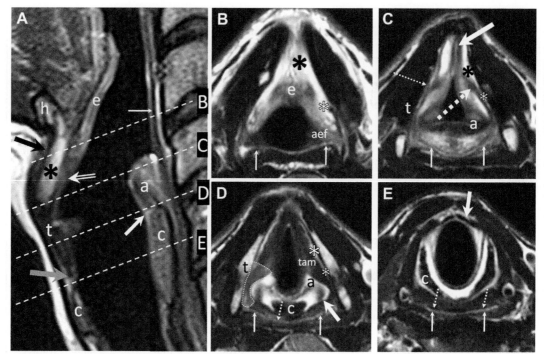

Fig. 1. Normal MR imaging anatomy of the larynx and hypopharynx (T2 images without fat saturation). Paramedian sagittal image (*A*) showing the hyoid bone (h), epiglottis (e), thyroid (t), cricoid (c), and arytenoid (a) cartilages and pre-epiglottic space (*asterisk*). Thick white arrow indicates the cricoarytenoid joint; thin white arrow indicates the posterior hypopharyngeal wall; black arrow indicates the thyrohyoid membrane; double white arrow indicates the thyroepiglottic ligament located inferiorly to the epiglottis; gray arrow indicates the cricothyroid membrane; and dashed white lines indicate the axial planes of images B to E. (*B*) Upper supraglottic region. The pre-epiglottic space (*black asterisk*) is located anteriorly to the epiglottis (e). No clear boundary with the paraglottic space (*white asterisk*) is present at this level. Aryepiglottic fold (aef), posterior hypopharyngeal wall (*thin arrows*). (*C*) Lower supraglottic region (false cord level). The pre-epiglottic space (*black asterisk*) lies laterally to the thyroepiglottic ligament (*thick white arrow*) and anteriorly to the paraglottic space (*white asterisk*). The thyroglottic ligament (*thin dashed arrow*) separates the pre-epiglottic space from the paraglottic space. Thyroarytenoid and aryepiglottic muscle fibers (*thick dashed arrow*) merge with the thyroglottic ligament. Arytenoid cartilage (a). Collapsed lumen of the piriform sinuses (*thin white arrows*). (*D*) True vocal cord level. The thyroarytenoid muscle (tam) makes up the bulk of the true vocal cords. Paraglottic space (*white asterisks*). Arytenoid cartilage (a) and cricoid cartilage (c) forming the cricoarytenoid joint (*thick arrow*). Thyroid cartilage (t). The area surrounded by the thin dashed contours is the TCAS. Dashed arrow points at the retrocricoarytenoid region of the hypopharynx and thin solid arrows point at the posterior hypopharyngeal wall. Note that the posterior parapharyngeal space is bordered posteriorly by the piriform sinuses. (*E*) Subglottic region. Cricoid cartilage (c). Cricothyroid membrane (*thick arrow*). Dashed arrows point at the retrocricoarytenoid region of the hypopharynx and solid thin arrows point at the posterior hypopharyngeal wall.

elastic and collagen tissue, and blood vessels.[31–33] Laterally, the paraglottic space is bordered by the thyrohyoid membrane, thyroid cartilage, and cricothyroid membrane, medially by the quadrangular membrane, laryngeal ventricle, aryepiglottic muscle, and thyroarytenoid muscle (which forms the bulk of the true vocal cords), posteriorly by the mucosa of the piriform sinuses and inferiorly by the conus elasticus. In the posterosuperior supraglottic region, there is no boundary between the paraglottic space and the pre-epiglottic space. However, in the posteroinferior supraglottic region, the thyroglottic ligament (a fibrous septum which fans out from the vocal ligament to the thyroid cartilage) separates the 2 spaces.[31–33] At the glottic level, the paraglottic space can be divided into an anterior part (two-thirds) and a posterior part (one-third) by a line extending laterally from the vocal process of the arytenoid to the thyroid lamina. The posterior paraglottic space is currently considered as part of the TCAS (see **Fig. 1**) and neoplastic invasion of TCAS is an important adverse prognostic factor in laryngeal cancer.[28,29,34]

The paraglottic space is best assessed on axial and coronal images. It is easily identified on MR imaging because of its high fat content and, therefore, has a high signal intensity on T1 and T2 (see **Fig. 1**). The normal paraglottic space may show some minor enhancement after iv. administration of gadolinium chelates as it contains blood vessels. MR imaging is superior to CT for assessing the narrow paraglottic space at the vocal cord level.[23,34,35]

The paraglottic space plays a pivotal role in submucosal tumor dissemination and it constitutes a "highway" for submucosal tumor spread. Invasion of the paraglottic space occurs whenever SCC arising in the laryngeal ventricle, false cords, or true vocal cords spreads laterally or whenever SCC of the piriform sinus spreads anteriorly. Key points of submucosal tumor spread along the paraglottic space include the following:

- Tumor spread in the paraglottic space typically occurs in a vertical direction (transglottic spread; **Fig. 2**).
- Lateral tumor spread from the paraglottic space results in thyroid cartilage invasion.
- Lateral tumor spread from the paraglottic space through the cricothyroid ligament

inferiorly and thyrohyoid membrane superiorly leads to invasion of extralaryngeal soft tissues (see **Fig. 2**).
- Tumor spread from the posterior paraglottic space leads to early involvement of the piriform sinus, cricoarytenoid joint, and posterior thyroarytenoid muscle.

Pre-epiglottic Space

The pre-epiglottic space plays an important role in the T classification of laryngeal cancers: if the pre-epiglottic space is invaded, SCC is classified as T3 according to AJCC/UICC guidelines.[8,9] Multiple authors have suggested that the degree of invasion of the pre-epiglottic space influences surgical options and to a moderate degree the likelihood of local recurrence after radio(chemo)therapy and open partial laryngectomy although others have questioned the impact of pre-epiglottic space invasion on local control after concurrent radiochemotherapy.[36-40]

The pre-epiglottic space mainly contains fatty tissue, some loose connective tissue, and blood vessels (see **Fig. 1**). Anteriorly, it is bounded by

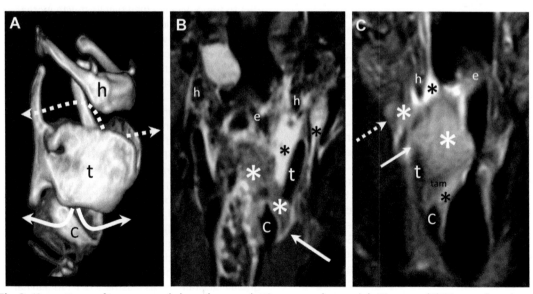

Fig. 2. Key patterns of tumor spread along the paraglottic space and pre-epiglottic space. (A) Diagram based on a 3D volume rendering reconstruction of laryngeal cartilages showing extralaryngeal patterns of spread through the cricothyroid membrane (*arrows*) and thyrohyoid membrane (*dashed arrows*). The following annotations apply to all figure parts: hyoid bone (h), thyroid cartilage (t), cricoid cartilage (c), epiglottis (e). (B) Coronal T2 STIR image showing a SCC with intermediate signal intensity (*white asterisks*), transglottic spread along the left paraglottic space and extension through the cricothyroid membrane into the extralaryngeal soft tissues (*arrow*). Note areas of very high signal intensity in the left supraglottic larynx and outside the larynx (*black asterisks*) corresponding to peritumoral inflammation. (C) Coronal T2 STIR image in another patient with a SCC (*white asterisks*) with moderately high signal intensity invading the pre-epiglottic space, paraglottic space, and right thyroarytenoid muscle (*tam*). Note lateral tumor spread through the thyrohyoid membrane into the soft tissues of the neck (*dashed arrow*) and destruction of the superior border of the right thyroid cartilage (*arrow*). Very high signal intensity areas (*black asterisks*) surrounding the tumor and corresponding to peritumoral inflammation.

the thyrohyoid membrane and thyroid cartilage, posteriorly by the epiglottis, cranially by the hyoepiglottic ligament, and caudally by the thyroepiglottic ligament.[31–33] It is important to bear in mind that the pre-epiglottic space extends not only anteriorly to but also posterolaterally to the epiglottis and the posterolateral border of the pre-epiglottic space on axial images is located at about the anteroposterior midpoint of the thyroid lamina.[33] The pre-epiglottic space is best seen on axial and sagittal images and it is easily identified on MR imaging and CT because of its high fat content (see **Fig. 1**) The normal pre-epiglottic space behaves like fatty tissue on MR imaging. Minor reticulated contrast enhancement of the pre-epiglottic space can be seen on high-resolution contrast-enhanced T1 because of the presence of blood vessels and loose connective tissue. Early invasion of the pre-epiglottic space occurs when SCC arising from the laryngeal surface of the epiglottis spreads in an anterior direction. Key points of submucosal tumor spread involving the pre-epiglottic space include the following:

- As there is no effective boundary posterosuperiorly between the pre-epiglottic space and paraglottic space, tumor spread from the pre-epiglottic space can result in paraglottic space invasion and vice versa
- Anterolateral tumor spread from the pre-epiglottic space through the thyrohyoid membrane results in invasion of extralaryngeal soft tissues (see **Fig. 2**).

Laryngeal Cartilages

Invasion of the thyroid and cricoid cartilages influences the T classification of laryngeal and hypopharyngeal cancers.[8,9] Laryngeal SCC with invasion of the inner cortex of the thyroid cartilage is classified as T3, whereas laryngeal SCC with invasion of the cricoid cartilage or invasion through the outer cortex of the thyroid cartilage is classified as T4a. In contrast, hypopharyngeal SCC invading the thyroid or cricoid cartilage is classified as T4a irrespective of the degree of cartilage invasion. In addition, invasion of the laryngeal cartilages affects prognosis after radiotherapy and influences the choice of surgery (total laryngectomy vs open partial laryngectomy or transoral laser microsurgery).[4,41]

The thyroid, cricoid and arytenoid cartilages (with the exception of the vocal process of the arytenoids which contains elastic fibrocartilage) are composed of hyaline cartilage (**Fig. 3**). Hyaline cartilage undergoes ossification with increasing age.[42] Ossified cartilage corresponds histologically to bone: it has an inner and outer cortex and a

marrow cavity with predominantly fatty tissue, some erythropoietic marrow and bone trabeculae (see **Fig. 3**). Although the normal ossification process of laryngeal cartilages tends to follow a predefined pattern and can result in complete ossification of the thyroid and cricoid cartilage, in most individuals, the central thyroid laminae and parts of the cricoid cartilage remain nonossified throughout life, and differences in ossification between right and left are common.[42,43] Furthermore, asymmetric ossification can be equally seen in normal arytenoid cartilages.[44]

The mechanism by which cancer invades laryngeal cartilages[45–47] involves the following steps:

- An inflammatory phase (with edema and increased vascularization) within the cartilage located in immediate tumor vicinity and before actual tumor invasion
- An osteoblastic phase with new bone formation
- An osteoclastic phase in which newly formed bone is eroded and frank invasion by tumor cells occurs.

Both early neoplastic cartilage invasion and inflammatory changes in the laryngeal cartilages due to tumor vicinity may manifest with increased cartilage ossification (sclerosis) at CT.[6] Therefore, the distinction between the normal mix of nonossified and ossified cartilage, sclerosis due to tumor invasion and sclerosis due to peritumoral inflammation is not possible with CT. Normal nonossified hyaline cartilage and ossified cartilage display characteristic signal intensities on MR imaging (see **Fig. 3**). Hyaline nonossified cartilage and the cortex of ossified cartilage are strongly hypointense on T1 and T2 and do not enhance after i.v. contrast administration, whereas the marrow cavity of ossified cartilage behaves like fatty marrow elsewhere in the body. On DWI, normal cartilages have a low signal on b1000 images and on ADC maps (see **Fig. 3**). These characteristic features on MR imaging and the increased capability of MR imaging to distinguish between tumor and peritumoral inflammatory changes (see below) greatly facilitate the assessment of laryngeal cartilage abnormalities and thus avoids diagnostic pitfalls related to CT.

MR IMAGING FINDINGS IN LARYNGEAL AND HYPOPHARYNGEAL CANCER
Tumor and Peritumoral Inflammation

Both primary and recurrent laryngeal and hypopharyngeal SCCs show characteristic signal intensity patterns on MR imaging: an intermediate signal intensity on T1, T2, and STIR and moderate

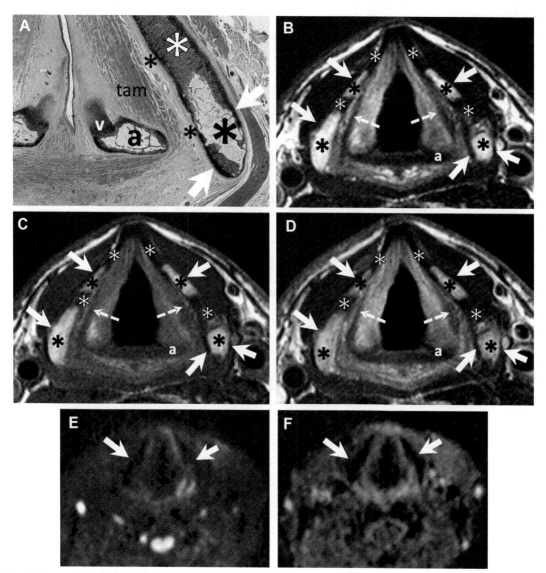

Fig. 3. Normal anatomy of the laryngeal cartilages. (*A*) Whole organ histologic slice at the false cord level. The thyroid cartilage is composed of hyaline nonossified cartilage (*white asterisk*) and of ossified cartilage, which has a cortex (*white arrows*) and a marrow cavity containing adipose tissue and bone trabeculae (*large black asterisk*). Small black asterisks indicate the posterior paraglottic space. Thyroarytenoid muscle fibers (tam) merged with the thyroglottic ligament laterally, body of the arytenoid cartilage (a) and vocal process (v). Axial T2 (*B*), T1 (*C*), contrast-enhanced T1 (*D*), b1000 (*E*), and ADC map (*F*) at the false cord level. Nonossified hyaline cartilage (*white asterisks in B, C,* and *D*) and cortex of ossified cartilage (*white arrows in B, C,* and *D*) with a very low signal intensity on all sequences. The marrow of ossified cartilage (*black asterisks in B, C,* and *D*) has the signal intensity of fat and does not enhance. b1000 image (*E*) and ADC map (*F*) show that cartilages have a low signal intensity (*arrows in E* and *F*). Dashed arrows in B, C, and D point at fibers of the thyroarytenoid muscle merging with the thyroglottic ligament.

contrast enhancement after iv. administration of gadolinium chelates[7,11] (**Fig. 4**). Primary laryngeal and hypopharyngeal SCCs can be mass-like, they can extend along the mucosal surfaces or they can be diffusely infiltrating at cross-sectional imaging, whereas recurrent SCCs tend to be located beneath an intact mucosa and they display a diffusely infiltrative invasion pattern with indistinct tumor margins (see **Fig. 4**; **Figs. 5** and **6**).[17,18,48,49] This difference can be explained by histologic characteristics as primary laryngeal and hypopharyngeal SCCs have a rather unicentric growth pattern while recurrent tumors have multicentric tumor foci disseminated over large

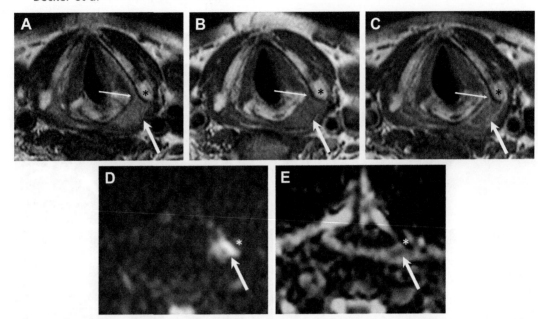

Fig. 4. Small primary SCC arising in the left piriform sinus with characteristic MR imaging features. Axial T2 (*A*), T1 (*B*), contrast-enhanced T1 (*C*), b1000 (*D*) and ADC map (*E*) at the vocal cord level show a mass in the apex of the left piriform sinus (*thick arrows* on all figure parts) with an intermediate signal intensity on T2, low signal intensity on T1 and moderate contrast enhancement. High signal on the b1000 image (*D*) and low signal on the ADC map (*E*) indicate restricted diffusion. Mean ADC was 1.03×10^{-3} mm²/s. The tumor shows most likely minimal invasion of the posterior paraglottic space (*thin arrow* in *A*, *B*, and *C*). Note a very thin hyperintense rim surrounding the tumor in C corresponding to peri-tumoral inflammation with increased vascularization. Asterisk on all figure parts shows a normal adjacent thyroid cartilage consisting of ossified cartilage.

anatomic areas beneath an intact mucosa.[18,48,49] Restricted diffusion is characteristic for both primary and recurrent SCCs and mean ADC values (calculated with b = 0 and b = 1000) are in the range of 0.9 to 1.3×10^{-3} mm²/s[19,50,51] (see **Figs. 4** and **6**). Correlation with histopathology has shown that mean ADC values in laryngeal and hypopharyngeal SCCs are significantly correlated with cellularity, stromal component, and nuclear-cytoplasmic ratio, and differences in ADC values between tumors can be mainly explained by variable amounts of tumor stroma components.[52]

Both primary and recurrent SCCs are often surrounded by variable degrees of peritumoral inflammation, which can accompany early and advanced cancers and may lead to overestimation of tumor size unless careful analysis of multiparametric MR imaging signal intensity is done (see **Fig. 2**; **Figs. 7** and **8**). These peritumoral inflammatory changes which precede tumor invasion of adjacent structures are characterized by a higher signal intensity on T2 and STIR and by a stronger contrast enhancement than the tumor itself. Also, on DWI peritumoral inflammation shows no restricted diffusion, and mean ADC values (calculated with b = 0 and b = 1000) are typically in the range of 1.4 to 1.9×10^{-3} mm²/s.

Using a multiparametric approach with the aforementioned diagnostic criteria, MR imaging with current state-of-the-art coils allows an improved distinction between tumor and peritumoral inflammatory changes, therefore facilitating a more precise evaluation of critical anatomic subsites. Although newer studies found a low CT sensitivity for the detection of neoplastic invasion of the paraglottic space,[35] older studies reported a high sensitivity of MR imaging and CT for the detection of neoplastic invasion of the pre-epiglottic space and paraglottic space.[53–55] However, as older studies have used different morphologic criteria that do not allow distinction between tumor and inflammation, the reported specificity of MR imaging and CT in the paraglottic space was low (around 50%), thus leading to overestimation of tumor spread in a considerable number of cases.[54–56] Nevertheless, using the aforementioned MR imaging criteria, which take differences in signal intensity, contrast enhancement, and DWI characteristics into consideration, it is currently possible to distinguish between tumor and inflammation in the paraglottic space and in the TCAS with a sensitivity of 100% and a specificity of 78%.[34] This area, which has important prognostic implications, is particularly difficult to evaluate on CT scans.[35] Although other

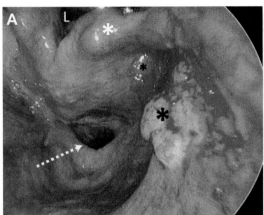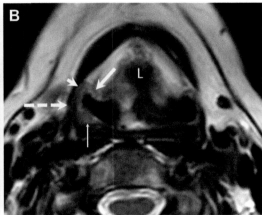

Fig. 5. Primary SCC arising in the right piriform sinus with a characteristic superficial pattern of spread. Endoscopic view (*A*) showing a right piriform sinus tumor involving the anterior wall of the piriform sinus (*small black asterisk*), the angle, the lateral wall (*large asterisks*), and with beginning spread on the posterior wall. Aryepiglottic fold (*large white asterisk*). Laryngeal lumen (L). Dashed arrow points at the esophageal verge. Note that as we are looking from above, the right piriform sinus appears on the right side of the image. Axial T2 image (*B*) shows the tumor with an intermediate signal intensity spreading along the anterior wall of the piriform sinus, that is, the posterior wall of the aryepiglottic fold (*thick arrow*), the angle (*short arrow*), the lateral wall (*dashed arrow*), and the posterior hypopharyngeal wall (*thin arrow*). Larynx (L). There is minimal invasion of the aryepiglottic fold fat (which is in continuity with the paraglottic space).

areas of the larynx, which contain higher amounts of fat, such as the pre-epiglottic space, are more easily evaluated with CT, it is worthwhile mentioning that currently there are no series in the literature systematically comparing the diagnostic performance of multiparametric DWI MR imaging with CT in the deep laryngeal spaces. Furthermore, because of the difficulty to obtain radiologic-pathologic correlation, most data in the literature are based on older studies, which have used older diagnostic criteria, and newer studies using the aforementioned criteria are based only on a limited number of cases.

Regarding the detection and staging of early SCC of the larynx and hypopharynx, data in the literature are scarce and do not allow to draw solid conclusions about the added value of MR imaging in T1 and T2 lesions.[57] Nevertheless, some authors have pointed out that MR imaging is clearly superior to CT in the preoperative staging of early glottic cancer.[58] It has even been suggested that DWI may detect changes in tumor size and shape before they become apparent at laryngostroboscopy and may help to distinguish laryngeal SCC from precursor lesions.[59]

Neoplastic Cartilage Invasion

Detection of neoplastic cartilage invasion at CT uses the criteria of sclerosis, erosion/lysis, and extralaryngeal spread.[6] Sclerosis is a sensitive but nonspecific sign of cartilage invasion,

especially in the thyroid cartilage (specificity = 40%).[6] In contrast, erosion/lysis and extralaryngeal spread are specific signs (specificity = 93%) but not sensitive as they are bound to the presence of more advanced invasion of laryngeal cartilages. In the presence of sclerosis alone, it is nearly impossible to decide, whether sclerosis corresponds to cartilage invasion, whether it is caused by peritumoral inflammation with bone remodeling, or whether it corresponds to asymmetric ossification. Furthermore, it has been shown that the positive predictive value of CT to detect major cartilage invasion and extralaryngeal spread is limited and varies between 53% and 81%[6,60,61] (**Fig. 9**). Another problem with CT is that nonossified cartilage can have similar attenuation values as SCC on contrast-enhanced CT rendering a correct radiologic interpretation difficult (**Fig. 10**). Applying the diagnostic criteria for tumor, inflammation, normal non-ossified, and normal ossified cartilage as explained earlier, MR imaging allows an improved diagnosis of cartilage abnormalities thus avoiding diagnostic pitfalls related to CT (see **Fig. 10**; **Figs. 11** and **12**). In summary, if a cartilage in the immediate tumor vicinity displays a moderately high signal intensity on T2, a moderate enhancement on contrast-enhanced T1 and restricted diffusivity, the cartilage should be regarded as invaded (see **Fig. 12**). However, if a cartilage in the immediate tumor vicinity displays a higher signal intensity on T2 and a stronger enhancement than the adjacent

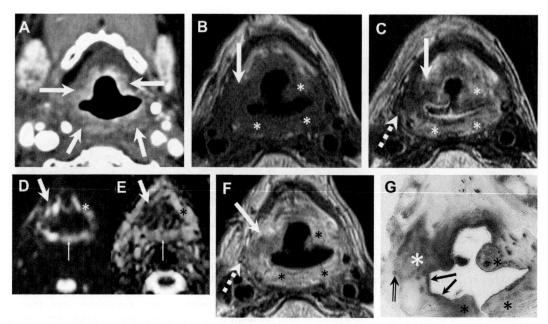

Fig. 6. Characteristic MR imaging findings in a recurrent supraglottic SCC after radiation therapy. The recurrent tumor was missed at initial endoscopy and CT but was correctly diagnosed at MR imaging. Axial contrast-enhanced CT at the supraglottic level (*A*) shows nonspecific, diffuse, and symmetric contrast enhancement surrounding the supraglottic larynx and the posterior hypopharyngeal wall (*arrows*). Findings were similar to those of a previous CT obtained 6 months earlier (not shown). Corresponding axial T1 (*B*), T2 (*C*), b1000 (*D*), ADC (*E*), and contrast-enhanced T1 (*F*) images obtained at the same level show a poorly defined, infiltrative lesion (*white arrows* in *B*, *C, D, E,* and *F*) involving the right aryepiglottic fold with invasion of the right pre-epiglottic and paraglottic space. The lesion has a low signal intensity on T1, intermediate signal intensity on T2, moderate enhancement and restricted diffusion strongly suggesting recurrent tumor. ADC was 1.12×10^{-3} mm^2/s. There is extralaryngeal spread through the thyrohyoid membrane (*dashed arrows* in *C* and *F*). The retropharyngeal space (*asterisks* in *B, C, F* and *thin arrows* in *D* and *E*) and the left aryepiglottic fold (*asterisks* on *B, C, D; E* and *F*) show edema with low signal intensity on T1, slightly higher signal intensity than the tumor on T2, no restricted diffusion, and stronger enhancement than the tumor on contrast-enhanced T1. Note also intermediate signal on T2 along the antero-posterior wall of the piriform sinus. This finding was considered suspicious of tumor involvement but could not be confirmed on the other MR imaging sequences. Corresponding whole organ histologic slice (*G*) confirms recurrent SCC. Tumor (*white asterisk*) invading the right pre-epiglottic and paraglottic space. Inflammatory edema (*black asterisks*). Neoplastic involvement of extralaryngeal soft tissues (*double arrow*) on the right. There was also superficial tumor spread along the mucosa of the right piriform sinus (*solid arrows*) as suspected on T2.

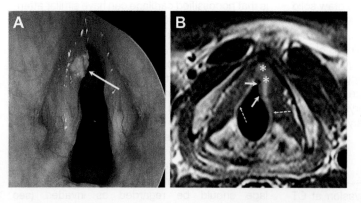

Fig. 7. T1a glottic SCC with peritumoral inflammatory changes. Endoscopic view (*A*) showing a small SCC (*arrow*) located in the anterior third of the left vocal cord. Vocal cord mobility was normal. Note that as we are looking from above, the left vocal cord appears on the left side of the image. Axial contrast-enhanced T1 image (*B*) shows the small and superficial tumor of the anterior left vocal cord with moderate enhancement (*solid arrows*). The tumor is surrounded by an area of stronger enhancement than the tumor itself (*asterisks*) corresponding to peritumoral inflammation. Note that tumor enhancement is also lower than the enhancement of the mucosa overlying the rest of the vocal cords (*dashed arrows*). The thyroarytenoid muscle and the paraglottic space are not invaded by the tumor.

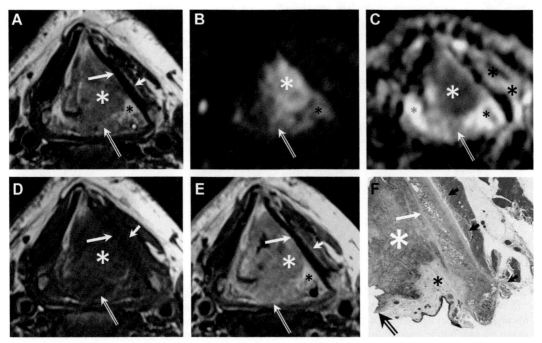

Fig. 8. Left supraglottic SCC with peritumoral inflammation and invasion of the paraglottic space. Axial T2 (*A*), b1000 (*B*), ADC (*C*), T1 (*D*), and contrast-enhanced T1 (*E*) obtained at the supraglottic level show a tumor arising from the left false cord with intermediate signal on T2, restricted diffusion, and moderate contrast enhancement (*white asterisk* on all figure parts). Tumor invasion of the retrocricoarytenoid region (*double arrow* on all figure parts) and of the anterior two-thirds of the left paraglottic space (*long solid arrow* on on *A, D* and *E*). The posterior left paraglottic space shows inflammation (*black asterisk* on all figure parts). The adjacent thyroid cartilage shows a low signal intensity on all sequences, which corresponds to normal nonossified hyaline cartilage. Note a thin rim of inflammation extending along the outer lamina of the left thyroid cartilage (*short arrows* on *A, D, E* and *large black asterisks* on *C*). Edema of the right posterior paraglottic space (*gray asterisk* on *C*). Detail from whole organ histologic slice (*F*) confirms all MR imaging findings. SCC (*white asterisk*) invading the anterior paraglottic space (*long white arrow*) and the retrocricoarytenoid region (*double arrow*). There was no invasion of the nonossified thyroid cartilage histologically. Inflammation in the right posterior paraglottic space (*black asterisk*) and of the strap muscles along the outer thyroid lamina (*short arrows*).

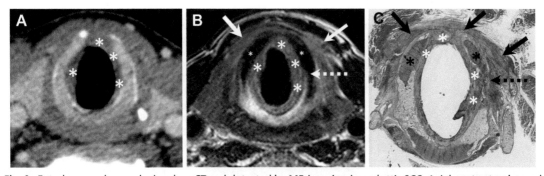

Fig. 9. Extralaryngeal spread missed on CT and detected by MR imaging in a glottic SCC. Axial contrast-enhanced CT (*A*) at the subglottic level shows nearly circumferential subglottic tumor spread (*asterisks*). The cricoid cartilage is poorly ossified and does not show signs of cartilage invasion. The extralaryngeal soft tissues were interpreted as normal. Corresponding T2 image (*B*) shows subglottic tumor spread (*large asterisks*). The anterior portion of the cricoid cartilage is composed of nonossified cartilage (*small asterisks*). Note an irregular contour on the left suspicious of cartilage invasion (*dashed arrow*). In addition, there is massive bilateral extralaryngeal tumor spread (*arrows*) not revealed by CT. Corresponding whole organ histologic slice (*C*) confirms MR imaging findings. Subglottic tumor (*white asterisks*). Nonossified cricoid cartilage (*black asterisks*). Invasion of nonossified hyaline cartilage (*dashed arrow*). Bilateral anterior extralaryngeal tumor spread (*arrows*) mainly occurring through the cricothyroid membrane.

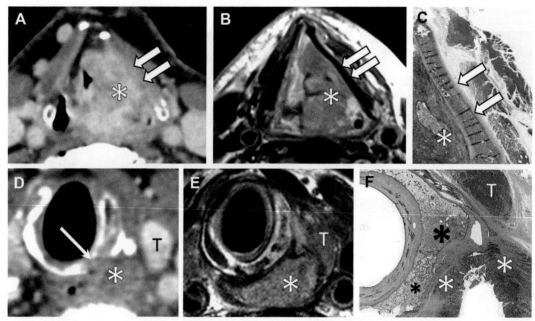

Fig. 10. Pitfalls related to similar attenuation values of SCC and nonossified hyaline cartilage on CT and avoided by MR imaging. Upper figure row (*A–C*) shows images of a patient with supraglottic SCC. Axial contrast-enhanced CT shows a tumor (*white asterisk*) invading the left paraglottic space and abutting the left thyroid lamina (*white arrows*). The thyroid lamina has similar attenuation values as the tumor. Cartilage invasion cannot be ruled out. Corresponding contrast-enhanced T1 image (*B*) shows that the tumor (*asterisk*), which invades the paraglottic space has an intermediate signal intensity, whereas the left thyroid lamina is strongly hypointense suggesting normal nonossified hyaline cartilage. (*C*) Detail from the corresponding histologic slice confirms MR imaging findings. There was tumor invasion of the paraglottic space but no invasion of the nonossified thyroid cartilage. Tumor (*asterisk*). Noninvaded hyaline cartilage (*white arrows*). Lower figure row (*D–F*) shows images of a patient with a piriform sinus tumor invading the esophageal verge. Axial, contrast-enhanced CT image (*D*) shows that the tumor (*asterisk*) is in close vicinity of the cricoid cartilage. The cricoid cartilage has an irregular ossification pattern and an area of osteolysis (*arrow*) is suspected. Thyroid gland (*T*). Corresponding T2 image obtained at the same level (*E*) shows the tumor with intermediate signal intensity (*asterisk*) surrounded by a hypointense rim. The posterior lamina of the cricoid cartilage shows a mix of ossified and nonossified portions and its cortex is preserved. Thyroid gland (*T*). Whole organ histologic slice (*F*) reveals absent invasion of the cricoid cartilage. The cricoid cartilage has an irregular ossification pattern with a mix of ossified (*small black asterisk*) and nonossified (*large black asterisk*) portions. Tumor invading the esophageal verge (*white asterisks*). Thyroid gland (*T*).

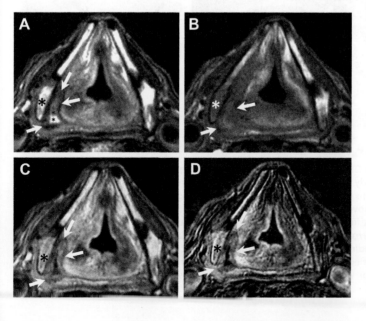

Fig. 11. Characteristic MR imaging features of cartilage inflammation. Patient with an SCC of the right piriform sinus. Axial T2 (*A*), T1 (*B*), contrast-enhanced T1 (*C*), and subtraction image obtained by subtracting T1 from contrast-enhanced T1 (*D*) show a piriform sinus tumor invading the anterior wall, the angle, the lateral wall, and the posterior wall of the piriform sinus (*arrows* on all figure parts). The tumor has an intermediate signal on T2, a low signal on T1, and a moderate enhancement on contrast-enhanced T1. Note that the thyroid cartilage in the immediate tumor vicinity (*asterisk* on all figure parts) shows a much higher signal intensity on T2 than the tumor, a similar low signal on T1, and a much stronger enhancement on T1. The difference in enhancement patterns is particularly well seen in D (subtraction image). Small asterisk in A indicates fluid retention in the right piriform sinus.

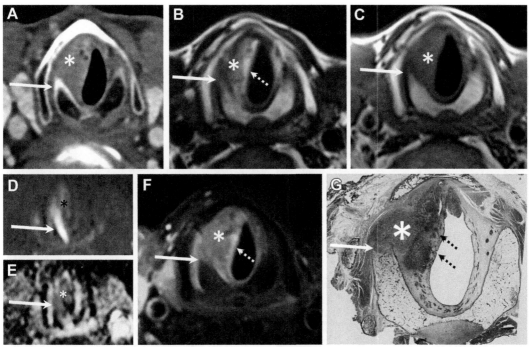

Fig. 12. MR imaging as a problem-solving tool for cartilage sclerosis on CT. Patient with a glottic SCC. Contrast-enhanced CT image (*A*) reveals subglottic tumor spread (*asterisk*) and sclerosis of the adjacent cricoid cartilage (*arrow*). Based on CT findings, it is difficult to decide whether sclerosis corresponds to neoplastic invasion or inflammation. Corresponding axial T2 (*B*), T1 (*C*), b1000 (*D*), ADC (*E*), and contrast-enhanced fat-saturated T1 (*F*) images show that the subglottic tumor has an intermediate signal intensity on T2, low signal intensity on T1, and moderately strong enhancement after iv. contrast (*asterisk* in *B*, *C*, and *F*). Note that the subglottic mucosa overlying the tumor has a stronger signal on T2 and a stronger enhancement than the tumor (*dashed arrows* in *B* and *F*). The adjacent cricoid cartilage, however, has similar signal intensities and similar contrast enhancement as the tumor (*arrows* in *B*, *C*, and *F*), suggesting neoplastic invasion. DWI shows restricted diffusion in the tumor (*asterisk* in *D* and *E*) and in the cricoid cartilage (*arrows* in *D* and *E*). Histologic slice (*G*) confirms subglottic submucosal tumor spread (*asterisk*) and neoplastic invasion of the cricoid cartilage (*arrow*). Inflammatory edema beneath the intact lateral subglottic mucosa (*dashed arrows*).

tumor, and if there is no restricted diffusion, the diagnosis of peritumoral cartilage inflammation should be made (see **Fig. 11**). It is worthwhile mentioning that DWI images are not always contributive to the diagnosis due to geometric distortion and lower spatial resolution. Therefore, if DWI images are of insufficient diagnostic quality, in the authors' experience, one should rely on standard morphologic MR imaging images.

DIFFERENTIATING TUMOR RECURRENCE FROM POST-TREATMENT CHANGES

Recurrence in laryngeal SCC is relatively common and depends on age, subsite, stage, histologic differentiation, and treatment modality. Although the recurrence rate is about 5% to 13% in T1 cancer, T3-T4 cancers have a recurrence rate of about 30% to 40%.[62,63] Recurrence most often occurs at the site of the primary tumor and about 90% of

recurrences occur within 3 years after primary treatment. In hypopharyngeal SCC, recurrence rates are even higher than in laryngeal SCC and they equally depend on subsite, stage, histologic differentiation, and primary treatment modality.[64] Early detection of recurrent disease plays a major role in a successful disease outcome. Endoscopic and clinical follow-up may overlook recurrent disease, especially after radiotherapy because of radiation-induced edema, fibrosis, or radiation-induced complications, for example, soft tissue necrosis or cartilage necrosis. Biopsy itself can substantially aggravate the situation by precipitating complications due to poor wound healing after biopsy.[17,65] Furthermore, as recurrences after radiotherapy tend to occur under an intact mucosa, endoscopic biopsy may also miss recurrent disease because of the necessity to obtain deep biopsies without being able to identify endoscopically the most appropriate site for tissue sampling.[7]

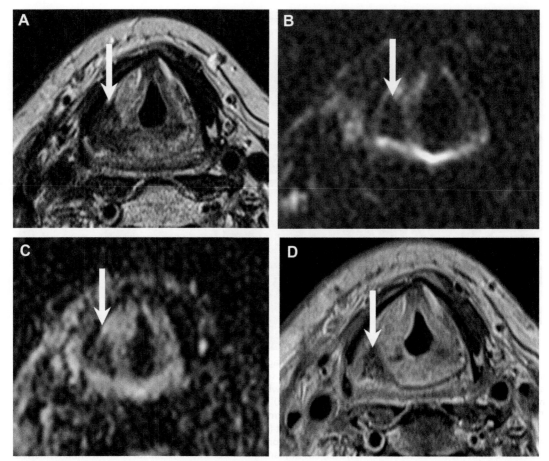

Fig. 13. Characteristic MR imaging features of late fibrosis/post-treatment scar tissue. MR imaging obtained 3 months after radiotherapy for an SCC of the piriform sinus. Axial T2 (*A*), b1000 (*B*), ADC (*C*), and contrast-enhanced T1 (*D*) show a well-defined strongly hypointense area on T2 (similar signal as muscle tissue) with minor contrast enhancement (*arrows* in *A* and *D*). Note low signal on b1000 and ADC map (*arrows* in *B* and *C*) because the tissue is very rich in collagen fibers (T2 blackout effect).

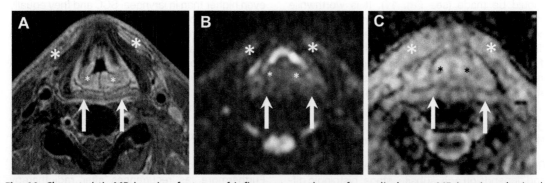

Fig. 14. Characteristic MR imaging features of inflammatory edema after radiotherapy. MR imaging obtained 3 months after radiotherapy for an SCC of the supraglottic larynx. Axial contrast-enhanced fat-saturated T1 (*A*), b1000 (*B*), and ADC (*C*) images show bilateral and symmetric swelling of the aryepiglottic folds with strong contrast enhancement and without restricted diffusion (*small asterisks* on all figure parts) suggesting inflammatory edema. Note also inflammatory edema in the prelaryngeal strap muscles (*large asterisks* on all figure parts), as well as in the hypopharynx and retropharyngeal space (*arrows*).

Several authors have demonstrated the added value of DWI for the detection of residual/recurrent head and neck cancer after radiotherapy in comparison to CT and for distinguishing residual/recurrent disease from benign post-treatment changes; however, they have pointed out that false-positive evaluations caused by late fibrosis/scar tissue still occurred.[15,66] Other authors found that major overlap of ADC values measured in benign post-treatment changes and in recurrent laryngeal cancer limited the ability of quantitative DWI to distinguish between the 2 entities.[67] Nevertheless, by carefully combining morphologic MR imaging criteria with DWI, a high diagnostic performance for distinguishing post-treatment residual/recurrent disease from benign changes after radiotherapy (in particular late fibrosis) can be achieved, the positive predictive value and the negative predictive value of DWI MR imaging being as high as 92% and 95%, respectively.[19] Both late fibrosis/mature scar and residual/recurrent disease have low ADC values (around 1×10^{-3} mm^2/s).[19] This diagnostic DWI pitfall can be avoided as their morphologic characteristics are different: recurrent SCC has a moderately high signal intensity on T2 (see **Fig. 6**); however, late fibrosis/mature scar typically displays a very low signal intensity on T2 (lower than or similar to the signal intensity of muscles) and often no or only minor contrast enhancement (**Fig. 13**).[12,19] Furthermore, mature scars/fibrosis tend to have a characteristic linear or triangular shape. Low ADC values in late fibrosis can be explained by the fact that mature scar tissue is mainly composed of densely packed collagen (T2 blackout effect). In contrast, radiation-induced edema typically manifests with symmetric soft tissue swelling of the larynx and hypopharynx, variable contrast enhancement, and no restricted diffusion (**Fig. 14**). Chondronecrosis after radiotherapy has a characteristic aspect on CT with air inclusions and fragmentation of sclerotic cartilages. However, in the presence of associated recurrent disease (in up to 30% of cases), distinguishing between chondronecrosis alone and chondronecrosis with tumor is less straightforward on CT. This diagnostic pitfall can be avoided by combining morphologic MR imaging sequences with DWI.[17] Nevertheless, necrotic debris, pus, and fungal infection in areas of chondronecrosis may also cause restricted diffusion and can be confounded with recurrent disease.

DIFFERENTIAL DIAGNOSIS

Less than 5% of laryngeal and hypopharyngeal tumors are of nonsquamous cell origin. Unlike primary SCC, they are often located beneath an

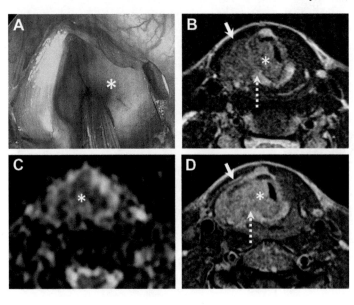

Fig. 15. Rosai-Dorman disease manifesting as a submucosal laryngeal tumor. The patient presented with increasing dyspnea and slight changes in voice quality over 3 months. Endoscopic view (A) showing an entirely submucosal lesion involving the right hemilarynx and leading to major subglottic obstruction (asterisk). Axial T2 (B), ADC (C), and contrast-enhanced T1 (D) obtained at the subglottic level show an infiltrative lesion involving the right subglottic region (asterisk) with an intermediate signal intensity on T2 and restricted diffusion (ADC = 0.7 × 10^{-3} mm^2/s). Homogeneous and relatively strong enhancement is seen in D. The lesion invades the thyroid cartilage and there is extralaryngeal tumor spread (arrows in B and D). Invasion of the right cricoid (dashed arrows in B and D). An enlarged level IV lymph node was equally seen (not shown). MR imaging suggested the probable diagnosis of lymphoma based on the low ADC, homogeneous enhancement, and the fact that the tumor was entirely submucosal. Biopsy revealed, however, Rosai Dorfman disease.

intact mucosa and sampling errors may occur with endoscopic biopsy.[7,68] The role of imaging mainly consists in confirming a submucosal tumor, determining the precise tumor extent, and guiding the endoscopist to the most appropriate biopsy site to avoid false-negative biopsies. Although some tumors, such as chondrosarcoma, lipoma, schwannoma, melanoma, paraganglioma or vascular lesions (hemangioma and vascular malformations) show characteristic imaging features at MR imaging allowing distinction from SCC,[7,68] other tumor types show overlapping features with SCC and only deep targeted biopsy can differentiate between SCC and non-SCC. Such tumors include adenoid cystic carcinoma, adenocarcinoma, rhabdomyosarcoma, and many more. When lymphoma first presents as a submucosal laryngeal lesion without associated adenopathy (rare presentation), the diagnosis can be quite challenging. However, although the very low ADC values (in the range of $0.5–0.8 \times 10^{-3}$ mm^2/s) may suggest the diagnosis of lymphoma, biopsy is always required as other rare conditions, such as Rosai Dorfman disease or IgG4 related disease may present with similar MR imaging features (**Fig. 15**). Nevertheless, as a

general rule, in patients with a suspected lesion beneath a completely intact mucosa at endoscopy and a tumor mass with similar imaging characteristics as SCC, the radiologist should suggest the diagnosis of an unusual histology.[7,68] It is also worthwhile mentioning that some non-neoplastic conditions, such as tuberculosis, may mimic SCC clinically and at morphologic MR imaging. The diagnosis can be quite challenging in nonendemic areas and in the absence of a known history of tuberculosis or predisposing factors. However, absent restriction of diffusion and pulmonary involvement (**Fig. 16**) in these cases are very helpful in suggesting the diagnosis and contributing to an adequate patient work-up.

WHAT THE REFERRING PHYSICIAN NEEDS TO KNOW

The major goal of radiology reports is to provide accurate, timely, and pertinent information. In many institutions, structured reporting is increasingly used for improved comprehensiveness, to avoid diagnostic errors by omitting key information, for a more consistent evaluation at multidisciplinary

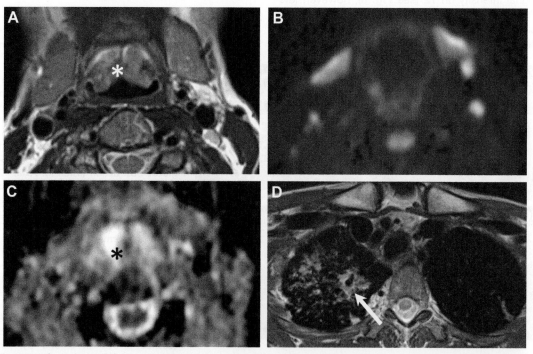

Fig. 16. Tuberculosis of the supraglottic larynx with pulmonary involvement. Patient presenting with hoarseness increasing over several months and some weight loss. Fiberoptic endoscopy showed a bulky and ulcerated lesion of the epiglottis. Before biopsy, an MR imaging was obtained. Axial T2 (*A*) shows an epiglottic lesion infiltrating the pre-epiglottic space (*asterisk*). Corresponding b1000 image (*B*) and ADC map (*C*) show no restriction of diffusivity (*asterisk* in *C*) suggesting an inflammatory lesion. ADC was 1.6×10^{-3} mm^2/s. Axial T2 image (from the same series as image *A*) at the level of the upper mediastinum (*C*) reveals characteristic right pulmonary involvement with cavern formation (*arrow*). The diagnosis of possible tuberculosis was suggested based on MR imaging findings. The diagnosis was confirmed.

tumor boards, for follow-up purposes, and for data collection and research. Structured reporting includes a structured format, consistent organization, and consistent terminology. Even if an IT-based structured reporting template is not available at a radiologist's institution, the following key information using standard terminology as described earlier should be included in every MR imaging report dealing with laryngeal and hypopharyngeal cancer:

- Which anatomic subsites of the larynx/hypopharynx are involved (the AJCC/TNM nomenclature should be used)?
- Is the pre-epiglottic space invaded?
- Is the paraglottic space invaded? If yes, which sites precisely?
- Are laryngeal cartilages invaded? If yes, to what degree (inner cortex vs through outer cortex)?
- Is there invasion of other structures beyond the larynx/hypopharynx, for example, strap muscles, soft tissues of the neck, carotid arteries, prevertebral space, or esophagus?
- Are there unilateral/bilateral lymph node metastases? What levels are involved?

In addition, at the authors' institution, the reporting radiologists also indicate how confident they are with respect to involvement of the key anatomic areas mentioned earlier, in particular if there are technical issues impairing a confident interpretation of imaging findings. Furthermore, when certain key findings are reported, we indicate the series and image numbers and we provide appropriately annotated key images. This procedure is especially useful for follow-up examinations and for coherent evaluation at multidisciplinary tumor boards. It is equally important to stress the fact that lack of appropriate clinical history related to previous treatment and lack of images from previous radiological examinations can lead to diagnostic uncertainty and, therefore, only a close cooperation with the referring physicians will ultimately lead to a high-quality radiologic report.

SUMMARY

The advent of high-resolution surface coils combined with parallel imaging techniques, more robust DWI techniques, and refined diagnostic criteria have been some of the most significant advances in oncologic imaging of the larynx and hypopharynx. Although MR imaging of the larynx and hypopharynx presents some technical challenges, advantages over CT outweigh disadvantages. Current state-of-the-art MR imaging allows a more precise assessment of submucosal tumor spread by detecting subtle soft-tissue abnormalities in anatomic areas that are more difficult to interpret on CT scans, such as the paraglottic space, the laryngeal cartilages, and the extralaryngeal soft tissues. Current MR imaging diagnostic criteria combining distinct signal intensity patterns on morphologic sequences with DWI features allow an improved discrimination between tumor, peritumoral inflammation and scar tissue, improved assessment of laryngeal cartilage abnormalities, and, ultimately, an increased precision for tumor delineation beyond the capability of multislice CT. Improved tumor delineation allows tailored treatment options, such as deciding between highly focused radiotherapy, transoral laser microsurgery, open partial laryngectomy, or total laryngectomy. Furthermore, MR imaging has a higher diagnostic performance than CT for the detection and precise depiction of post-treatment recurrent disease.

CLINICS CARE POINTS

- Both primary and recurrent laryngeal and hypopharyngeal SCCs have characteristic MR imaging features, which include an intermediate signal intensity on T1, T2, and T2 STIR, moderate contrast enhancement after iv. administration of gadolinium chelates and ADC values less than 1.3×10^{-3} mm^2/s

- Careful analysis of multiparametric MR imaging signal intensity allows distinction between tumor and peritumoral inflammation as inflammation has a higher signal intensity on T2 and T2 STIR and a stronger contrast enhancement than the tumor itself.[11,34,58] Also, on DWI, peritumoral inflammation shows no restriction of diffusion and ADC values are in general above 1.3×10^{-3} mm^2/s.

- Applying the current diagnostic MR imaging criteria for tumor, inflammation, normal non-ossified and normal ossified cartilage, multiparametric MR imaging allows an improved diagnosis of cartilage abnormalities, thus avoiding diagnostic pitfalls related to CT.[11]

- The combination of morphologic MR imaging and DWI criteria allows improved detection of post-treatment recurrent disease and superior differentiation between residual tumor, late fibrosis, and post-treatment edema.[12,17,19] Although recurrent SCC has an intermediate T2 signal and low ADC values, late fibrosis/scar tissue is characterized by very low T2 signal and low ADC values. In contrast, post-treatment edema has high T2 signal and high ADC values.[12,17,19]

DISCLOSURE

The radiologic-pathologic correlation used to illustrate this article was part of a research project funded by the Swiss national Science Foundation (SNSF) under grant No 320030_173091/1.

REFERENCES

1. Nocini R, Molteni G, Mattiuzzi C, Lippi G. Updates on larynx cancer epidemiology. Chin J Cancer Res 2020;32(1):18–25.
2. Petersen JF, Timmermans AJ, van Dijk BAC, et al. Trends in treatment, incidence and survival of hypopharynx cancer: a 20-year population-based study in the Netherlands. Eur Arch Otorhinolaryngol 2018;275(1):181–9.
3. Bradley PJ. Epidemiology of hypopharyngeal cancer. Adv Otorhinolaryngol 2019;83:1–14.
4. Jones TM, De M, Foran B, et al. Laryngeal cancer: United Kingdom National Multidisciplinary guidelines. J Laryngol Otol 2016;130(S2):S75–82.
5. Gilbert K, Dalley RW, Maronian N, et al. Staging of laryngeal cancer using 64-channel multidetector row CT: comparison of standard neck CT with dedicated breath-maneuver laryngeal CT. AJNR Am J Neuroradiol 2009;31:251–6.
6. Becker M, Zbaren P, Delavelle J, et al. Neoplastic invasion of the laryngeal cartilage: reassessment of criteria for diagnosis at CT. Radiology 1997;203(2):521–32.
7. Becker M, Burkhardt K, Dulguerov P, et al. Imaging of the larynx and hypopharynx. Eur J Radiol 2008; 66(3):460–79.
8. Amin MB, Edge SB, Greene FL, et al, editors. AJCC cancer staging manual. 8th edition. New York: Springer-Verlag; 2017.
9. Brierley JD, Gospodarowicz MK, Wittekind C, editors. TNM classification of malignant tumours. Hoboken: Wiley Blackwell; 2017.
10. Becker M, Zbaren P, Laeng H, et al. Neoplastic invasion of the laryngeal cartilage: comparison of MR imaging and CT with histopathologic correlation. Radiology 1995;194(3):661–9.
11. Becker M, Zbaren P, Casselman JW, et al. Neoplastic invasion of laryngeal cartilage: reassessment of criteria for diagnosis at MR imaging. Radiology 2008;249(2):551–9.
12. Ravanelli M, Farina D, Rizzardi P, et al. MR with surface coils in the follow-up after endoscopic laser resection for glottic squamous cell carcinoma: feasibility and diagnostic accuracy. Neuroradiology 2013;55:225–32.
13. Preda L, Conte G, Bonello L, et al. Diagnostic accuracy of surface coil MRI in assessing cartilaginous invasion in laryngeal tumours: do we need contrast-agent administration? Eur Radiol 2017; 27(11):4690–8.
14. Vandecaveye V, De Keyzer F, Nuyts S, et al. Detection of head and neck squamous cell carcinoma with diffusion weighted MRI after (chemo)radiotherapy: correlation between radiologic and histo- pathologic findings. Int J Radiat Oncol Biol Phys 2007;67: 960–71.
15. Abdel Razek AA, Kandeel AY, Soliman N, et al. Role of diffusion- weighted echo-planar MR imaging in differentiation of residual or recurrent head and neck tumors and posttreatment changes. AJNR Am J Neuroradiol 2007;28:1146–52.
16. Thoeny HC, De Keyzer F, King AD. Diffusion-weighted MR imaging in the head and neck. Radiology 2012;263:19–32.
17. Varoquaux A, Rager O, Dulguerov P, et al. Diffusion-weighted and PET/MR imaging after radiation therapy for malignant head and neck tumors. Radiographics 2015;35(5):1502–27.
18. Becker M, Varoquaux AD, Combescure C, et al. Local recurrence of squamous cell carcinoma of the head and neck after radiochemotherapy: diagnostic performance of FDG-PET/MRI with diffusion weighted sequences. Eur Radiol 2018;28(2): 651–63.
19. Ailianou A, Mundada P, de Perrot T, et al. MRI with diffusion weighted imaging for the detection of post-treatment head and neck squamous cell carcinoma: why morphological MRI criteria matter. Am J Neuroradiol AJNR 2018. https://doi.org/10.3174/ ajnr.A5548.
20. Casselman JW. High resolution imaging of the skull base and larynx. In: Schoenberg SO, Dietrich O, Reiser MF, editors. Parallel imaging in clinical MR applications. Berlin, Heidelberg, New York: Springer Science & Business Media; 2007. p. 199–208.
21. Ljumanovic R, Langendijk JA, van Wattingen M, et al. MR imaging predictors of local control of glottic squamous cell carcinoma treated with radiation alone. Radiology 2007;244:205–12.
22. Verduijn GM, Bartels LW, Raaijmakers CP, Terhaard CH, Pameijer FA, van den Berg CA. Magnetic resonance imaging protocol optimization for delineation of gross tumor volume in hypopharyngeal and laryngeal tumors. Int J Radiat Oncol Biol Phys 2009;74(2):630–6.
23. Maroldi R, Ravanelli M, Farina D. Magnetic resonance for laryngeal cancer. Curr Opin Otolaryngol Head Neck Surg 2014;22(2):131–9.
24. Ruytenberg T, Verbist BM, Vonk-Van Oosten J, et al. Improvements in high resolution laryngeal Magnetic Resonance Imaging for preoperative transoral laser microsurgery and radiotherapy considerations in early lesions. Front Oncol 2018;8:216. https://doi. org/10.3389/fonc.2018.00216.
25. Hermans R, Van den Bogaert W, Rijnders A, et al. Predicting the local outcome of glottic squamous cell carcinoma after definitive radiation therapy:

value of computed tomography-determined tumour parameters. Radiother Oncol 1999;50(1):39–46.

26. Dagan R, Morris CG, Bennett JA, Mancuso AA, Amdur RJ, Hinerman RW, Mendenhall WM. Prognostic significance of paraglottic space invasion in T2N0 glottic carcinoma. Am J Clin Oncol 2007; 30(2):186–90.

27. Lee JH, Machtay M, McKenna MG, et al. Radiotherapy with 6-megavolt photons for early glottic carcinoma: potential impact of extension to the posterior vocal cord. Am J Otolaryngol 2001;22: 43–54.

28. Succo G, Crosetti E, Bertolin A, et al. Treatment for T3 to T4a la- ryngeal cancer by open partial horizontal laryngectomies: prognos- tic impact of different pathologic tumor subcategories. Head Neck 2018; 40:1897–908.

29. Lucioni M, Lionello M, Guida F, et al. The thyro-cricoarytenoid space (TCAS): clinical and prognostic implications in laryngeal cancer. Acta Otorhinolaryngol Ital 2020;40(2):106–12.

30. Peretti G, Piazza C, Mora F, et al. Reasonable limits for transoral laser microsurgery in laryngeal cancer. Curr Opin Otolaryngol Head Neck Surg 2016;24(2): 135–9.

31. Reidenbach MM. The paraglottic space and trans-glottic cancer: anatomical considerations. Clin Anat 1996;9:244–51.

32. Reidenbach MM. Borders and topographic relationships of the paraglottic space. Eur Arch Otorhinolaryngol 1997;254:193–5.

33. Sato K. Spaces of the Larynx. In: Functional histoanatomy of the human larynx. Singapore: Springer; 2018. https://doi.org/10.1007/978-981-10-5586-7_20.

34. Ravanelli M, Paderno A, Del Bon F, et al. Prediction of posterior paraglottic space and cricoarytenoid unit involvement in endoscopically t3 glottic cancer with arytenoid fixation by magnetic resonance with surface coils. Cancers (Basel) 2019;11(1):67.

35. Benazzo M, Sovardi F, Preda L, et al. Imaging accuracy in preoperative staging of T3-T4 laryngeal cancers. Cancers (Basel) 2020;12(5):1074.

36. Joo YH, Park JO, Cho KJ, et al. Relationship between preepiglottic space invasion and lymphatic metastasis in supracricoid partial laryngectomy with cricohyoidopexy. Clin Exp Otorhinolaryngol 2014;7(3):205–9.

37. Suoglu Y, Guven M, Kiyak E, et al. Significance of pre-epiglottic space invasion in supracricoid partial laryngectomy with cricohyoidopexy. J Laryngol Otol 2008;122(6):623–7.

38. Lee WT, Rizzi M, Scharpf J, et al. Impact of preepiglottic space tumor involvement on concurrent chemoradiation therapy. Am J Otolaryngol 2010;31(3): 185–8.

39. Ljumanović R, Langendijk JA, Schenk B, et al. Supraglottic carcinoma treated with curative radiation therapy: identification of prognostic groups with MR imaging. Radiology 2004;232(2):440–8.

40. Smits HJG, Assili S, Kauw F, et al. Prognostic imaging variables for recurrent laryngeal and hypopharyngeal carcinoma treated with primary chemoradiotherapy: a systematic review and meta-analysis. Head Neck 2021;43(7):2202–15.

41. Obid R, Redlich M, Tomeh C. The treatment of laryngeal cancer. Oral Maxillofac Surg Clin North Am 2019;31(1):1–11.

42. Becker M, Leuchter I, Platon A, et al. Imaging of laryngeal trauma. Eur J Radiol 2014;83(1):142–54.

43. Hatley W, Samuel E, Evison G. The pattern of ossification in the laryngeal cartilages: a radiological study. Br J Radiol 1965;38:585–91.

44. Zan E, Yousem DM, Aygun N. Asymmetric mineralization of the arytenoid cartilages in patients without laryngeal cancer. AJNR Am J Neuroradiol 2011; 32(6):1113–8.

45. Bennett A, Carter RL, Stamford IF, et al. Prostaglandin-like material extracted from squamous cell carcinomas of the head and neck. Br J Cancer 1980;41:204–8.

46. Gallo A, Mocetti P, De Vincentiis M, et al. Neoplastic infiltration of laryngeal cartilages: histocytochemical study. Laryngoscope 1992;102:891–5.

47. Gregor RT, Hammond K. Framework invasion by laryngeal carcinoma. Am J Surg 1987;154:452–8.

48. Zbaren P, Nuyens M, Curschmann J, et al. Histologic characteristics and tumor spread of recurrent glottic carcinoma: analysis on whole-organ sections and comparison with tumor spread of primary glottic carcinomas. Head Neck 2007;29(1): 26–32.

49. Zbaren P, Christe A, Caversaccio MD, et al. Pretherapeutic staging of recurrent laryngeal carcinoma: clinical findings and imaging studies compared with histopathology. Otolaryngol Head Neck Surg 2007;137(3):487–91.

50. Zhang SC, Zhou SH, Shang DS, Bao YY, Ruan LX, Wu TT. The diagnostic role of diffusion-weighted magnetic resonance imaging in hypopharyngeal carcinoma. Oncol Lett 2018;15(4):5533–44.

51. Varoquaux A, Rager O, Lovblad KO, et al. Functional imaging of head and neck squamous cell carcinoma with diffusion-weighted MRI and FDG PET/CT: quantitative analysis of ADC and SUV. Eur J Nucl Med Mol Imaging 2013;40(6):842–52.

52. Driessen JP, Caldas-Magalhaes J, Janssen LM, et al. Diffusion-weighted MR imaging in laryngeal and hypopharyngeal carcinoma: association between apparent diffusion coefficient and histologic findings. Radiology 2014;272(2):456–63.

53. Loevner LA, Yousem DM, Montone KT, et al. Can radiologists accurately predict preepiglottic space invasion with MR imaging? AJR Am J Roentgenol 1997;169(6):1681–7.

54. Zbaren P, Becker M, Lang H. Staging of laryngeal cancer: endoscopy, computed tomography and magnetic resonance versus histopathology. Eur Arch Otorhinolaryngol 1997;254(Suppl 1):S117–22.

55. Zbären P, Becker M, Laeng H. Pretherapeutic staging of hypopharyngeal carcinoma: clinical findings, computed tomography, and magnetic resonance imaging compared with histopathologic evaluation. Arch Otolaryngol Head Neck Surg 1997;123: 908–13.

56. Banko B, Djukic V, Milovanovic J, Kovac J, Novakovic Z, Maksimovic R. MRI in evaluation of neoplastic invasion into preepiglottic and paraglottic space. Auris Nasus Larynx 2014;41(5):471–4.

57. van Egmond SL, Stegeman I, Pameijer FA, et al. Systematic review of the diagnostic value of magnetic resonance imaging for early glottic carcinoma. Laryngoscope Investig Otolaryngol 2018;3(1): 49–55.

58. Allegra E, Ferrise P, Trapasso S, et al. Early glottic cancer: role of MRI in the preoperative staging. Biomed Res Int 2014;2014:890385. https://doi.org/10.1155/2014/890385.

59. Shang DS, Ruan LX, Zhou SH, et al. Differentiating laryngeal carcinomas from precursor lesions by diffusion-weighted magnetic resonance imaging at 3.0 T: a preliminary study. PLoS One 2013;8:e68622.

60. Beitler JJ, Muller S, Grist WJ, et al. Prognostic accuracy of computed tomography findings for patients with laryngeal cancer undergoing laryngectomy. J Clin Oncol 2010;28:2318–22.

61. Li B, Bobinski M, Gandour-Edwards R, et al. Overstaging of cartilage invasion by multidetector CT scan for laryngeal cancer and its potential effect on the use of organ preservation with chemoradiation. Br J Radiol 2011;84(997):64–9.

62. Li P, Hu W, Zhu Y, Liu J. Treatment and predictive factors in patients with recurrent laryngeal carcinoma: a retrospective study. Oncol Lett 2015; 10(5):3145–52.

63. Induction chemotherapy plus radiation compared with surgery plus radiation in patients with advanced laryngeal cancer. The department of veterans affairs laryngeal cancer study group. N Engl J Med 1991; 324:1685–90.

64. Tsai YT, Chen WC, Chien CY, et al. Treatment patterns and survival outcomes of advanced hypopharyngeal squamous cell carcinoma. World J Surg Oncol 2020;18:82. https://doi.org/10.1186/s12957-020-01866-z.

65. Becker M, Schroth G, Zbären P, et al. Long-term changes induced by high-dose irradiation of the head and neck region: imaging findings. Radiographics 1997;17(1):5–26.

66. Vaid S, Chandorkar A, Atre A, et al. Differentiating recurrent tumours from post-treatment changes in head and neck cancers: does diffusion-weighted MRI solve the eternal dilemma? Clin Radiol 2017; 72:74–83.

67. Tshering Vogel DW, Zbaeren P, Geretschlaeger A, et al. Diffusion-weighted MR imaging including biexponential fitting for the detection of recurrent or residual tumour after (chemo)radiotherapy for laryngeal and hypopharyngeal cancers. Eur Radiol 2013;23: 562–9.

68. Becker M, Moulin G, Kurt AM, et al. Non-squamous cell neoplasms of the larynx: radiologic-pathologic correlation. Radiographics 1998;18(5):1189–209.

MR imaging of Nasal and Paranasal Sinus Malignant Neoplasms

Daniel Thomas Ginat, MD, MS

KEYWORDS

• MRI • Nasal • Paranasal sinus • Malignant • Neoplasms

KEY POINTS

- MR imaging plays an important role in defining the extent of sinonasal tumors for staging, particularly assessing intracranial and orbital invasion, as well as perineural spread and lymph node metastases.
- MR imaging is useful for differentiating tumor from mucosal thickening and secretions.
- Although most sinonasal tumors appear nonspecific on MR imaging and a pathologic tissue diagnosis is ultimately necessary, some tumors can display characteristic features.

INTRODUCTION

Sinonasal malignancies are relatively uncommon, with an overall incidence of less than 1 per 100,000 individuals.[1] Nevertheless, the location of sinonasal cancers with respect to critical neurovascular structures, including the orbit, brain, cranial nerves, and carotid arteries, makes surgical resection technically difficult.[2] Thus, accurate delineation of the tumors and regional anatomy via radiologic imaging are crucial for treatment planning. This article reviews the MR imaging protocols, staging, and imaging features related to malignant sinonasal neoplasms, along with pearls and pitfalls.

IMAGING PROTOCOL

T2-weighted and precontrast and postcontrast T1-weighted thin sections of up to 3 mm in at least 2 orthogonal planes with coverage of the skull base are essential to include in a sinonasal MR imaging protocol.[3] The use of fat suppression, particularly based on frequency selective fat-suppression techniques, is debatable, as the skull base and sinonasal regions are prone to artifacts related to failure of fat suppression at bone-air-soft tissue interfaces. However, this can be mitigated using the multipoint DIXON technique, which provides better image quality with uniform fat suppression and shorter scan time compared with short tau inversion recovery and spectral presaturation with inversion recovery T1-weighted techniques.[4] Diffusion-weighted imaging can be included in the protocol for helping to differentiate malignant from benign tumors.[5] Indeed, malignant sinonasal tumors tend to have significantly lower diffusivity than benign tumors and inflammatory lesions, excluding areas of bulk necrosis.[6]

STAGING

The American Joint Committee on Cancer (AJCC) staging system is based on anatomic findings and is commonly referenced for TNM classification.[7] The AJCC tumor staging is available for nasal cavity and ethmoid sinus cancers (**Table 1**) and maxillary sinus cancers (**Table 2**),[8] which considers the extent of the tumor, particularly whether there are bone erosions, intraorbital or intracranial

Department of Radiology, University of Chicago, Pritzker School of Medicine, 5841 South Maryland Avenue, Chicago, IL 60637, USA
E-mail address: dtg1@uchicago.edu

Magn Reson Imaging Clin N Am 30 (2022) 73–80
https://doi.org/10.1016/j.mric.2021.07.003
1064-9689/22/© 2021 Elsevier Inc. All rights reserved.

mri.theclinics.com

Table 1
Nasal cavity and ethmoid sinus cancer American Joint Committee on Cancer staging

Tx	Primary tumor cannot be assessed
Tis	Carcinoma in situ
T1	Tumor only in the nasal cavity or 1 ethmoid sinus, with or without bony invasion
T2	Tumor invading multiple subsites in a single region or extending to involve an adjacent region within the nasoethmoidal complex, with or without bony invasion
T3	Tumor extends to invade the medial wall or floor of the orbit, maxillary sinus, palate, or cribriform plate
T4a	Moderately advanced local disease: tumor invades any of the following: anterior orbital contents, skin of the nose or cheek, minimal extension to the anterior cranial fossa, pterygoid plates, sphenoid or frontal sinuses
T4b	Tumor invades any of the following: orbital apex, dura, brain, middle cranial fossa, cranial nerves other than maxillary division of trigeminal nerve (V2), nasopharynx, or clivus

Table 2
Maxillary sinus cancer American Joint Committee on Cancer staging

Tx	Primary tumor cannot be assessed
Tis	Carcinoma in situ
T1	Tumor only in maxillary sinus mucosa, does not invade into bone
T2	Tumor invades bone, including extension into the hard palate and/or middle nasal cavity
T3	Tumor invades the posterior wall of the maxillary sinus, subcutaneous issues, floor, or medial wall of the orbit, pterygoid fossa, or ethmoid sinuses
T4a	Moderately advanced local disease: tumor invades the anterior orbital contents, skin of the cheek, pterygoid plates, infratemporal fossa, cribriform plate, or sphenoid or frontal sinuses
T4b	Very advanced local disease: tumor invades any of the following: orbital apex, dura, brain, middle cranial fossa, cranial nerves other than maxillary division of trigeminal nerve (V2), nasopharynx, or clivus

extension, and trigeminal nerve involvement. In addition, the AJCC staging for regional lymph node metastases is based on number, size, and distribution of affected lymph nodes (**Table 3**). Overall, the 5-year prognosis ranges from 35% for stage 4 and 63% for stage 1 sinonasal cancers.[9] Besides the AJCC, several other staging systems are available for sinonasal cancers, including the Kadish staging system, which is tailored for esthesioneuroblastoma (**Table 4**).[10]

Computed tomography and MR imaging are complementary for assessing sinonasal malignancies, along with clinical evaluation. MR imaging is advantageous for differentiating enhancing tumor from nonenhancing secretions, which can otherwise have variable signal characteristics (**Fig. 1**), which in turn enables more precise size measurement. Furthermore, MR imaging, particularly coronal postcontrast T1-weighted sequences, is useful for delineating intracranial and intraorbital tumor extension (**Fig. 2**). Likewise, postcontrast T1-weighted sequences are useful for identifying perineural tumor spread, in which there is thickening and abnormal enhancement along the affected nerve (**Fig. 3**).

Table 3
Regional lymph node American Joint Committee on Cancer staging

Nx	Regional nodes cannot be assessed
N0	No regional lymph node metastasis
N1	Metastasis in a single ipsilateral lymph node ≤3 cm in greatest dimension
N2a	Metastasis in single ipsilateral lymph node >3 cm but not >6 cm in greatest dimension
N2b	Metastasis in multiple ipsilateral lymph nodes, none >6 cm in greatest dimension
N2c	Metastasis in bilateral or contralateral lymph nodes, none >6 cm in greatest dimension
N3	Metastasis in a lymph node >6 cm in greatest dimension

Table 4
Modified Kadish esthesioneuroblastoma staging system

Stage	Feature
A	Tumor confined to the nasal cavity
B	Tumor in the nasal and paranasal cavities
C	Tumor extends locally beyond the nasal and paranasal cavities, including the skull base, intracranial compartment, or orbit
D	Distant disease, either to regional lymph nodes or to distant metastasis

MR imaging can also readily depict regional lymph node metastases, particularly retropharyngeal lymph nodes, which have a relatively high incidence of involvement with sinonasal malignancies and can be considered abnormal when measuring greater than 5 mm in short axis or appear heterogeneous (**Fig. 4**).[11] The retropharyngeal lymph nodes are best depicted on axial fat-suppressed T2- or postcontrast T1-weighted MR imaging sequences.

DIFFERENTIAL DIAGNOSIS

There is a wide variety of histologic types of sinonasal malignancies (**Table 5**), the most common of which is squamous cell carcinoma.[12] Certain tumors have rather unique predisposing factors. In particular, intestinal-type adenocarcinoma is associated with long-term exposure to hardwood dusts and to a lesser extent textile and metal dust exposure.[13] Otherwise, beyond the presence of aggressive features, sinonasal malignant neoplasms generally have nonspecific conventional MR imaging features, with few particularly distinguishing features among the various tumors. Nevertheless, some of these neoplasms can be associated with notable radiologic features, which are described and depicted for the following selected tumors:

- *Esthesioneuroblastoma:* Although not invariably present, cystic spaces on MR imaging along the intracranial margin of a sinonasal mass are suggestive of esthesioneuroblastoma (**Fig. 5**).[14]
- *Melanoma:* Sinonasal melanoma can display high T1 signal owing to the presence of melanin or hemorrhage (**Fig. 6**). Nevertheless, other types of tumors can also display high T1 signal. However, the additional finding of a septate pattern on precontrast T1-weighted MR imaging can help suggest melanoma.[15]

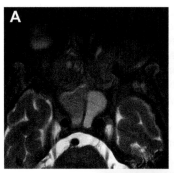
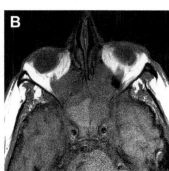
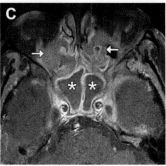

Fig. 1. Axial fat-suppressed T2-weighted (*A*), T1-weighted (*B*), and fat-suppressed postcontrast T1-weighted (*C*) MR images show infiltrative carcinoma involving the bilateral ethmoid sinuses (*arrows*) with associated obstructed secretions (*asterisks*) in the bilateral sphenoid sinuses. The secretions have variable signal characteristics but do no enhance.

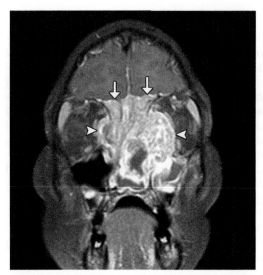

Fig. 2. Coronal postcontrast T1-weighted MR image shows a sinonasal alveolar rhabdomyosarcoma with intracranial (*arrows*) and bilateral orbital (*arrowheads*) extension.

- *Lymphoma versus carcinoma:* The diffusion-weighted imaging characteristics differ among malignant neoplasms. For example, the apparent diffusion coefficient (ADC) values of sinonasal lymphoma are significantly lower than for squamous cell and undifferentiated sinonasal carcinomas (**Fig. 7**).[16] Furthermore, the percentages of total tumor area with low ADC values of lymphoma are significantly greater than for the carcinomas.
- *Solitary fibrous tumor:* In accordance with their borderline/low-grade malignant status, solitary fibrous tumors tend to be well defined with potential bone remodeling. The tumor enhances avidly, but heterogeneously because of areas of dense collagen or entrapment of mucoserous glands from the surrounding sinonasal mucosa.[17] This can result in a chocolate-chip-cookie appearance on

postcontrast T1-weighted images (**Fig. 8**).[18] The tumors mainly display low or intermediate signal in T2-weighted sequences.

CLINICS CARE POINTS

There are several potential clinicoradiologic confounders that can be encountered with sinonasal malignancies, including the following:

- *Mucosal thickening:* Sinonasal mucosal thickening is often present around the tumors. The mucosa typically enhances to a greater degree than the "evil gray" of malignant neoplasms on MR imaging (**Fig. 9**).
- *Dural reaction:* The presence of intracranial tumor extension can lead to reactive changes in the dura.[19] This manifests as mild diffuse thickening and enhancement of the affected dura. The degree of enhancement of the reactive dura is typically greater than that of the neoplasm on MR imaging (**Fig. 10**).
- *Inverted papilloma with malignant transformation:* Inverted papilloma is a benign tumor that can occasionally transform into carcinoma. In such cases, biopsy can potentially miss the malignant component, which might otherwise be evident on imaging. Features suggestive of malignant transformation of inverted papilloma include prominent bone erosions, necrosis, and the loss of cerebriform appearance on MR imaging (**Fig. 11**).[20]
- *Concurrent infection and malignancy:* Patients with sinonasal malignancies can present with superimposed sinusitis, and the neoplasm can be missed even with tissue sampling. The presence of underlying enhancing tissue with extension beyond the margins of the sinonasal cavities on MR imaging should raise the possibility of malignant tumor (**Fig. 12**).[21] Alternatively, invasive sinusitis can also display aggressive imaging features that potentially mimic malignancy.

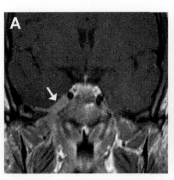
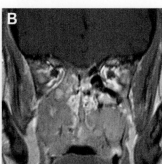

Fig. 3. Coronal postcontrast T1-weighted MR images (*A, B*) show tumor (*arrow*) along the course of the V3 trigeminal nerve branch with extension into the cavernous sinus from sinonasal adenoid cystic carcinoma that involves the hard palate.

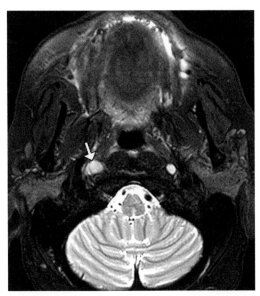

Fig. 4. Axial fat-suppressed T2-weighted MR image shows an enlarged right retropharyngeal lymph node (*arrow*) owing to metastasis from a right maxillary sinus carcinoma.

Table 5
Sinonasal malignancy World Health Organization 2017 histologic classification

Group	Histology

Carcinomas	• Keratinizing squamous cell carcinoma
	• Nonkeratinizing squamous cell carcinoma
	• Spindle cell (sarcomatoid) squamous cell carcinoma
	• Lymphoepithelial carcinoma
	• Sinonasal undifferentiated carcinoma
	• NUT carcinoma
	• Neuroendocrine carcinoma
	• Adenocarcinoma
	    ○ Intestinal-type adenocarcinoma
	    ○ Nonintestinal-type adenocarcinoma

Teratocarcinosarcoma	

Sarcomatous/mesenchymal soft tissue tumors	• High grade
	    ○ Fibrosarcoma
	    ○ Undifferentiated pleomorphic sarcoma
	    ○ Leiomyosarcoma
	    ○ Rhabdomyosarcoma
	    ○ Angiosarcoma
	    ○ Malignant peripheral nerve sheath tumor
	    ○ Biphenotypic sinonasal sarcoma
	    ○ Synovial sarcoma
	• Borderline/low grade
	    ○ Sinonasal glomangiopericytoma
	    ○ Solitary fibrous tumor

Hematolymphoid tumors	• Extranodal NK/T-cell lymphoma • Extraosseous plasmacytoma
Neuroectodermal/melanocytic tumors	• Ewing sarcoma/primitive neuroectodermal tumors • Olfactory neuroblastoma • Mucosal melanoma

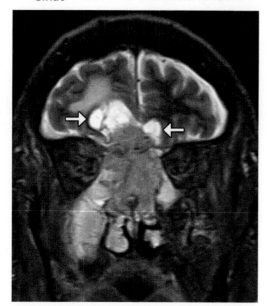

Fig. 5. Coronal fat-suppressed T2-weighted MR image shows an esthesioneuroblastoma with intracranial extension associated with margins cysts (*arrows*). (*Courtesy of* Jason Johnson MD.)

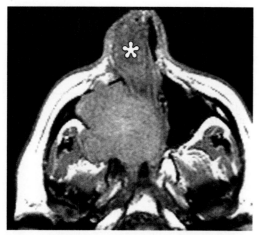

Fig. 6. Axial T1-weighted MR image shows an intrinsically hyperintense right sinonasal melanoma with extension beyond the sinus margins. There is also nasal packing material (*) for epistaxis.

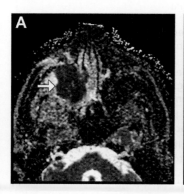
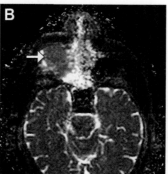

Fig. 7. Axial ADC maps from 2 different patients show lower diffusivity in the right maxillary lymphoma (*A*) than in the right maxillary sinus squamous cell carcinoma (*B*) (*arrows*).

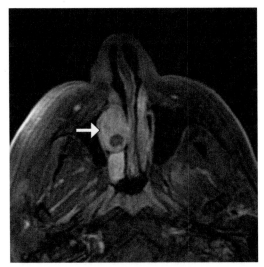

Fig. 8. Axial postcontrast T1-weighted MR image shows an avidly enhancing right nasal cavity solitary fibrous tumor (*arrow*) with areas of low signal, producing a chocolate-chip-cookie appearance.

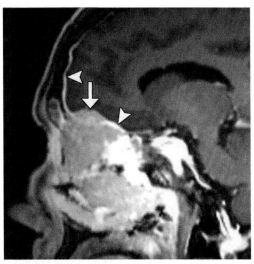

Fig. 10. Sagittal postcontrast T1-weighted MR image shows a sinonasal carcinoma with intracranial extension (*arrow*) and adjacent reactive dura (*arrowheads*), which enhances more avidly than the tumor.

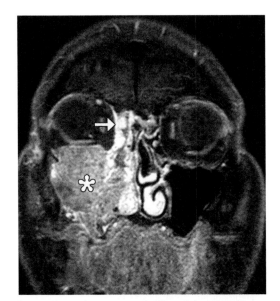

Fig. 9. Coronal postcontrast T1-weighted MR image shows a right maxillary sinus carcinoma (*) with invasion of the right orbit, cheek, and nasal cavity. There is mucosal thickening in the adjacent right ethmoid sinuses (*arrow*), which was erroneously interpreted as tumor extending toward the skull base by an inexperienced radiologist. Notice how the neoplasm enhances less avidly than the mucosa.

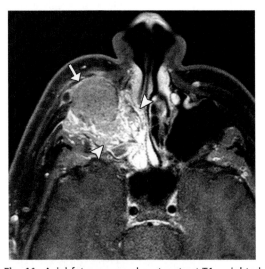

Fig. 11. Axial fat-suppressed postcontrast T1-weighted MR image shows a right maxillary sinus inverted papilloma with malignant transformation consisting of a hypoenhancing component with extension beyond the sinus margins (*arrow*) and a component with a cerebriform pattern (*arrowheads*).

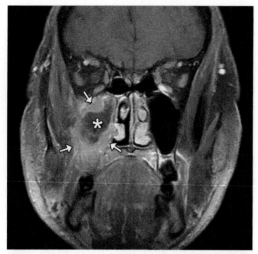

Fig. 12. Coronal postcontrast T1-weighted MR image shows a right maxillary sinus carcinoma appearing as a circumferential rind of enhancing soft tissues with extension beyond the sinus margins (*arrows*) and fluid with the antrum (*). The patient was originally diagnosed with fungal sinusitis.

SUMMARY

MR imaging examinations consisting of thin-section multiplanar sequences without and with contrast as well as diffusion-weighted imaging are useful for characterizing malignant sinonasal tumors. In particular, MR imaging is well adapted for identifying orbital and intracranial extensions, as well as perineural and regional lymph node involvement, which is relevant for staging. In addition, MR imaging can detect findings suggestive of malignant neoplasm in otherwise clinically unsuspected cases.

REFERENCES

1. Dutta R, Dubal PM, Svider PF, et al. Sinonasal malignancies: a population-based analysis of site-specific incidence and survival. Laryngoscope 2015;125(11):2491–7.

2. Carlton DA, David Beahm D, Chiu AG. Sinonasal malignancies: endoscopic treatment outcomes. Laryngoscope Investig Otolaryngol 2019;4(2):259–63.

3. Borges A. Imaging of the central skull base. Neuroimaging Clin North Am 2009;19(4):669–96.

4. Gaddikeri S, Mossa-Basha M, Andre JB, et al. Optimal fat suppression in head and neck MRI: comparison of multipoint Dixon with 2 different fat-suppression techniques, spectral presaturation and inversion recovery, and STIR. AJNR Am J Neuroradiol 2018;39(2):362–8.

5. Taha MS, El Fiky LM, Taha TM, et al. Utility of apparent diffusion coefficient in characterization of different sinonasal pathologies. Am J Rhinol Allergy 2014;28(5):181–6.

6. Sasaki M, Eida S, Sumi M, et al. Apparent diffusion coefficient mapping for sinonasal diseases: differentiation of benign and malignant lesions. AJNR Am J Neuroradiol 2011;32(6):1100–6.

7. Amin MB, Edge SB, Greene FL, et al, editors. AJCC cancer staging manual. New York: Springer; 2017.

8. Desai DD, Brandon BM, Perkins EL, et al. Staging of sinonasal and ventral skull base malignancies. Otolaryngol Clin North Am 2017;50(2):257–71.

9. Mortuaire G, Camous D, Vandenhende-Szymanski C, et al. Local extension staging of sinonasal tumours: retrospective comparison between CT/MRI assessment and pathological findings. Clin Otolaryngol 2017;42(5):988–93.

10. Chao KS, Kaplan C, Simpson JR, et al. Esthesioneuroblastoma: the impact of treatment modality. Head Neck 2001;23:749–57.

11. Sai A, Shimono T, Yamamoto A, et al. Incidence of abnormal retropharyngeal lymph nodes in sinonasal malignancies among adults. Neuroradiology 2014; 56(12):1097–102.

12. El-Naggar AK, Chan JKC, Grandis JR, et al, editors. WHO classification of head and neck tumours: WHO classification of tumours, vol. 9, 4th edition. Geneva: International Agency for Research on Cancer; 2017.

13. Leivo I. Intestinal-type adenocarcinoma: classification, immunophenotype, molecular features and differential diagnosis. Head Neck Pathol 2017;11(3):295–300.

14. Som PM, Lidov M, Brandwein M, et al. Sinonasal esthesioneuroblastoma with intracranial extension: marginal tumor cysts as a diagnostic MR finding. AJNR Am J Neuroradiol 1994;15(7):1259–62.

15. Kim YK, Choi JW, Kim HJ, et al. Melanoma of the sinonasal tract: value of a septate pattern on precontrast T1-weighted MR imaging. AJNR Am J Neuroradiol 2018;39(4):762–7.

16. Gencturk M, Ozturk K, Caicedo-Granados E, et al. Application of diffusion-weighted MR imaging with ADC measurement for distinguishing between the histopathological types of sinonasal neoplasms. Clin Imaging 2019;55:76–82.

17. Yang BT, Song ZL, Wang YZ, et al. Solitary fibrous tumor of the sinonasal cavity: CT and MR imaging findings. AJNR Am J Neuroradiol 2013;34(6):1248–51.

18. Ginat DT, Bokhari A, Bhatt S, et al. Imaging features of solitary fibrous tumors. AJR Am J Roentgenol 2011;196(3):487–95.

19. Ahmadi J, Hinton DR, Segall HD, et al. Surgical implications of magnetic resonance-enhanced dura. Neurosurgery 1994;35(3):370–7.

20. Yan CH, Tong CCL, Penta M, et al. Imaging predictors for malignant transformation of inverted papilloma. Laryngoscope 2019;129(4):777–82.

21. Ginat DT, Johnson DN, de Souza J, et al. Concurrent fungus ball and squamous cell carcinoma of the maxillary sinus. Eur Ann Otorhinolaryngol Head Neck Dis 2016;133(2):153–4.

Artificial Intelligence and Deep Learning of Head and Neck Cancer

Ahmed Abdel Khalek Abdel Razek, MD[a,†,]*, Reem Khaled, MD[a], Eman Helmy, MD[a], Ahmed Naglah, PhD[b], Amro AbdelKhalek, MD[c], Ayman El-Baz, PhD[b]

KEYWORDS

• Head and neck cancer • Radiomics • Artificial intelligence • Texture analysis

KEY POINTS

- Artificial intelligence (AI) is the simulation of human intelligence by machines to solve problems and learn solutions for new problems.
- Machine learning is an application of AI that enables obtaining meaningful data from examples.
- Deep learning is an improvement of artificial neural networks. It is characterized by having additional layers leading to better abstraction and more trusted data predictions.
- Radiomics extracts quantitative imaging features from medical images. Applications in head and neck tumors include tumor characterization, grading, staging, prediction of prognosis, and post-treatment sequels.
- Texture analysis is a technique that captures the spatial heterogeneity in intensity levels of pixels and quantifies their grey-level pattern within digital images.

INTRODUCTION

Imaging has an essential role in the diagnosis, staging, and management of head and neck cancer (HNC). Conventional computed tomography (CT) and magnetic resonance imaging (MRI) are widely used in imaging of HNC to provide detailed information about anatomy and pathology. Functional MR imaging modalities are concerned with the functional and physiologic assessment of tumors, these modalities include diffusion MR imaging, diffusion tensor imaging, dynamic susceptibility perfusion contrast MR imaging, arterial spin labeling, MR spectroscopy, and positron emission tomography.[1–5] Computerized image analysis has been used for diagnostic decision support a long time ago, but the advances in computational power and software engineering in the last decade have led to accelerated development and expanded potential to be applied to radiology problems.[6] Artificial intelligence (AI) has been introduced to the field of medical imaging with promising capabilities including lesions identification, image segmentation, data analysis, radiomic features extraction, prioritizing reporting and study triage, and image reconstruction.[7] Several studies have discussed the use of AI and DL in the evaluation of patients with HNC regarding differentiating

[a] Department of Diagnostic Radiology, Mansoura University, Elgomheryia Street, Mansoura 35512, Egypt; [b] BioImaging Laboratory, Department of Bioengineering, University of Louisville, J.B. Speed School of Engineering, Lutz Hall, 200 E Shipp Avenue, Louisville, KY 40208, USA; [c] Internship at Mansoura University Hospital, Mansoura Faculty of Medicine, Elgomheryia Street, Mansoura 35512, Egypt

[†] Deceased

* Corresponding author. Department of Diagnostic Radiology, Faculty of Medicine, Mansoura University, Elgomhoria Street, Mansoura, Egypt 35512.

E-mail address: arazek@mans.edu.eg

Magn Reson Imaging Clin N Am 30 (2022) 81–94
https://doi.org/10.1016/j.mric.2021.06.016

benign from malignant lesions, grading and staging of malignant lesions, prognostication, and posttreatment response.[6–10]

BASIC BACKGROUND
Artificial Intelligence

AI is the simulation of human intelligence by machines to be capable of solving problems and learning solutions for new problems.[11] AI is rapidly developing overtime and moved from experiments to implementations in different fields, including medicine. Since radiology has gone digital, adoption of these computational techniques and merging of AI with radiology workflow will significantly improve the quality, efficiency, and depth of radiology tasks with better impact on patient care and radiology practice.[12] In 1956, McCarthy created the term as a branch of computer science referring to making computers imitate humans' intelligence. It makes machines smarter and more valuable, and the renewed focus of interest in AI started in 2000[13,14] (**Fig. 1**).

Machine Learning

Machine learning (ML) is a subset of AI, based on a reverse training process to detect pathologic attributes and extract meaningful databases from radiological images, which is a constituent of human intelligence. Quantitative algorithms will perform repetitive and well-defined tasks constantly that cannot be performed by humans[15] (**Fig. 2**). These algorithms depend on the selection of features from the data on which they are applied.[16] Computational methods divide ML into supervised, unsupervised, and reinforcement learning methods. In a supervised learning model, the machine is trained using well-labeled data input. Data output is mostly labeled by human experts and used as ground truth for the algorithm. While in unsupervised learning, data labels are not provided to the learning algorithm. In reinforcement learning, a certain task is performed by a computer program in a dynamic environment and receives feedback in terms of positive and negative reinforcement. The optimal ML model finds the hidden structure in the data and separates data into clusters or groups[17] (**Fig. 3**).

Artificial Neural Networks

Artificial Neural Networks (ANNs) are mathematical artificial neurons mimicking the human neural architecture. ANNs are composed of a series of units or nodes termed "artificial neurons," and these neurons are organized in layers and connected with each other through a weighted connection. This weight indicates the strength of the connections between layers. The arrangement of layers begins with an "input" layer, then a single or multiple "hidden" layers, and lastly the "output" layer. Data travel from the input layer after traversing the hidden layers several times through the weighted links and finally transferred to the last layer to provide the network's output and accomplish the task[18] (**Fig. 4**).

Deep Learning

Deep learning (DL) is a major step forward of ANNs, by applying more layers that permit higher levels of abstraction and intricate relationships to improve predictions from data. Currently, DL is the most important ML method in the general imaging and computer vision domains.[19] The former ANNs were typically a few (<5) layers deep. With the advent of powerful computational techniques and proper update of the weights, modifications in the use of convolutional neural networks (CNNs) and applying multiple neural layers typically more than 20 lead to enhancing the robustness of DL[15] (**Fig. 5**). The use of DL algorithms is increasingly conducted in everyday tasks. Radiologists will have the time to focus on intellectually demanding tasks. Also, radiologists and DL algorithms can work together to achieve higher performance than either alone. Eventually, DL algorithms may replace radiologists entirely or at least in their capacity of image interpretation.[20]

Radiomics

Radiomics is a new field that captures imaging patterns from radiological images and extracts a large number of features that are used in clinical decision-support systems for diagnosis, prognostication, and treatment response assessment. Moreover, it is considered an important biomarker in oncology as it determines certain attributes such as intratumor heterogeneity, geometry, and texture to classify tumors or subtypes.[21,22] The basic concept is the generation of mineable and trustful data from images. Radiomics involves five main steps; in the beginning, the image preprocessing step including acquisition and reconstruction, followed by lesion segmentation which is the most essential step. The next step is the extraction and qualification of features. The last steps include analysis of the chosen data followed by the creation of databases and data sharing.[23] Radiomics is a promising tool that possibly will augment image interpretation and build a storage of big data that will improve the productivity and efficiency of the radiologists' workflow[24] (**Figs. 6 and 7**).

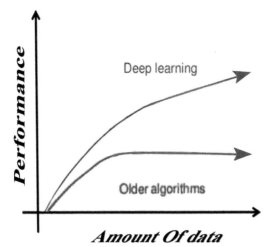

Fig. 1. Artificial intelligence versus humans. In the past, present, and future (in the near future), human intelligence can be imitated by intelligent machines in many areas. It will significantly improve the quality, value, and depth of radiology's impact on patient care and population health and will revolutionize radiologists' workflows.

Texture Analysis

Texture analysis (TA) is a technique for evaluating the relationships between adjacent pixels or voxels' position and their spatial arrangement of intensities of signal features in digital images.[25] Textural features are derived from different image-analysis techniques that depict the unique signal intensities or patterns and quantify intratumor heterogeneity

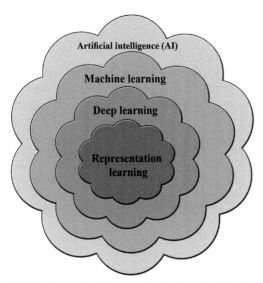

Fig. 2. Artificial intelligence fields. The artificial intelligence fields include machine learning, deep learning, and representation learning.

noninvasively. These features cannot be perceived by the human visual system. It is useful in lesion segmentation, characterization, and longitudinal disease monitoring.[26,27] Some texture characteristics of lesions such as heterogeneity, homogeneity, presence of solid and cystic parts, septations, vascularity, and contrast energy may be similar to those perceived by radiologists. Radiology TA methods are not limited to 2D image-based approaches, but the use of 3D image-based approaches has been developed also.[28]

TA can be applied by various techniques, based on either structural, statistical, model, or transform-based analyses techniques. The most commonly used is the statistical technique, either through commercially available or in-house software tools.[29] The main categories of texture parameters often used include (1) a statistical class such as histogram, absolute gradient, run-length matrix, co-occurrence matrix; (2) model class such as autoregressive model; and (3) transform class such as wavelets. Different quantitative histogram parameters are derived from the pixel values in digital images including mean, standard deviation (SD), skewness, and kurtosis.[30–32] **Table 1** shows histogram parameters.

CLINICAL APPLICATIONS
Head and Neck Tumors

Differentiation of malignant from benign head and neck tumors
Differentiation between benign and malignant head and neck tumors is crucial before treatment planning. Determination of pathologic grade of malignant tumors is important in prognosis and survival. Yet, CT and MR imaging may fail to solve the problem in differentiation between different entities in some cases.[33] Applying TA can assist in differentiating benign from malignant head and neck tumors, provided one specific machine with a defined protocol is used.[34] Radiomics-based ML is a novel method that has the potential to help recognize common lesions in the anterior skull base before the operation.[35] The radiomic nomogram including the clinical model and radiomic signature is a simple, effective, and reliable method used in differentiating paranasal sinuses tumors, prognosis, and patient risk stratification that is important for treatment strategy.[36]

Head and Neck Cancer

Grading of HNC
Determination of pathologic grade of HNC before therapy is an important predictive prognostic factor particularly in the clinical management of the patient. A CT-based radiomic features study achieved an

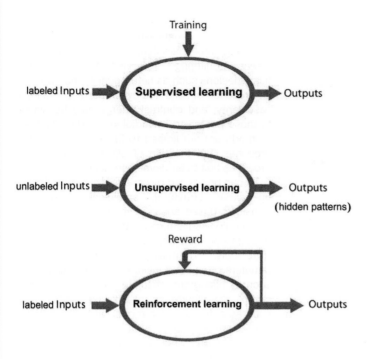

Fig. 3. Categories of machine learning. In a supervised learning model, the machine is trained using well-labeled data input. Data output is mostly labeled by human experts and used as ground truth for the algorithm. In unsupervised learning, data labels are not provided to the learning algorithm. In reinforcement learning, a certain task is carried out by a computer program in a dynamic environment and receives feedback in terms of positive and negative reinforcement. The optimal machine learning model finds the hidden structure in the data and separates data into clusters or groups.

area under the curve (AUC) of 0.75 in predicting the histopathologic characteristics of tumor grade in HNC noninvasively.[37] Another MR-based radiomics features study was useful for noninvasive discrimination of histopathologic tumor grade between the poorly differentiated HNC and well/moderately differentiated HNC patients by using the quantitative parameters of fat-suppressed T2 weighted-image (T2WI).[38] Apparent diffusion coefficient (ADC)-based radiomics also was able to discriminate between low- and high-grade HNC with an AUC of 0.82.[39]

Staging of HNC
Preoperative staging of HNC is mandatory for individual therapeutic strategies and can be assessed by MR-based radiomics features to discriminate stage I-II HNC from stage III-IV HNC. A study was performed for the distinction between stage I-II and III-IV HNC; combined T2W and contrast enhanced T1 weighted image were selected for extraction of radiomics features. This study was useful in the preoperative staging as a noninvasive and quantitative method and has achieved a good performance in the distinction between stage I-II and III-IV HNC with an AUC of 0.828 and 0.850 for the training cohort and 0.853 and 0.849 for the testing cohort, respectively.[40]

Prognosis of HNC
The prognostication of HNC depends on the histologic grade, staging of the tumor, and metastasis into cervical lymph nodes (LNs).[41] Nomograms

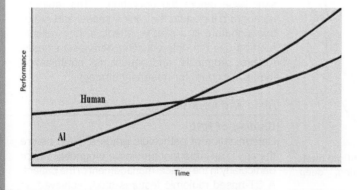

Fig. 4. Artificial neural network with neurons similar to those within a brain. It is formed by a series of units or nodes termed "artificial neurons." These neurons are organized in layers and connected with each other through a weighted connection.

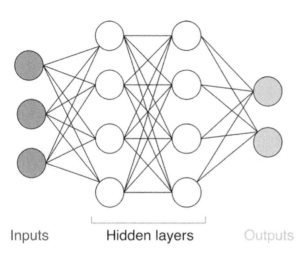

Inputs   Hidden layers   Outputs

Fig. 5. Deep learning performance. Deep learning has a better performance by increasing the amount of data by the use of neural networks with many layers.

based on combined radiomic signature and clinical TNM stage demonstrated promising noninvasive preoperative prognostication of patients with HNC in clinical practice.[42] A study based on an MRI-radiomic model on a group of patients with oral cancer and another group with oropharyngeal cancer has achieved an AUC of 0.69 to 0.71 in overall survival (OS) and 0.70 to 0.74 in relapse-free survival (RFS) in the validation cohort, respectively. After combining the radiomic and clinical features, the best models were reached and yielded AUCs of 0.72 to 0.81 in (OS) and 0.74 to 0.78 in (RFS) for oral cancer and oropharyngeal cancer, respectively. Integrated model results exceeded the clinical standard prognostic models alone.[43]

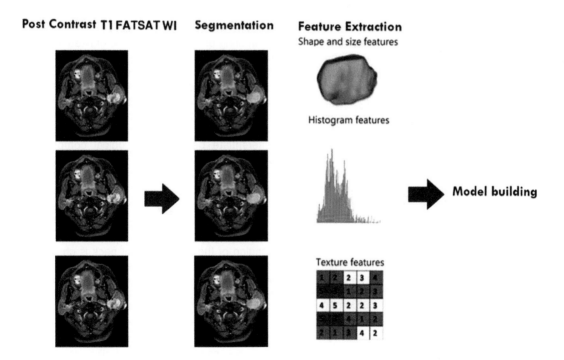

Fig. 6. Workflow of radiomics. First, MRI imaging acquisition is obtained, then image segmentation was performed on contrast T1-WI, then feature extraction within the defined tumor regions, measuring tumor intensity, shape, and texture, and finally radiomic model building.

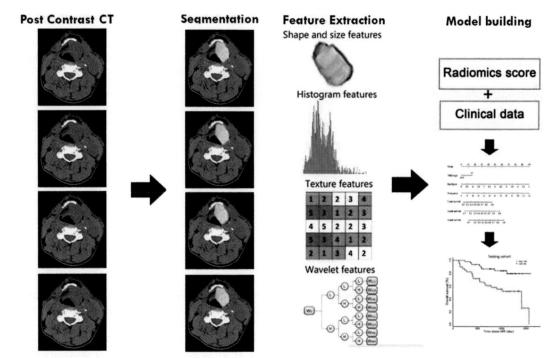

Fig. 7. Workflow of radiomics. First, CT imaging acquisition is obtained, then image segmentation was performed on contrast-enhanced CT images followed by features extraction from within the defined tumor regions, measuring tumor intensity, shape, texture, and wavelet filter, and finally radiomic model building.

Radiogenomics of HNC

Genetic information and radiomic features of HNC can significantly affect patients' survival. It was found that squamous cell carcinoma of the head and neck (HNSCC) is associated with various genetic biomarkers such as human papillomavirus (HPV) status and somatic mutations including TP53, KMT2D, and FAT1. TP53 and FAT1 variants were frequently found in HPV-negative tumors. Both radiomic and genomic features might affect the treatment decision, prognosis, and therapeutic response.[44] A study extracted radiomic features from CT images of 20 patients with HNSCC after radio-chemotherapy and found no significant correlation between radiomic features of heterogeneity and TP53 or KMT2D mutation variants. A significant decrease of radiomic intratumor heterogeneity was found in patients with FAT1 mutations and smaller primary tumor volumes. The somatic mutation gene in FAT1 is an important prognostic marker that showed improved OS and a beneficial outcome after surgery.[44]

Prediction response to therapy

Tumor segmentation is an important step before the planning of radiotherapy (RT) to delineate the organs-at-risks and to contour all tumor components including solid enhancing part and necrotic core. Currently, DL automated segmentation tools based on CT provide fast and reliable contouring of the whole-volume of head and neck tumors. In addition, it provides more time-saving and better quality of RT planning.[45] Also, radiomic markers can be used to predict response after chemotherapy in metastatic LNs in HNC. A study used multivariable pretreatment quantitative ultrasound (US) radiomic features of metastatic LNs to differentiate between radiological complete responders versus partial responders with an accuracy of 87.5% in predicting treatment response.[46]

After treatment (monitoring after radiotherapy)

Imaging of the posttreatment neck is challenging because of its complex appearance that may lead to suboptimal reporting, inadequate interpretation, and no standardized guidelines for further management.[47,48] Radiomic texture methods have been used to assess the potential capacity in longitudinal monitoring of tumor response. However, the same methods are also used in the detection of normal tissue physiologic changes after RT doses. Several studies used textural features extracted from CT images to study

Table 1
Definitions of histogram parameters

Parameter	Definition
Mean	Average value of the pixels within the region of interest
SD	Determine how much different or variable are the values from the average (mean value). A low SD: the data points tend to be very close to the mean A high SD: the data points are spread out over a large range of values
Skewness	Estimate symmetry of the histogram. • A zero measure indicates symmetric distribution of values on both sides of the mean • A negative skew: the histogram tail on the left side is longer than the right side. • A positive skew: the tail on the right side is longer than the left side.
Kurtosis	Measure peakedness of the histogram. • A zero value indicates normal distribution. • Positive kurtosis: Its value is greater than zero with tall and more peaked histogram than a normal distribution. • Negative kurtosis: Its value is less than zero with more flat histogram than a normal distribution.

Ref.[30]

variations in parotid glands during and after RT of HNC. They observed a decrease in parotid volume and tissue heterogeneity that was correlated with pretreatment dosimetric parameters, which could indicate a relationship between dose plan and structural changes after RT.[49]

Predicting thyroid cartilage invasion
Accurate prediction of thyroid cartilage invasion from HNC is still lower. Consequently, a study used preoperative CT-based radiomic features to obtain better accuracy in predicting thyroid cartilage invasion. A classifier comprising logistic regression algorithms was applied together with the support vector machine-based synthetic minority oversampling method, and the classifier had a higher AUC reaching 0.905 that exceeded the radiologists' performance.[50]

Head and Neck Lymphoma

Differentiation of ocular adnexal lymphoma from idiopathic orbital inflammation
Differentiation between idiopathic orbital inflammation (IOI) and ocular adnexal lymphoma (OAL) is important because of different treatment plans for each disease and different prognoses. IOI responds positively to corticosteroids in most cases, while OAL is treated by low-dose radiation therapy.[51] MR-based radiomics could be used to aid in improving the diagnostic accuracy in differentiating OAL and IOI. A study achieved AUCs of 0.74 and 0.73 in the training and testing cohorts, respectively.[52] Another study used histogram analysis of ADC maps combined with conventional MRI feature of orbital preseptal space affection, and the logistic model reached an AUC of 0.939 in differentiating between IOI and OAL.[53]

Differentiation sinonasal primary lymphomas from HNC
MRI-based radiomics features can improve the discrimination between sinonasal lymphomas and SCCs with subsequent improvement in treatment strategies for oncology patients. A study achieved high diagnostic performance in differentiating the two diseases with AUC values of 0.94 for the primary cohort and 0.85 for the testing cohort.[54]

Differentiation nasopharyngeal carcinoma and lymphoma
Lymphoma is the second frequently encountered nasopharyngeal neoplasm after nasopharyngeal carcinoma (NPC).[55] Each disease has different biological behavior, plan of therapy, and prognosis. Discrimination between NPC and nasopharyngeal lymphoma (NPL) by conventional MRI is difficult because of overlapping morphologic imaging features.[56] The mean ADC value of both diseases showed a significant difference in several previous studies. However, quantitative ADC analysis depends on measuring a single region of interest (ROI) within the largest tumor section, which may lead to underestimation of the whole-tumor characteristics.[57] A recent study used the histogram analysis of ADC maps that measures distributed ADC values of the whole tumor for better reflection of the biological heterogeneity of a tumor. Among all ADC parameters, the highest performance of uniformity was achieved (AUC = 0.768), while the 10th percentiles of ADC gained an AUC of 0.725 in the differentiation between NPC and NPL.[58]

Nasopharyngeal Carcinoma

Differentiation NPC from benign lesions

NPC is a disease with distinctive clinical behavior, epidemiology, and histopathology which is different from that of HNSCC.[59] Differentiation between early NPC and normal adenoid tissue is challenging. Studies extracted some quantitative textural features from nasopharyngeal CT in patients with NPC and patients with normal adenoid tissue and showed a statistically significant difference. This difference is attributed to the basic architectural variations between the two tissue types on a microscopic level.[60]

Staging of NPC (T staging)

Precise staging of NPC is crucial before using suitable therapy strategies. Applying DL approach based on MR images can perform automated T staging for NPC accurately. It was found that the use of DL in T staging is similar to the traditional TNM T staging in its prognostic performance.[61] A study was carried out on patients with primary NPC without distant metastasis (DM) and before therapy. After extraction of the imaging features and building a predictive model for DM, it was found that this model can be used as a visual prognostic predictor for DM in patients with NPC. Moreover, it can allow better management decisions by assisting in the patients' stratification according to their risk of DM.[62]

Prediction of progression-free survival of NPC

The prognostic predictors of progression-free survival (PFS) in patients with NPC are based on textural features such as the tumor volume and its uniform contrast enhancement before treatment. Some features help in better prediction of PFS in patients with NPC including small tumor size, homogenous CE-T1W in a primary lesion, as well as the overall staging.[63]

Prediction of recurrence of NPC

The prediction of poor survival in patients with NPC because of loco-regional recurrence and or metastasis is essential for treatment design and counseling for the patients and their families. A study was carried on patients with NPC undergoing therapy showed that MRI-based texture features are independent predictors of recurrence yielding an AUC of about 0.79.[64]

Cervical Lymph Nodes

Differentiation metastatic from reactive nodes

Differentiation of malignant from benign cervical LNs and delineation of malignant cervical LNs as metastatic or lymphoma are essential because of different therapeutic approaches, staging, and prognosis.[65,66] It is a great challenge to differentiate between metastatic and tumor-free cervical LNs. Metastatic LNs are considered the major risk factor resulting frequently in recurrence and poor OS in HNC. Some radiomic models have been built to aid early treatment strategies and predict LN status. A study was carried out on patients with papillary thyroid carcinoma and aimed to predict LN metastasis. This was based on preoperative thyroid US images as noninvasive radiomic features. Selected features favoring metastatic LNS were a complex echo pattern, posterior region homogeneity, and macrocalcification or multiple calcifications. This study achieved an AUC of 0.78 for the model-based group and an AUC of 0.72 for the independent validation group.[67]

Differentiation of metastatic from lymphomatous nodes

Characterization of malignant LNs into either metastatic or lymphomatous nodes is crucial before treatment. Regarding cervical lymphadenopathy, TA has achieved a great role in different ways. A study used the whole-lesion histogram analysis of ADC maps in neck nodes to discriminate lymphoma from metastatic SCC of an unknown origin. The highest diagnostic performance was given by the ADCmean and ADCmedian values demonstrating a strong diagnostic accuracy and high specificity.[68]

Detection of extracapsular spread of metastatic lymph node

Medical imaging before surgery provides helpful information for clinical staging and determination of the degree of neck LN dissection during the operation, in addition to the status of extracapsular spread (ECS).[69] A study was performed on patients with known oral cavity cancer; magnetic resonance texture analysis (MRTA) was used to improve the prediction of ECS. The study compared the diagnostic accuracy of first-order textural features such as entropy, kurtosis, and skewness with the conventional MRI attributes of ECS including central necrosis, irregular margin, local invasion, and flare sign. It was found that combined first-order MRTA and conventional imaging features may enhance the prediction accuracy up to 79%.[70]

Salivary Gland Tumors

Differentiating benign from malignant salivary tumors

Selection of the surgical choice of parotid tumors depends on the tumor histologic type. Therefore, preoperative characterization of parotid tumors is required before treatment design. Total parotidectomy is used to treat malignant tumors, and the facial nerve may be sacrificed.[71,72] Histogram analysis is a novel technique that analyzes parametric maps; it depends on the distribution of pixels providing valuable data about the tumor heterogeneity. Currently, it is recognized as a helpful tool for tumor diagnosis, grade, stage, and prognosis in different diseases.[73] Moreover, histogram analysis serves as an objective technique that offers additional data helpful in the distinction of common parotid gland tumors such as pleomorphic adenomas (PAs), Warthin tumors (WTs), and salivary gland malignancy through analysis of the ADC maps. The most helpful parameters are Skewness and ADCmean.[74] A study applied TA and ADC to differentiate between benign and malignant parotid tumors as well as between PAs and WTs; radiomic features were extracted from conventional MRI (T1WI and CE-T1WI). Radiologists may benefit from the use of ADC values and texture features in the delineation of parotid lesions. Further prospective studies with the use of TA are still required to establish the performance of this technique in clinical use.[75]

Prediction of xerostomia in NPC

Xerostomia occurs as a result of radiation-induced parotid damage in patients with NPC under RT. The importance of ADC histogram analysis in the evaluation of xerostomia has been successfully evaluated. A study found a decrease in parotid volume, skewness, and kurtosis after RT but with an elevation of all other ADC histogram values. In the prediction of late xerostomia degrees, early mean alteration of certain ADC histogram values is useful.[76]

In this study, the increased parotid SD is a sign of the larger distribution of ADC values. The SD is increased as a result of the heterogeneous microstructure of irradiated glands with increased acinar cell necrosis and inflammatory cell infiltrates. The peak of the histogram was shifted from the low ADC area toward the relatively high ADC area because of acinar cell necrosis leading to a decrease in skewness. Also, kurtosis was decreased as expected, and this was attributed to the heterogeneous distribution of the ADC values of the parotid gland with flattened histogram peak.[77] The dynamic microstructural change of the radiation-induced parotid damage over time is assessed by the whole volume histogram analysis. There is a progressive elevation of SD, 75th, and 90th percentiles of parotid glands over 4 months after RT which could be explained by the repair of parotid ducts and occurrence of fibrosis. Although it is a time-consuming procedure, it can offer added data that could not be received from routine techniques. The simple mean ADC values calculated by circular ROIs remained without alteration.[76]

Prediction of cancer death risk from salivary cancer

Malignant salivary gland tumors have a variable histologic microstructure with different sizes of cell nests, tissue types, and viscosities of the extracellular components. Consequently, the ADC histogram exhibits divergent values according to the histologic subtypes and components.[78] Therefore, the whole tumor ADC value of the measured area may not represent the heterogeneous microstructure and mask the focal tiny areas within the tumor that might have ADC values relevant to the aggressiveness and sensitivity to cancer therapy.[79] A study assessed the value of ADC measurement according to the percentage of tumor area to classify different types of salivary gland tumors. Moreover, multiparametric ADC histogram analysis such as skewness, kurtosis, and ADC percentiles showed effective prognosis and survival of patients with HNC.[77]

Thyroid Gland Nodules

Differentiation benign from malignant thyroid nodules

Nodular thyroid is a common disease that accounts for 4%–7% of the population on palpation and 10%–40% on the sonographic examination. Thyroid cancer is an uncommon disease when compared to the common nodular thyroid disease. The discrimination between the two diseases is essential because of different prognosis and treatment outcomes.[80] Applications of computer-aided diagnosis (CAD) systems have been developed to assist radiologists in performing more accurate and faster medical data examinations with less diagnostic errors. CAD systems were the forerunners for ML techniques which are increasingly being introduced to radiology tasks because of their potential ability in extracting complex characteristics from biomedical information. For example, CAD systems can help in the detection and analysis of thyroid diseases to distinguish between lesions and aid in patient's classification automatically.[81]

A study has applied CAD systems and extracted textural features from combined T2WI and ADC values using CNN, achieving high performance in differentiating benign from malignant thyroid nodules, accuracy of 0.87, specificity 0.97, and sensitivity 0.69.[82] In another novel study, combined DWI and ADC values were used to extract textural features with the multi-input CNN method to diagnose thyroid cancer with an accuracy of 0.88.[83]

Aggressiveness and subtyping of thyroid cancer

TA is an emerging noninvasive modality that can help in the characterization of thyroid cancer and the prediction of histopathological types. A preliminary study applied MRTA-extracted radiomic features from standard T1 and T2 WIs and found significant statistical relations between MRTA features and histopathologic parameters.[84] A previous work derived TA from ADC measurements only and yielded a sensitivity of 92% and specificity of 96% indicating the role of TA in stratification of patients with thyroid cancer.[85]

Immunohistochemistry of thyroid nodules

Immunohistochemistry (IHC) features are useful in the prediction of the nature of thyroid nodules and subsequently improving patients' diagnosis and prognosis. A recent study investigated TA features derived from CT images preoperatively with the prediction of IHC characteristics of thyroid nodules. The results showed high correlations between imaging and IHC markers. The best performance predictive model gained accuracy of 82.5% in the training cohort and 85% in the validation cohort. However, TA is suggested to be used as an added noninvasive method predicting IHC features not to replace IHC examinations.[86]

Cervical nodal metastasis in thyroid cancer

Nodal metastasis is the major risk factor associated with recurrence and poor OS in patients with thyroid cancer. Radiomics model used the preoperative US thyroid images and can be applied as a noninvasive prediction model to identify metastatic LNs with an accuracy of 71%. Features suggesting LN metastasis by US images include heterogeneous internal echogenicity, posterior region homogeneity, and macrocalcification or multiple calcifications. This LN status prediction model serves in optimizing therapeutic plans, disease prognostication, and treatment outcomes.[67]

Soft-tissue Tumors

Differentiation of malignant from benign soft-tissue tumors

The use of radiomics in imaging of musculoskeletal system has been recognized recently. Radiomics is a fast consistent low-cost method that extracts the characteristic imaging features noninvasively. It is able to determine tumor heterogeneity and texture to classify tumors or subtypes. Radiomics has been incorporated into ML in the evaluation of soft-tissue masses. Recent researches introduced ML in the discrimination between malignant and benign soft-tissue tumors,

grading of soft-tissue sarcomas (STS), and prediction of patients' survival in high-grade sarcomas.[87]

Differentiation of benign peripheral neurogenic tumors from soft-tissue sarcomas

The most common benign peripheral neurogenic tumors (BPNTs) are schwannomas and neurofibromas, while STSs are rare tumors. STSs can be mistaken for BPNTs; therefore, it is important to discriminate between both entities before the operation to avoid inadequate marginal resection. A study found that all whole-tumor ADC histogram parameters except kurtosis and entropy had a significant difference between BPNTs and STSs with high accuracy rather than conventional MRI and ADC values.[88]

Differentiation of rhabdomyosarcoma and infantile hemangioma

Differentiation between tissue sarcoma (RMS) and infantile hemangioma (IH) clinically or radiologically alone is sometimes problematic. The added value of TA in distinguishing both diseases in infants is to alleviate the diagnosis without any invasive procedures and to depict subtle pathologic changes. A study applied MRI-based TA to differentiate between RMS and IH with the extraction of several texture features, particularly the gray-level zone length matrix. The study achieved sensitivity and specificity of 93% and 87%, respectively, in distinguishing RMS from IH. Further studies are needed to confirm its reproducibility and feasibility. TA is a promising noninvasive diagnostic tool in children with uncertain clinical findings.[89]

Reflecting Ki67 index in soft-tissue sarcoma

Ki67 Proliferation index is a very important histopathological marker used in the prognosis of different malignancies. In sarcomas, it can help distinguish between low-grade and high-grade sarcomas, estimate the response to neoadjuvant RT, and predict overall patient survival. A study derived texture features from T1- and T2-weighted images of several STS and correlated these features with proliferation index Ki67. The best correlation achieved AUC reaching up to 0.90 denoting that proliferation index Ki67 could be used as a biological marker in STS.[90]

Identification of paragangliomas

Head and neck paragangliomas (PGLs) are the most common nonepithelial neck tumors and usually originate from the paraganglia in carotid artery bifurcation. This similar anatomic distribution and nonspecific presentation make difficult clinical distinctions of PGLs from other neck masses. Preoperative percutaneous biopsy from PGLs is difficult because of the risk of adrenergic crisis and bleeding from the hypervascular tumor.[91] TA was applied in a study to differentiate between PGLs and other neck masses. Features were selected from T2-weighted fat-saturated DIXON images and obtained an AUC of 0.855 with high accuracy in defining PGLs from other neck masses and in developing a statistical classification model.[92]

Prediction succinate dehydrogenase mutation in PGLs

Genetic predisposition of head and neck PGLs is estimated in about 35% of cases. Familial PGL, pheochromocytoma, thyroid, and ovarian cancers are associated with succinate dehydrogenase (SDH) gene mutation.[93] Detecting SDH mutation is clinically significant because of the higher risk of developing malignancy and recurrence.[94] A study used 2D TA derived from both T2WI and CE-T1WI MRI to predict SDH mutation status in PGLs of the head and neck. Only T2-based predictive textures were statistically significant with an AUC of 0.71 and accuracy of 70.8%. TA is a noninvasive technique that can aid in further genetic workup.[95]

CLINICS CARE POINTS

- Artificial intelligence (AI) methods are rapidly developing overtime with different promising subsets such as machine learning, deep learning, and radiomics.
- Integration of AI with radiology workflow improves diagnosis and monitoring of treatment response.
- This article summarizes the clinical applications of AI in head and neck cancer including differentiation, grading, staging, prognosis, genetic profile, and monitoring after treatment.
- Further studies are required to establish powerful methodology as well as coupling of genetic and radiologic profiles to be validated in the clinical use.

DISCLOSURE

The authors have nothing to disclose.

REFERENCES

1. Razek AAKA, Tawfik AM, Elsorogy LGA, et al. Perfusion CT of head and neck cancer. Eur J Radiol 2014; 83:537–44.
2. Razek AA, Elkhamary S, Al-Mesfer S, et al. Correlation of apparent diffusion coefficient at 3T with prognostic parameters of retinoblastoma. Am J Neuroradiol 2012;33:944–8.
3. Razek AA, Mossad A, Ghonim M. Role of diffusion-weighted MR imaging in assessing malignant versus benign skull-base lesions. Radiol Med 2011;116: 125–32.
4. Bergamino M, Nespodzany A, Baxter LC, et al. Preliminary assessment of intravoxel incoherent motion diffusion-weighted MRI (IVIM-DWI) metrics in Alzheimer's disease. J Magn Reson Imaging 2020;52: 1811–2186.
5. Razek AAKA, Ashmalla GA, Gaballa G, et al. Pilot study of ultrasound parotid imaging reporting and data system (PIRADS): inter-observer agreement. Eur J Radiol 2015;84:2533–8.
6. Maleki F, Le WT, Sananmuang T, et al. Machine learning applications for head and neck imaging. Neuroimaging Clin N Am 2020;30:517–29.
7. Currie G, Hawk KE, Rohren E, et al. Machine learning and deep learning in medical imaging: intelligent imaging. J Med Imaging Radiat Sci 2019;50:477–87.
8. Resteghini C, Trama A, Borgonovi E, et al. Big data in head and neck cancer. Curr Treat Options Oncol 2018;19:1–15.
9. Werth K, Ledbetter L. Artificial intelligence in head and neck imaging: a glimpse into the future. Neuroimaging Clin N Am 2020;30:359–68.
10. Jethanandani A, Lin TA, Volpe S, et al. Exploring applications of radiomics in magnetic resonance imaging of head and neck cancer: a systematic review. Front Oncol 2018;8:131.
11. Fazal MI, Patel ME, Tye J, et al. The past, present and future role of artificial intelligence in imaging. Eur J Radiol 2018;105:246–50.
12. Tang A, Tam R, Cadrin-Chênevert A, et al. Canadian association of radiologists white paper on artificial intelligence in radiology. Can Assoc Radiol J 2018; 69:120–35.
13. Briganti G, Le Moine O. Artificial intelligence in medicine: today and tomorrow. Front Med 2020;7: 27.
14. Boon IS, Au Yong T, Boon CS. Assessing the role of artificial intelligence (AI) in clinical oncology: utility of machine learning in radiotherapy target volume delineation. Medicines 2018;5:131.
15. Erickson BJ, Korfiatis P, Akkus Z, et al. Machine learning for medical imaging. Radiographics 2017; 37:505–15.
16. Bengio Y, Courville A, Vincent P. Representation learning: a review and new perspectives. IEEE Trans Pattern Anal Mach Intell 2013;35:1798–828.
17. Choy G, Khalilzadeh O, Michalski M, et al. Current applications and future impact of machine learning in radiology. Radiology 2018;288:318–28.

18. Gore JC. Artificial intelligence in medical imaging. Magn Reson Imaging 2020;68:A1–4.

19. Esteva A, Robicquet A, Ramsundar B, et al. A guide to deep learning in healthcare. Nat Med 2019;25:24–9.

20. Mazurowski MA, Buda M, Saha A, et al. Deep learning in radiology: an overview of the concepts and a survey of the state of the art with focus on MRI. J Magn Reson Imaging 2019;49:939–54.

21. Lambin P, Leijenaar RT, Deist TM, et al. Radiomics: the bridge between medical imaging and personalized medicine. Nat Rev Clin Oncol 2017;14:749.

22. Parmar C, Grossmann P, Bussink J, et al. Machine learning methods for quantitative radiomic biomarkers. Sci Rep 2015;5:13087.

23. Kumar V, Gu Y, Basu S, et al. Radiomics: the process and the challenges. Magn Reson Imaging 2012;30:1234–48.

24. Gillies RJ, Kinahan PE, Hricak H. Radiomics: images are more than pictures, they are data. Radiology 2015;278:563–77.

25. Castellano G, Bonilha L, Li L, et al. Texture analysis of medical images. Clin Radiol 2004;59:1061–89.

26. Kassner A, Thornhill R. Texture analysis: a review of neurologic MR imaging applications. Am J Neuroradiol 2010;31:809–16.

27. Varghese BA, Cen SY, Hwang DH, et al. Texture analysis of imaging: what radiologists need to know. Am J Roentgenol 2019;212:520–8.

28. Summers RM. Texture analysis in radiology: Does the emperor have no clothes? Abd Radiol 2017;42:342–5.

29. Lubner MG, Smith AD, Sandrasegaran K, et al. CT texture analysis: definitions, applications, biologic correlates, and challenges. Radiographics 2017;37:1483–503.

30. Miles KA, Ganeshan B, Hayball MP. CT texture analysis using the filtration-histogram method: what do the measurements mean? Cancer Imaging 2013;13:400.

31. Parmar C, Velazquez ER, Leijenaar R, et al. Robust radiomics feature quantification using semiautomatic volumetric segmentation. PLoS One 2014;9:e102107.

32. de Leon AD, Kapur P, Pedrosa I. Radiomics in kidney cancer: MR imaging. Magn Reson Imaging Clin N Am 2019;27:1–13.

33. Razek AAKA, Elsorogy LG, Soliman NY, et al. Dynamic susceptibility contrast perfusion MR imaging in distinguishing malignant from benign head and neck tumors: a pilot study. Eur J Radiol 2011;77:73–9.

34. Fruehwald-Pallamar J, Hesselink J, Mafee M, et al. Texture-based analysis of 100 MR examinations of head and neck tumors–is it possible to discriminate between benign and malignant masses in a multicenter trial? Rofo 2016;188:195–202.

35. Zhang Y, Shang L, Chen C, et al. Machine-learning classifiers in discrimination of lesions located in the anterior skull base. Front Oncol 2020;10:752.

36. Zhang H, Wang H, Hao D, et al. An MRI-based radiomic nomogram for discrimination between malignant and benign sinonasal tumors. J Magn Reson Imaging 2021;53:141–51.

37. Mukherjee P, Cintra M, Huang C, et al. CT-based radiomic signatures for predicting histopathologic features in head and neck squamous cell carcinoma. Radiol Imaging Cancer 2020;2:e190039.

38. Fujima N, Homma A, Harada T, et al. The utility of MRI histogram and texture analysis for the prediction of histological diagnosis in head and neck malignancies. Cancer Imaging 2019;19:1–10.

39. Ren J, Qi M, Yuan Y, et al. Radiomics of apparent diffusion coefficient maps to predict histologic grade in squamous cell carcinoma of the oral tongue and floor of mouth: a preliminary study. Acta Radiol 2021;62:453–61.

40. Ren J, Tian J, Yuan Y, et al. Magnetic resonance imaging based radiomics signature for the preoperative discrimination of stage I-II and III-IV head and neck squamous cell carcinoma. Eur J Radiol 2018;106:1–6.

41. Razek AAKA, Nada N. Arterial spin labeling perfusion-weighted MR imaging: correlation of tumor blood flow with pathological degree of tumor differentiation, clinical stage and nodal metastasis of head and neck squamous cell carcinoma. Eur Arch Otorhinolaryngol 2018;275:1301–7.

42. Yuan Y, Ren J, Shi Y, et al. MRI-based radiomic signature as predictive marker for patients with head and neck squamous cell carcinoma. Eur J Radiol 2019;117:193–8.

43. Mes SW, van Velden FH, Peltenburg B, et al. Outcome prediction of head and neck squamous cell carcinoma by MRI radiomic signatures. Eur Radiol 2020;30:6311–21.

44. Zwirner K, Hilke FJ, Demidov G, et al. Radiogenomics in head and neck cancer: correlation of radiomic heterogeneity and somatic mutations in TP53, FAT1 and KMT2D. Strahlenther Onkol 2019;195:771–9.

45. Zhu W, Huang Y, Zeng L, et al. AnatomyNet: deep learning for fast and fully automated whole-volume segmentation of head and neck anatomy. Med Phys 2019;46:576–89.

46. Tran WT, Suraweera H, Quaioit K, et al. Predictive quantitative ultrasound radiomic markers associated with treatment response in head and neck cancer. Future Sci OA 2020;6:FSO433.

47. Razek AAKA, Abdelaziz TT. Neck imaging reporting and data system: what does radiologist want to know? J Comput Assist Tomogr 2020;44:527–32.

48. Razek AAKA, Gaballa G, Ashamalla G, et al. Dynamic susceptibility contrast perfusion-weighted magnetic resonance imaging and diffusion-

weighted magnetic resonance imaging in differentiating recurrent head and neck cancer from postradiation changes. J Comput Assist Tomogr 2015;39:849–54.

49. Wong AJ, Kanwar A, Mohamed AS, et al. Radiomics in head and neck cancer: from exploration to application. Transl Cancer Res 2016;5:371.

50. Guo R, Guo J, Zhang L, et al. CT-based radiomics features in the prediction of thyroid cartilage invasion from laryngeal and hypopharyngeal squamous cell carcinoma. Cancer Imaging 2020;20:1–11.

51. Eissa L, Razek AAKA, Helmy E. Arterial spin labeling and diffusion-weighted MR imaging: utility in differentiating idiopathic orbital inflammatory pseudotumor from orbital lymphoma. Clin Imaging 2021;71:63–8.

52. Guo J, Liu Z, Shen C, et al. MR-based radiomics signature in differentiating ocular adnexal lymphoma from idiopathic orbital inflammation. Eur Radiol 2018;28:3872–81.

53. Ren J, Yuan Y, Wu Y, et al. Differentiation of orbital lymphoma and idiopathic orbital inflammatory pseudotumor: combined diagnostic value of conventional MRI and histogram analysis of ADC maps. BMC Med Imaging 2018;18:1–8.

54. Wang X, Dai S, Wang Q, et al. Investigation of MRI-based radiomics model in differentiation between sinonasal primary lymphomas and squamous cell carcinomas. Japn J Radiol 2021. https://doi.org/10.1007/s11604-021-01116-6.

55. MacDermed D, Thurber L, George TI, et al. Extranodal nonorbital indolent lymphomas of the head and neck: relationship between tumor control and radiotherapy. Int J Radiat Oncol Biol Phys 2004;59:788–95.

56. Kato H, Kanematsu M, Kawaguchi S, et al. Evaluation of imaging findings differentiating extranodal non-Hodgkin's lymphoma from squamous cell carcinoma in naso-and oropharynx. Clin Imaging 2013;37:657–63.

57. Just N. Improving tumour heterogeneity MRI assessment with histograms. Br J Cancer 2014;111:2205–13.

58. Lian S, Zhang C, Chi J, et al. Differentiation between nasopharyngeal carcinoma and lymphoma at the primary site using whole-tumor histogram analysis of apparent diffusion coefficient maps. Radiol Med 2020;125:647–53.

59. Abdel Khalek Abdel Razek A, King A. MRI and CT of nasopharyngeal carcinoma. Am J Roentgenol 2012;198:11–8.

60. Tsai A, Buch K, Fujita A, et al. Using CT texture analysis to differentiate between nasopharyngeal carcinoma and age-matched adenoid controls. Eur J Radiol 2018;108:208–14.

61. Yang Q, Guo Y, Ou X, et al. Automatic T staging using weakly supervised deep learning for nasopharyngeal carcinoma on MR images. J Magn Reson Imaging 2020;52:1074–82.

62. Zhang L, Dong D, Li H, et al. Development and validation of a magnetic resonance imaging-based model for the prediction of distant metastasis before initial treatment of nasopharyngeal carcinoma: a retrospective cohort study. EBioMedicine 2019;40:327–35.

63. Mao J, Fang J, Duan X, et al. Predictive value of pretreatment MRI texture analysis in patients with primary nasopharyngeal carcinoma. Eur Radiol 2019;29:4105–13.

64. Raghavan Nair JK, Vallières M, Mascarella MA, et al. Magnetic resonance imaging texture analysis predicts recurrence in patients with nasopharyngeal carcinoma. Canad Assoc Radiol J 2019;70:394–402.

65. Razek AAKA, Gaballa G. Role of perfusion magnetic resonance imaging in cervical lymphadenopathy. J Comput Assist Tomogr 2011;35:21–5.

66. Razek AAKA, Helmy E. Multi-parametric arterial spin labeling and diffusion-weighted imaging in differentiation of metastatic from reactive lymph nodes in head and neck squamous cell carcinoma. Eur Arch Otorhinolaryngol 2021;278:2529–35.

67. Liu T, Zhou S, Yu J, et al. Prediction of lymph node metastasis in patients with papillary thyroid carcinoma: a radiomics method based on preoperative ultrasound images. Technol Cancer Res Treat 2019;18. 1533033819831713.

68. Vidiri A, Minosse S, Piludu F, et al. Cervical lymphadenopathy: can the histogram analysis of apparent diffusion coefficient help to differentiate between lymphoma and squamous cell carcinoma in patients with unknown clinical primary tumor? Radiol Med 2019;124:19–26.

69. Ho T-Y, Chao C-H, Chin S-C, et al. Classifying neck lymph nodes of head and neck squamous cell carcinoma in MRI images with radiomic features. J Digit Imaging 2020;33:613–8.

70. Frood R, Palkhi E, Barnfield M, et al. Can MR textural analysis improve the prediction of extracapsular nodal spread in patients with oral cavity cancer? Eur Radiol 2018;28:5010–8.

71. Abdel Razek AA, Samir S, Ashmalla GA. Characterization of parotid tumors with dynamic susceptibility contrast perfusion-weighted magnetic resonance imaging and diffusion-weighted MR imaging. J Comput Assist Tomogr 2017;41:131–6.

72. Razek AAKA. Multi-parametric MR imaging using pseudo-continuous arterial-spin labeling and diffusion-weighted MR imaging in differentiating subtypes of parotid tumors. Magn Reson Imaging 2019;63:55–9.

73. Xu X-Q, Ma G, Wang Y-J, et al. Histogram analysis of diffusion kurtosis imaging of nasopharyngeal carcinoma: correlation between quantitative

parameters and clinical stage. Oncotarget 2017;8: 47230–8.

74. Abdel Razek AAK, Gadelhak BN, El Zahabey IA, et al. Diffusion-weighted imaging with histogram analysis of the apparent diffusion coefficient maps in the diagnosis of parotid tumours. Int J Oral Maxillofac Surg 2021. https://doi.org/10.1016/j.ijom.2021.03.019.

75. Fruehwald-Pallamar J, Czerny C, Holzer-Fruehwald L, et al. Texture-based and diffusion-weighted discrimination of parotid gland lesions on MR images at 3.0 Tesla. NMR Biomed 2013;26: 1372–9.

76. Zhou N, Guo T, Zheng H, et al. Apparent diffusion coefficient histogram analysis can evaluate radiation-induced parotid damage and predict late xerostomia degree in nasopharyngeal carcinoma. Oncotarget 2017;8:70226–38.

77. King AD, Chow K-K, Yu K-H, et al. Head and neck squamous cell carcinoma: diagnostic performance of diffusion-weighted MR imaging for the prediction of treatment response. Radiology 2013;266:531–8.

78. Chen P, Dong B, Zhang C, et al. The histogram analysis of apparent diffusion coefficient in differential diagnosis of parotid tumor. Dentomaxillofac Radiol 2020;49:20190420.

79. Murase R, Sumida T, Kawamura R, et al. Suppression of invasion and metastasis in aggressive salivary cancer cells through targeted inhibition of ID1 gene expression. Cancer Lett 2016;377:11–6.

80. Razek AA, Sadek A, Kombar O, et al. Role of apparent diffusion coefficient values in differentiation between malignant and benign solitary thyroid nodules. Am J Neuroradiol 2008;29:563–8.

81. Li L-N, Ouyang J-H, Chen H-L, et al. A computer aided diagnosis system for thyroid disease using extreme learning machine. J Med Syst 2012;36: 3327–37.

82. Naglah A, Khalifa F, Khaled R, et al. Novel MRI-based CAD system for early detection of thyroid cancer using multi-input CNN. Sensors 2021;21: 3878.

83. Naglah A, Khalifa F, Khaled R, et al. Thyroid cancer computer-aided diagnosis system using MRI-based multi-input CNN model. In: Proceedings of the 2021 IEEE 18th International Symposium on Biomedical Imaging (ISBI 2021), Nice, France, 13–16 April 2021. Piscataway, NJ, USA: IEEE; 2021. p. 1691–4.

84. Meyer H-J, Schob S, Höhn AK, et al. MRI texture analysis reflects histopathology parameters in thyroid cancer–a first preliminary study. Transl Oncol 2017;10:911–6.

85. Brown AM, Nagala S, McLean MA, et al. Multi-institutional validation of a novel textural analysis tool for preoperative stratification of suspected thyroid tumors on diffusion-weighted MRI. Magn Reson Med 2016;75:1708–16.

86. Gu J, Zhu J, Qiu Q, et al. Prediction of immunohistochemistry of suspected thyroid nodules by use of machine learning–based radiomics. Am J Roentgenol 2019;213:1348–57.

87. Wang H, Zhang J, Bao S, et al. Preoperative MRI-based radiomic machine-learning nomogram may accurately distinguish between benign and malignant soft-tissue lesions: a two-center study. J Magn Reson Imaging 2020;52:873–82.

88. Nakajo M, Fukukura Y, Hakamada H, et al. Whole-tumor apparent diffusion coefficient (ADC) histogram analysis to differentiate benign peripheral neurogenic tumors from soft tissue sarcomas. J Magn Reson Imaging 2018;48:680–6.

89. Sarioglu FC, Sarioglu O, Guleryuz H, et al. MRI-based texture analysis for differentiating pediatric craniofacial rhabdomyosarcoma from infantile hemangioma. Eur Radiol 2020;30:5227–36.

90. Meyer H-J, Renatus K, Höhn AK, et al. Texture analysis parameters derived from T1-and T2-weighted magnetic resonance images can reflect Ki67 index in soft tissue sarcoma. Surg Oncol 2019;30:92–7.

91. Rijken JA, de Vos B, van Hest LP, et al. Evolving management strategies in head and neck paragangliomas: A single-centre experience with 147 patients over a 60-year period. Clin Otolaryngol 2019; 44:836–41.

92. Ghosh A, Malla SR, Bhalla AS, et al. Texture analysis of routine T2 weighted fat-saturated images can identify head and neck paragangliomas–A pilot study. Eur J Radiol Open 2020;7:100248.

93. Srirangalingam U, Walker L, Khoo B, et al. Clinical manifestations of familial paraganglioma and phaeochromocytomas in succinate dehydrogenase B (SDH-B) gene mutation carriers. Clin Endocrinol 2008;69:587–96.

94. Boedeker CC, Neumann HP, Maier W, et al. Malignant head and neck paragangliomas in SDHB mutation carriers. Otolaryngol Head Neck Surg 2007;137: 126–9.

95. Naganawa S, Kim J, Yip SS, et al. Texture analysis of T2-weighted MRI predicts SDH mutation in paraganglioma. Neuroradiology 2021;63:547–54.

Magnetic Resonance Imaging of Perineural Spread of Head and Neck Cancer

Tougan Taha Abdelaziz, MD[a],*, Ahmed Abdel Khalek Abdel Razek, MD[b],†

KEYWORDS

- Perineural tumor spread • Squamous cell carcinoma • MR imaging • PET-MR imaging

KEY POINTS

- Primary imaging findings of perineural tumor spread (PNTS) are thickening, nodularity, complete enhancement of the nerve and obliteration of the pad fat.
- Secondary imaging findings of PNTS are muscular denervation and superior muscular aponeurotic system changes.
- Squamous cell carcinoma and adenoid cystic carcinomas represent the highest incidence of PNTS in head and neck cancers.
- Targeted pre-contrast and postcontrast fat-suppressed magnetic resonance (MR) imaging technique is the most appropriate modality for a suspected case of PNTS.
- Hybrid PET-MR and PET-CT are problem-solving techniques, in posttreatment surveillance and in advanced disease, with a concern about nodal or distant metastasis.

BACKGROUND

A distinctive feature of head and neck cancer (HNC) is using cranial nerves (CNs) and their peripheral branches as a conduit for tumoral growth away from the primary site of the tumor.[1] Following the nerve invasion, the tumoral cells pursue the sheath to reach deeper connections of the nerve. Perineural invasion (PNI) is a term used to define the microscopic diagnosis that may be beyond the scope of the different radiological imaging modalities. It is described as either the infiltration of at least 33% of the nerve circumference or the presence of tumoral cells within the nerve sheath (usually for small-caliber nerves near the site of primary tumor).[2] In contrast, perineural tumor spread (PNTS) defines the macroscopic growth of tumor cells along the nerve that can be detected radiologically and clinically (usually for large-caliber nerves beyond the primary tumor site).[3]

Pathogenesis of Perineural Spread

PNTS is a separate pathologic entity of tumoral spread that can occur in the absence of other types of spread. Recent studies have proved that PNTS is not simple migration through low-resistance planes because of the presence of several collagenous layers and basement membranes that separate the nerve from the surroundings. Moreover, only certain types of tumors favor PNTS more than others. This difference was explained by PNTS being mostly the result of a complex interaction between specific tumoral

---

[a] Department of Diagnostic Radiology, Ain Shams Faculty of Medicine, 56 Ramses St, Abbasia, Cairo 1158, Egypt; [b] Department of Diagnostic Radiology, Mansoura University, Elgomheryia Street, Mansoura 35512, Egypt

† Deceased

* Corresponding author.

E-mail address: togantaha@med.asu.edu.eg

Magn Reson Imaging Clin N Am 30 (2022) 95–108

https://doi.org/10.1016/j.mric.2021.06.017

cell types, stromal elements, and the nerves that facilitate the invasion of the collagenous tissue and the spread along the nerve sheath complex through increasing the production or activity of some chemicals or the expression of certain cell surface receptors.[2,4–8]

Histologic and Regional Subtypes

Although PNTS has a low prevalence in cases of squamous cell carcinoma (SCC), SCC has the highest incidence of PNTS in all HNC. Adenoid cystic carcinoma (ACC), which most commonly arises from the minor salivary glands, is well known for having the highest incidence of PNTS; however, it represents only 1% to 3% of all HNC.[8–11] Other tumors that show a high incidence of PNTS are mucoepidermoid carcinoma, desmoplastic type of melanoma, and extranodal lymphoma.[12]

The primary site of origin of the tumor plays an important role, with an increased incidence of PNTS with tumors originating in the skull base, skin, and paranasal sinuses. In addition, any tumor, regardless of its histologic or regional subtype, can spread along the nerves if it involves a specific anatomic site rich in neural structures, as in the pterygopalatine fossa, cavernous sinus, or masticator space tumors.[3]

Anatomic Consideration

The tumor usually propagates in a retrograde direction (proximal) carrying the disease to the brainstem. Less often, PNTS can occur in a antegrade pattern (distal) through nerve branches and interconnections (**Fig. 1**).[2]

The trigeminal and facial nerves are the most frequently involved nerves in PNTS because they have the most extensive regional spread and proximity to the anatomic regions and tumor types that show a high incidence of PNTS. Nevertheless, because of rich neural interconnections in the head and neck regions, any nerve could potentially be affected.[13]

Fortunately, the first head and neck neural pathways cross a particular fatty zone at their skull base course. These pads of fats are essential for the diagnosis of PNTS, because fat signal and density are easily detected in T1-weighted imaging (T1WI) and computed tomography (CT) respectively. Obliteration of this fat is considered as an easily detectable and early sign of nerve infiltration (**Fig. 2**).[11] Understanding the CNs' anatomy is critical to identify the different patterns of PNTS. Any segment of the nerve could be infiltrated; however, the most involved are the peripheral and skull base segments.

The trigeminal nerve is the largest CN, and its main trunk arises from the lateral pons to enter the Meckel cave containing the gasserian ganglion. Distal to the ganglion, the nerve trifurcates into its main 3 branches:

The ophthalmic division (V1) passes along the lateral wall of the cavernous sinus to the superior orbital fissure and passes anteriorly within the orbit along the orbital roof, superior to the superior rectus and superior levator palpebrae muscles. Then it gives 3 branches that are involved in PNTS: the nasociliary, lacrimal, and frontal nerves carry tumor mostly of cutaneous origin (SCC, melanoma, and basal cell carcinoma) and ACC from the lacrimal gland.[9,11]

Maxillary division (V2) courses caudal to V1 in the lateral wall of the cavernous sinus, leaving the skull base through the foramen rotundum to

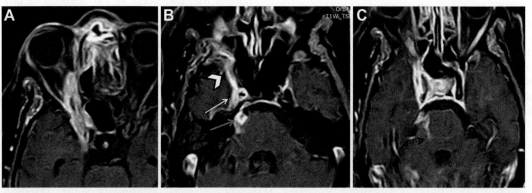

Fig. 1. Retrograde and antegrade patterns of PNTS along V1, trigeminal nerve trunk, and V2 in a case of anterior ethmoidal SCC. (*A–C*) Axial contrast-enhanced T1-weighted imaging (CET1WI) shows a retrograde PNTS along the nasociliary branch of V1 forming an enhancing mass at the right orbital apex (*black arrow*). Extension of tumor cells to the cavernous sinus and Meckel cave (*white arrow*). Tumor cells extend in an antegrade direction to the V2 (*arrowhead*) and retrograde direction to zone 3 of the trigeminal nerve trunk in the prepontine cistern (*gray arrow*) and intra-axial fascicular course (*dotted arrow*).

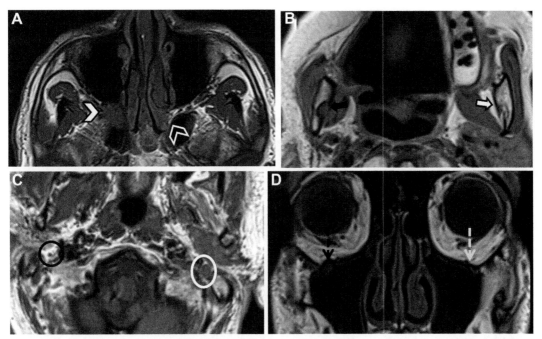

Fig. 2. Obliterated fat pad around infiltrated nerve. (*A–C*) Axial noncontrast T1WI shows obliterated fat pad at the infiltrated right pterygopalatine fossa (PPF) (*white arrowhead*) compared with the normal one (*black arrowhead*), infiltration of the fat pad at the right mandibular foramen (*black arrow*) as opposed to contralateral normal fat signal (*white arrow*), and the infiltrated and enlarged left facial nerve obliterating the surrounding fat pad in the stylomastoid foramen (*white circle*) contrasting the right normal nerve (*black circle*). (*D*) Coronal T1WI shows an infiltrated right infraorbital fat pad around the invaded nerve (*dashed black arrow*). Note the normal left nerve and surrounding fat (*white dashed arrow*).

enter the pterygopalatine fossa (PPF), which acts as a branching point for V2 and is considered one of the essential crossroad regions for PNTS where the nerve branches communicate with the palate, face, and sinonasal cavity. V2 branches carry tumor cells from the midface via the infraorbital nerve, tumors of the palate via the greater and lesser palatine nerves, and tumors of the maxillary sinus usually follow the superior alveolar nerve. Tumor cells can follow any of these routes reaching the PPF, the gasserian ganglion, and middle cranial fossa.[9,11]

The mandibular nerve (V3) bypasses the cavernous sinus, carrying both motor and sensory fibers, leaving the skull base through the foramen ovale to enter the masticator space. It carries tumors from the lower lip and chin through the mental nerve, passing in a retrograde direction to the inferior alveolar and finally the mandibular nerve. Tumors arising from the parotid and skin of the lateral aspect of the face can follow the auriculotemporal nerve, before joining the V3. Tumors of the masticator space, nasopharynx, and buccal mucosa can follow the V3.[9,11]

The facial nerve (VII) exits the skull base through the stylomastoid foramen. The main extracranial nerve trunk passes in the parotid gland, where it gives its terminal branches. Most tumors passing along the VII CN are of parotid origin or skin cancers invading the parotid. On imaging, the obliteration of the fat pad at the stylomastoid foramen signals a facial nerve disorder.[9,11]

Bilateral PNTS can occur, albeit in rare conditions, as multifocal cutaneous SCC, or cross over across the front of the face.[14]

Trigeminofacial nerve anastomosis sites are known to cause broader extension of the HNC. The most involved nerves are the auriculotemporal nerve, a branch of V3 that joins the facial nerve at the parotid gland (**Fig. 3**). The vidian nerve is another important nerve interconnection site, formed by the confluence of the superficial petrosal nerve (from geniculate ganglion of the facial nerve) and the deep greater petrosal nerve (from sympathetic plexus on internal carotid artery). The vidian nerve carries preganglionic fibers to the sphenopalatine ganglion in the PPF. The postganglionic parasympathetic fibers pass through the V1 and V2 branches of the trigeminal nerves.[15]

Other less known but essential anastomosis sites are between the infraorbital nerve of V2 and the buccal and zygomatic branches of VII, the

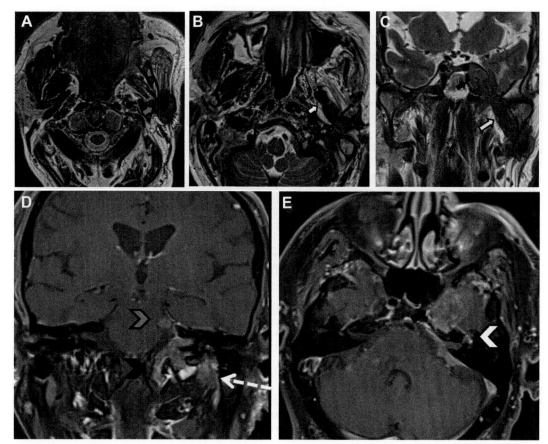

Fig. 3. Trigeminal-facial interconnection in parotid ACC. (*A, B*) Axial T2-weighted imaging (T2WI) shows primary parotid tumor (*gray arrow*) with infiltration of the auriculotemporal nerve (*solid white arrow*). (*C*) Coronal T2WI shows the continuous infiltration of the auriculotemporal nerve, V3, and gasserian ganglion (*black arrow*). (*D*) Coronal CET1WI shows continuous infiltration of the facial nerve passing from the parotid up to the cisternal course (*dashed white arrow*), spread to the cervical plexus (*black arrowhead*), and the infiltration of the trigeminal nerve trunk (*gray arrowhead*). (*E*) Axial CET1WI shows infiltration of the gasserian ganglion (*black arrow*) and geniculate ganglion(*white arrowhead*). Note denervation changes at the masseter and pterygoid muscles.

supraorbital nerve of V1 with the temporal branches of the facial nerve, the zygomaticofacial nerve, a branch of V2 and the zygomatic branch of the facial nerve, the mental nerve (a branch of V3), and the facial nerve.[16]

The cavernous sinus and Meckel cave are additional axes for the PNTS in between the trigeminal nerve branches (see **Fig. 1**).[17]

Zonal Staging of Perineural Tumor Spread

The zonal classification system described by Williams and colleagues,[18] which describes the radiological and histologic disease extension, is widely accepted and used by head and neck multidisciplinary teams because it defines the severity of the disease process and allows standardized management. This system describes zone 1 for the CNs extending from the peripheral course up to the skull base foramina. Zone 2 describes the

extension of the disease to the gasserian and geniculate ganglia for the fifth and seventh CNs respectively, and zone 3 is referred to as the prepontine cistern and brain stem course in the fifth CN and to the internal auditory canal and cerebellopontine angle cistern in the seventh CN. Extension of the disease beyond the gasserian and geniculate ganglia (zone 3) assumes an inoperable stage.[19]

Clinical Manifestations

About 40% to 45% of patients are asymptomatic, although the disease is visible on imaging. Besides, the presenting symptoms may be not specific to the PNTS and can occur in various benign conditions, such as neuritis, vascular stroke, schwannoma, temporomandibular joint disorder, and vascular compression syndrome.[20]

Several clinical storylines may be encountered in the diagnosis of PNTS: (1) at the time of the initial diagnosis of the HNC, symptoms are almost not apparent and even masked by the primary tumor; (2) recurrence of the previously treated tumor, in which the PNTS could be the only manifestation of the recurrent disease; (3) multiple CN distributions may point to a central affection, such as cavernous sinus or leptomeningeal disease; (4) nonspecific pain, numbness, or muscle weakness in the absence of a known primary tumor.[17]

For this reason, radiologists must put the PNTS in the diagnostic checklist, even in reporting unrelated conditions such as nonspecific facial pain, headache, or sinusitis. Mapping the CNs in the nonfocused imaging study is challenging and may lead to overlooked findings. Dankbaar and colleagues[9] pointed to easily detected signs such as the obliteration of the fat pads around the nerves and subsequent denervation changes in the related muscles, and these are 2 clues that could be detected in the nonfocused examination and alert the radiologist to the possible nerve infiltration, requiring more targeted examination to clarify the disease origin and extension.

IMAGING TECHNIQUES

Imaging forms a crucial component of the initial diagnosis of HNC, PNTS, and further posttreatment surveillance protocols. The challenging point is early diagnosis of the disease process at the level of peripheral nerves before it reaches the skull base regions, thus allowing curative therapy.

Magnetic Resonance Imaging

Targeted MR imaging technique using 1.5 T or, better, 3 T is the most appropriate modality for a suspected case of PNTS. At our institution, the protocols are tailored according to the clinical scenario; patients with vague facial pain or muscle weakness with no known primary should be imaged with 2 fields of view. The larger one extends from the sella turcica to the root of the neck to obtain an overview of the expected disorder in the head and neck region. Then a targeted field of view extending from the roof of the orbit to the lower border of the submandibular gland in the axial plane and extending from the anterior orbital margin to the posterior border of the temporal bone in the coronal plane to cover the trigeminal and facial nerves distribution. The field of view may be modified to cover a known primary in another clinical scenario.

T1WI without fat suppression is essential to better evaluate the pad of fat surrounding the questionable nerves, using the high T1 signal of the fat as a natural contrast in the skull base region, and avoiding the susceptibility artifacts frequently seen in saturated sequences. T2-weighted imaging (T2WI) with and without fat-suppression sequences, are essential to identify the subsequent denervation changes that may affect the supplied muscles. The key sequences are contrast-enhanced T1WI with fat suppression; axial two-dimensional images with a slice thickness of 2 mm; and three-dimensional isotropic sequence with axial, coronal, and sagittal reformat, used to visualize the involved nerve directly.

Axial spin-echo echo-planar diffusion weight imaging (DWI) uses 2 b values: b = 0 and 1000 s/mm^2. This type of diffusion is designed to reduce the field of view within the imaging plane, decreasing the geometric distortion and eliminating phase wrap artifacts that are suitable for the head and neck region, particularly the skull base and expected pathway of CNs. Qualitative evaluation of the DWI signal in b1000 and corresponding apparent diffusion coefficient (ADC) map, and quantitative evaluation with the calculation of the ADC value in ADC map, putting the region of interest on the most robust, hypointense lesion are performed. Multiple factors determine ADC value, either technical, such as the type of machine or magnetic field heterogenicity; air; bone and air interface; and slice thickness; or other factors related to the tumor histologic type; for example, lymphoma shows lower diffusion coefficient value than SCC, and the degree of tumor differentiation is lower in poorly differentiated than well-differentiated tumors.[21]

Computed Tomography

CT shows the change of size and shape of the neural foramina. However, some investigators have reported that CT has a limited role in early disease detection, considering the erosion of neural foramina or bulky mass as late signs. Besides, CT is used when there is a concern about osteoradionecrosis or in contraindications to MR imaging, as in the case of implants that will move or malfunction in the magnetic field, and patients who cannot tolerate long MR imaging sequences because of dyspnea or obstructed secretion expected in patients with HNC. CT-guided biopsy is an additional indication in equivocal cases.[14]

Hybrid Imaging

Including PET-CT and PET-MR imaging is a problem-solving technique, especially in posttreatment surveillance and in advanced disease, when there is a concern about nodal or distant metastasis. However, the essential role of high-quality morphologic imaging with higher soft tissue resolution for the detection of the PNTS in HNC hinders the PET-CT and favors a focused head and neck PET-MR imaging technique.[22]

In PET-MR imaging, after adjusting the blood glucose level of the patient (<150 mg/dL), injection of body weight–adapted activity of F^{18}-fluoro-deoxyglucose (FDG) (1 mCi/10 kg body weight) was performed, resulting in an activity of 6.5 ± 2 mCi. PET was performed in list mode for 20 minutes for the head and neck region. Then PET images were reconstructed and fused with the targeted contrast-enhanced MR imaging sequences. Morphologic evaluation of the primary tumor site, related CNs, and expected nerve interconnection regions was done in conventional MR imaging sequences then correlated with the FDG uptake and the maximum standardized uptake value in PET-MR images.

IMAGING FINDINGS

As a practical approach, the imaging findings are classified as follows.

Primary Signs

Primary signs are related to direct invasion of the nerve by the tumor cells, manifested as (1) thickening, nodularity, or enlargement of the nerve with complete enhancement, which occurs because of disruption of the blood-nerve barrier (**Fig. 4**).[23] (2) Nerve infiltration can be discontinuous in imaging, referred to as skipped metastasis. Although it is continuous on the histopathologic level, this could be explained by the variability of the tumor load along the course

of the nerve. For that reason, scrutinizing the whole nerve course is essential to avoid underdiagnosis of the disease extension (**Fig. 5**). (3) Obliteration of the specific pad of fat around the nerves attributed to tumor growth and surrounding inflammatory changes (see **Fig. 2**). (4) Enlargement or possible erosions of the neural foramina and bony canals. (5) Cavernous sinus infiltration with the bulge of its lateral wall and accentuated enhancement (see **Fig. 1B**). Signal changes in the conventional noncontrast sequences are also noted. Obliteration of the fluid signal and enhancement at the Meckel cave are signs of gasserian ganglion infiltration (**Fig. 6A, B**). (6) Enhancement of the dura related to the involved nerve, thickening, and enhancement of the cisternal and fascicular course of the nerve are all signs of central tumor infiltration (see **Fig. 1C**). (7) Diffusion restriction in the morphologically abnormal nerve (**Fig. 6C**).[21] (8) The linear abnormal FDG uptake in the head and neck region, corresponding with CNs or their branches, should raise suspicion for PNTS, especially with morphologically abnormal nerve (**Fig. 6D, E**). In the case of discordant morphologic-metabolic data, the increased PET uptake is more significant.[24]

Secondary Signs

1. Muscular denervation: denervation changes of the related muscles, commonly the mastication muscles secondary to V3 infiltration (see **Fig. 4A, B**), muscles of the facial expression secondary to facial nerve invasion, and tongue sequelae of hypoglossal nerve affection. The denervation changes of the muscles pass 3 pathologic stages with corresponding MR imaging features: first, the acute stage during the first month, during which the muscle is

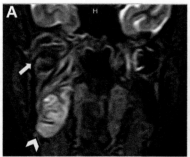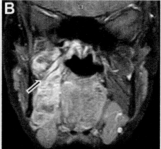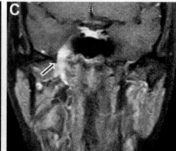

Fig. 4. Direct and indirect signs of PNTS along V3 in primary maxillary SCC. (*A*) Coronal T2WI with fat suppression shows the denervation changes of the pterygoid muscles showing edema (*white arrow*) and postcontrast enhancement as indirect signs of V3 disorder. Note the regional malignant lymph node (*arrowhead*). (*B, C*) Coronal CET1WI shows direct visualization of the infiltrated V3 in its masticator space course and continuous up to the foramen ovale and gasserian ganglion (*black arrows*).

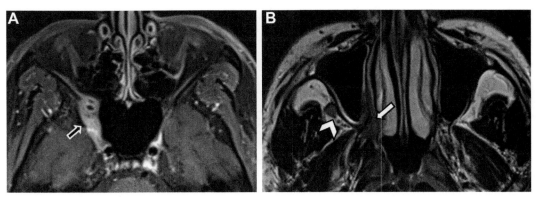

Fig. 5. Continuous and skipped PNTS infiltration along V2 in primary palatal mucoepidermoid carcinoma. (A) Axial CET1WI shows an infiltrated right V2 extending cordlike to the foramen rotundum (*black arrow*). (B) Axial T2WI shows a skipped retroantral nodular lesion (*arrowhead*). Note infiltrated sphenopalatine nerve at the corresponding foramen (*white arrow*).

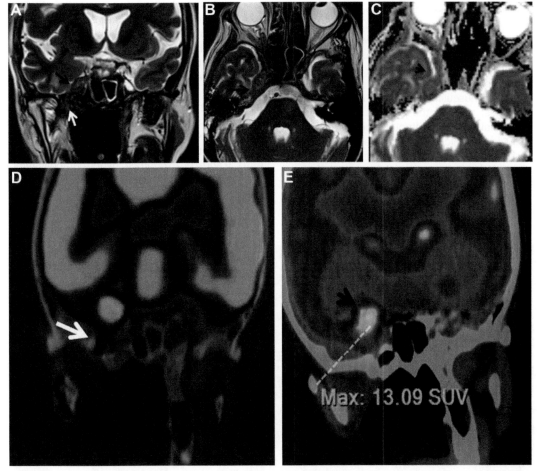

Fig. 6. Functional imaging in a treated primary maxillary SCC, presented with tumor recurrence and PNTS along trigeminal nerve branches. (A) Coronal T2WI shows infiltration of V3 passing through the foramen ovale (*white arrow*) retrograde extension to the Meckel cave and the trigeminal ganglion (*solid black arrow*). (B) Axial T2WI reveals an antegrade PNTS along V1 toward the orbital apex (*dashed arrow*). (C) ADC map reveals diffusion restriction of the infiltrated nerves. (D, E) Coronal PET-CT shows increased FDG uptake in the foramen ovale (*white arrow*) and Meckel cave (*black arrow*) in the recurrent viable tumor.

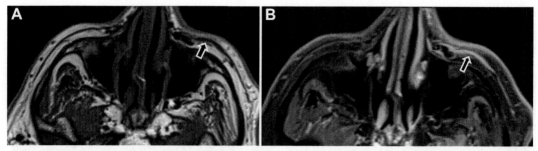

Fig. 7. An abnormal SMAS as an indirect sign of PNTS in primary parotid ACC with PNTS along the facial nerve branches. (*A*) Axial noncontrast and (*B*) postcontrast T1WI show thickening and abnormal enhancement of the SMAS (*arrows*) contrasting the normal contralateral side.

enlarged with edematous T2 signal and accentuated postcontrast enhancement. Second, the subacute denervation changes, which persist up to 20 months and in which the muscle shows the standard size, with still detected T2 hyperintensity and accentuated postcontrast enhancement (however, more fatty deposition leads to T1 hyperintensity as well). Third, the last denervation changes are the chronic stage, in which there is muscle atrophy with more fatty infiltration.[13]

2. Superior muscular aponeurotic system (SMAS) changes: most of the peripheral branches of the facial nerve pass through the SMAS, which explains the thickening and/or enhancement of this system when the peripheral nerves are loaded with tumor cells, giving secondary signs to the radiologist (**Fig. 7**).[25]

Postoperative Imaging Appearance

Postoperative evaluation for treated HNC is usually challenging secondary to the big dilemma of posttreatment changes versus residual or recurrent disease. One of the expected findings following surgery for PNTS is an enhancing nodule at the site of the resected nerve, termed a stump neuroma, which occurs secondary to disorganized nerve growth at the surgical site. Follow-up is important because stability of this nodule is reassuring (**Fig. 8**), whereas any increase in size suggests progressive tumor spread.[26] The hybrid imaging is useful in the evaluation of tumor response to treatment, and decreased FDG uptake corresponds to a diminished viable tumor (**Figs. 9** and **10**). In contrast, hypermetabolic tumor cells or increased uptake correlate with the

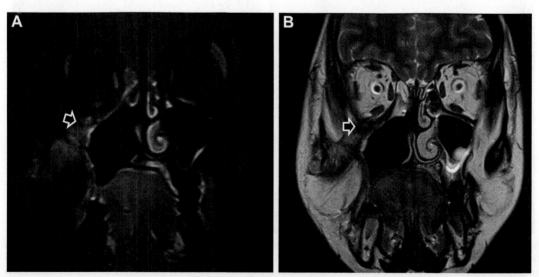

Fig. 8. Inferior orbital nerve stump neuroma after maxillectomy for maxillary osteosarcoma. (*A*) Coronal CET1WI and (*B*) T2WI show nodular thickening and enhancement of the right inferior orbital nerve (*arrows*). Stability in the follow-up was reassuring for postsurgical neuroma.

presence of viable tumor tissue (see **Figs. 6**D, E and **10A**).

IMAGING PITFALLS AND DIFFERENTIAL DIAGNOSIS

The full-thickness pathologic enhancement of the nerve should be differentiated from the peripheral enhancement that may be seen in normal nerves (target sign) and attributed to enhancement in the perineural venous plexus. Crescent-shaped enhancement at the caudal aspect of the Meckel cave related to the gasserian ganglion is a normal finding and should be differentiated from the PNTS, which is usually more globular.[27,28]

Normal anatomic variation of the size of the venous structures is seen along the body. Of particular importance is a discrepancy of the pterygoid venous plexus that results in asymmetric enhancement of the infratemporal fossa and parapharyngeal fat space, mimicking PNTS along the auriculotemporal nerve. Correlation with T2WI differentiates between infiltrated nerve and vascular signal void.[29]

Inadequate fat suppression in postcontrast fat-suppressed sequences, which usually occur at air-bone interface regions, in addition to dental

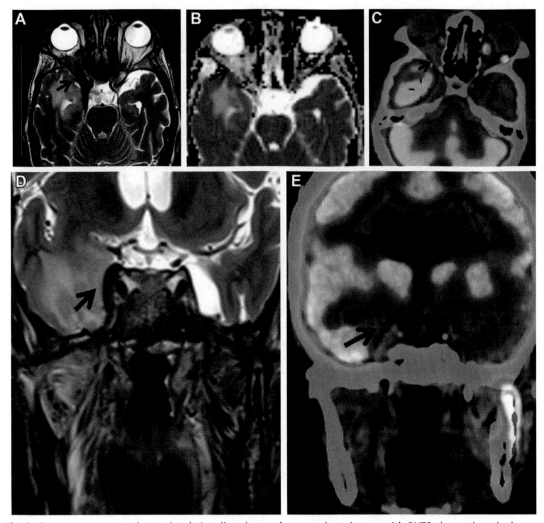

Fig. 9. Treatment response in previously irradiated nasopharyngeal carcinoma with PNTS along trigeminal nerve branches. (*A*) Axial T2WI shows orbital apex mass secondary to PNTS along V1. (*B*) ADC map reveals no diffusion restriction. (*C*) Axial PET-CT displays a metabolically inactive mass with no FDG uptake. (*D*) Coronal T2WI shows tumor spread to the lateral wall of the cavernous sinus (*arrows*) displaying a low T2 signal suggestive of posttreatment fibrosis matching the lack of FDG uptake in coronal PET-CT (*E*). Note the right temporal lobe postirradiation injury (*C*) and left mandible osteoradionecrosis (*E*) complicating previous irradiation.

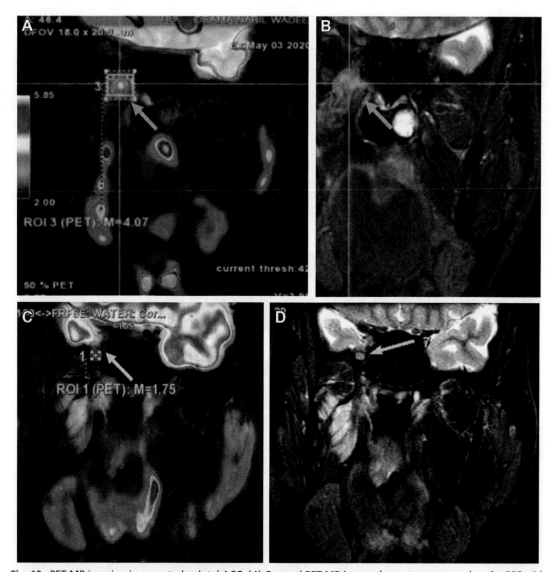

Fig. 10. PET-MR imaging in operated palatal ACC. (*A*) Coronal PET-MR image shows tumor spread to the PPF with increased FDG uptake (*orange arrow*). (*B*) Coronal T2 fat suppression reveals an infiltrated PPF with nodular thickening and abnormal signal (*orange arrow*). (*C*) Coronal PET-MR image at the level of V2 displays posttreatment neuritis with low FDG uptake (*yellow arrow*). (*D*) Coronal T2 fat suppression shows enlarged V2 at foramen rotundum with increase T2 signal (*yellow arrow*).

filling artifacts giving false impressions of postcontrast enhancement may lead to misinterpretation of PNTS so correlation with other sequences is recommended.

Postirradiation neuritis is encountered with accentuated nerve enhancement in the radiation port displaying stability or even regression in further follow-up.

The peripheral course of the nerve (zone1) being affected could be related to infectious or inflammatory processes, mostly from sinonasal, orbit, or skull base lesions, where the primary source of the disease is well detected (**Figs. 11** and **12**). Another neoplastic process of zone 1 is usually caused by benign tumor of the nerve sheath, such as neurofibroma and schwannoma (**Fig. 13**), although the latter is more often encountered in zone 2 because it arises from the junction between glial and Schwann cells. Zone 2 infiltration is usually manifested by cavernous sinus symptoms, affecting the sixth and third CNs; however, in PNTS, the predominant symptoms affect the fifth CN. Cavernous sinus infiltration could be attributed to multiple

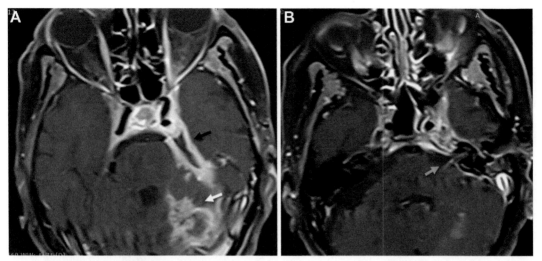

Fig. 11. Petrous apicitis and facial neuritis. (*A, B*) Axial CET1WI show petrous apex inflammatory process with abnormal enhancement extending to the Meckel cave and cavernous sinus associated with meningeal enhancement (*black arrows*), associated facial neuritis with linear enhancement (*gray arrow*), and left cerebellar hemisphere infarction with gyriform enhancement (*white arrow*).

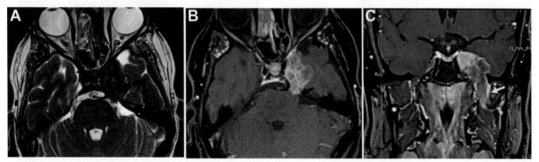

Fig. 12. Perineural spread along CN V and V3 of aspergillosis. (*A*) Axial T2WI shows fungus spread to the Meckel cave and gasserian ganglion with characteristic low T2 signal (*black arrow*). (*B*) Axial CET1WI shows enhancement of the fungal infiltration extending to the trigeminal nerve trunk (*black arrow*). (*C*) Coronal CET1W shows perineural fungal spread along V3 through the foramen ovale (*white arrow*).

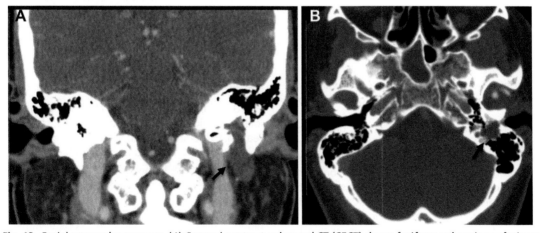

Fig. 13. Facial nerve schwannoma. (*A*) Coronal contrast-enhanced CT (CECT) shows fusiform enhancing soft tissue mass along the descending mastoid segment of the facial nerve passing the stylomastoid foramen to the parotid gland (*arrow*). (*B*) Axial CECT shows smooth widening of the facial nerve canal (*arrow*).

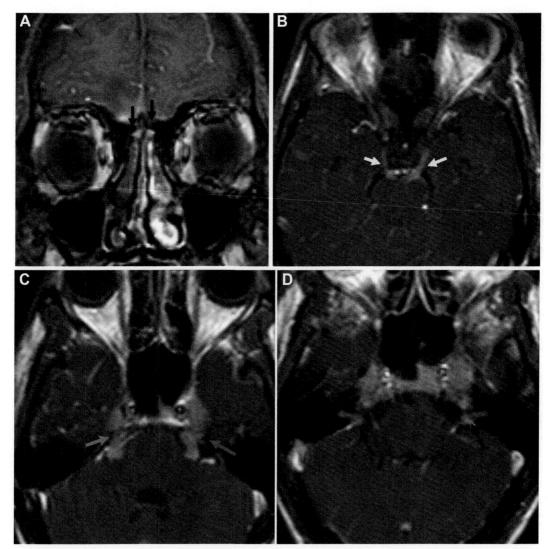

Fig. 14. Non-Hodgkin lymphoma with leptomeningeal spread. (*A*) Coronal CET1WI shows infiltration of the olfactory nerves (*black arrows*). (*B–D*) Axial CET1WI shows infiltration of the oculomotor nerves (*white arrows*), trigeminal nerves (*gray arrows*), facial and vestibulocochlear nerves (*dashed arrows*). The infiltrated nerves are thickened and enhancing with contrast.

disorders, such as meningioma, schwannoma, inflammatory pseudotumor, and granulomatous disease.

Other causes of disruption of the blood-brain barrier, such as ischemia, inflammation, or demyelination, can cause central nerve (zone3) enhancement. Isolated zone 3 infiltration is not an expected pattern of PNTS in this situation; granulomatous disease such as sarcoidosis, viral neuritis, leptomeningeal carcinomatosis, and extracerebral lymphoma (**Fig. 14**) are within the diagnostic consideration.[13]

SUMMARY

PNTS is a distinctive feature of HNC. Different clinical scenarios could be encountered; for this reason, PNTS should be included in the diagnostic checklist. Contrast-enhanced MR imaging is the most appropriate imaging modality for detection of PNTS. CT is mainly used when MR imaging is contraindicated or could not be tolerated by the patient. Hybrid imaging is a problem-solving technique used especially in posttreatment surveillance.

CLINICS CARE POINTS

- PNTS should be considered in the diagnostic checklist, even in reporting unrelated conditions as nonspecific facial pain.
- The histological type of the tumor, and the primary site of origin plays an important role, with an increased incidence of PNTS.
- Specific anatomical site rich in neural structures as in pterygopalatine fossa, cavernous sinus, or masticator space tumors should be radiologically investigated when PNTS is considered.
- Thickening, nodularity or enlargement of the nerve with complete enhancement, obliteration of specific pad of fat around the nerves, enlargement or possible erosions of the neural foramina and bony canals, diffusion restriction in morphologically abnormal nerve and abnormal 18F-FDG uptake in the head and neck region, corresponding to CNs or their branches are primary signs for PNTS.
- Secondary signs of PNTS are muscular denervation and SMAS thickening and enhancement.

DISCLOSURE

This article received no funding or financial support. All coauthors declare that they have no conflicts of interest.

REFERENCES

1. Fowler BZ, Crocker IR, Johnstone PA. Perineural spread of cutaneous malignancy to the brain: a review of the literature and five patients treated with stereotactic radiotherapy. Cancer 2005;103:2143–53.
2. Liebig C, Ayala G, Wilks JA, et al. Perineural invasion in cancer: a review of the literature. Cancer 2009;115:3379–91.
3. Johnston M, Yu E, Kim J. Perineural invasion and spread in head and neck cancer. Expert Rev Anticancer Ther 2012;12:359–71.
4. Marchesi F, Piemonti L, Mantovani A, et al. Molecular mechanisms of perineural invasion, a forgotten pathway of dissemination and metastasis. Cytokine Growth Factor Rev 2010;21:77–82.
5. Gattenlöhner S, Stühmer T, Leich E, et al. Specific detection of CD56 (NCAM) isoforms for the identification of aggressive malignant neoplasms with progressive development. Am J Pathol 2009;174:1160–71.
6. Homrich M, Gotthard I, Wobst H, et al. Cell Adhesion Molecules and Ubiquitination-Functions and Significance. Biology 2015;5:1.
7. Chandra P, Purandare N, Shah S, et al. Common patterns of perineural spread in head-neck squamous cell carcinoma identified on fluoro-deoxyglucose positron emission tomography/computed tomography. Indian J Nucl Med 2016;31:274–9.
8. Barrett AW, Speight PM. Perineural invasion in adenoid cystic carcinoma of the salivary glands: a valid prognostic indicator? Oral Oncol 2009;45:936–40.
9. Dankbaar JW, Pameijer FA, Hendrikse J, et al. Easily detected signs of perineural tumour spread in head and neck cancer. Insights Imaging 2018;9:1089–95.
10. Abdel Razek AAK, Mukherji SK. State-of-the-Art Imaging of Salivary Gland Tumors. Neuroimaging Clin N Am 2018;28:303–17.
11. Shimamoto H, Chindasombatjaroen J, Kakimoto N, et al. Perineural spread of adenoid cystic carcinoma in the oral and maxillofacial regions: evaluation with contrast-enhanced CT and MRI. Dentomaxillofac Radiol 2012;41:143–51.
12. Paes FM, Singer AD, Checkver AN, et al. Perineural spread in head and neck malignancies: clinical significance and evaluation with 18F-FDG PET/CT. Radiographics 2013;33:1717–36.
13. Brea Álvarez B, Tuñón Gómez M. Perineural spread in head and neck tumors. Radiologia 2014;56:400–12.
14. Gandhi M, Sommerville J. The Imaging of Large Nerve Perineural Spread. J Neurol Surg B Skull Base 2016;77:113–23.
15. Tsutsumi S, Ono H, Ishii H, et al. Visualization of the vidian canal and nerve using magnetic resonance imaging. Surg Radiol Anat 2018;40:1391–6.
16. Yang HM, Won SY, Kim HJ, et al. Sihler staining study of anastomosis between the facial and trigeminal nerves in the ocular area and its clinical implications. Muscle Nerve 2013;48:545–50.
17. Badger D, Aygun N. Imaging of Perineural Spread in Head and Neck Cancer. Radiol Clin North Am 2017;55:139–49.
18. Williams LS, Mancuso AA, Mendenhall WM. Perineural spread of cutaneous squamous and basal cell carcinoma: CT and MR detection and its impact on patient management and prognosis. Int J Radiat Oncol Biol Phys 2001;49:1061–9.
19. Baulch J, Gandhi M, Sommerville J, et al. 3T MRI evaluation of large nerve perineural spread of head and neck cancers. J Med Imaging Radiat Oncol 2015;59:578–85.
20. Mazziotti S, Gaeta M, Blandino A, et al. Perineural spread in a case of sinonasal sarcoidosis: case report. AJNR Am J Neuroradiol 2001;22:1207–8.
21. Varoquaux A, Rager O, Dulguerov P, et al. Diffusion-weighted and PET/MR Imaging after Radiation

Therapy for Malignant Head and Neck Tumors. Radiographics 2015;35:1502–27.

22. Kirchner J, Schaarschmidt BM, Sauerwein W, et al. 18 F-FDG PET/MRI vs MRI in patients with recurrent adenoid cystic carcinoma. Head Neck 2019;41:170–6.

23. Maroldi R, Farina D, Borghesi A, et al. Perineural tumor spread. Neuroimaging Clin N Am 2008;18:413.

24. Antoch G, Stattaus J, Nemat AT, et al. Non-small cell lung cancer: dual-modality PET/CT in preoperative staging. Radiology 2003;229:526–33.

25. Panizza BJ. An overview of head and neck malignancy with perineural spread. J Neurol Surg B Skull Base 2016;77:81–5.

26. Sommerville J, Gandhi M. Postoperative imaging and surveillance in large nerve perineural spread. J Neurol Surg B Skull Base 2016;77:182–92.

27. Hong HS, Yi BH, Cha JG, et al. Enhancement pattern of the normal facial nerve at 3.0 T temporal MRI. Br J Radiol 2010;83:118–21.

28. Yousry I, Moriggl B, Schmid UD, et al. Trigeminal ganglion and its divisions: detailed anatomic MR imaging with contrast-enhanced 3D constructive interference in the steady-state sequences. AJNR Am J Neuroradiol 2005;26:1128–35.

29. Kirsch CFE, Schmalfuss IM. Practical Tips for MR Imaging of Perineural Tumor Spread. Magn Reson Imaging Clin N Am 2018;26:85–100.

Posttreatment Magnetic Resonance Imaging Surveillance of Head and Neck Cancers

Colin Zuchowski, MD[a,1], Jordan Kemme, MD[a,1], Ashley H. Aiken, MD[a], Kristen L. Baugnon, MD[a], Ahmed Abdel Khalek Abdel Razek, MD[b,†], Xin Wu, MD[a,*]

KEYWORDS

- Head and neck cancer • MR imaging surveillance • Sinonasal • Nasophayrnx • Orbits
- Salivary glands • Cutaneous malignancies

KEY POINTS

- Magnetic resonance (MR) offers superior soft tissue contrast, which is most useful in the surveillance of head and neck neoplasms with high propensities for intraorbital invasion, intracranial invasion, or perineural disease spread.
- Neoplasms arising from the sinonasal cavities, nasopharynx, orbits, parotid and minor salivary glands, and the skin have the highest likelihood of involving these areas, and thus benefit from MR imaging surveillance.
- High-quality pretreatment and baseline posttreatment MR imaging are helpful in distinguishing posttreatment changes and treated neoplasm from active residual or recurrent disease.
- Diffusion-weighted and perfusion-weighted imaging may increase confidence in this distinction, although their applications in the head and neck remain predominantly investigational.

INTRODUCTION

Complex multimodality treatment strategies are used to treat head and neck (HN) cancer, including surgery, radiation therapy, and/or chemotherapy.[1] Imaging plays an important role in the early detection of locoregional recurrence, persistent disease, metastases, and second primary neoplasms, which has been shown to improve therapeutic outcome.[2] Although guidelines exist for HN cancer surveillance imaging, there is no consensus on optimal modality or interval.[2] With a variety of imaging technologies available, including computed tomography (CT), magnetic resonance (MR) imaging, and PET, it has become increasingly challenging for the referring team to request the most appropriate study for posttreatment surveillance.[3]

The superior soft tissue contrast resolution inherent to MR imaging adds value to the evaluation of the orbit, skull base, intracranial, and deep face spaces, as well as the detection of perineural disease spread (PNS).[3,4] Therefore, the main HN cancer subsites surveilled by MR imaging are the sinonasal cavities, salivary glands, nasopharynx, orbits, and the skull base. In contrast, cancers of the oral cavity, oropharynx, larynx, and hypopharynx are more commonly surveilled by a combination of CT and PET imaging because

[a] Department of Radiology and Imaging Sciences, Emory University School of Medicine, 1364 Clifton Road Northeast, Suite BG20, Atlanta, GA 30322, USA; [b] Department of Diagnostic Radiology, Mansoura University, Elgomheryia Street, Mansoura 35512, Egypt
[1] Equal contribution.
[†] Deceased
[*] Corresponding author.
E-mail address: xin.wu@emory.edu

Magn Reson Imaging Clin N Am 30 (2022) 109–120
https://doi.org/10.1016/j.mric.2021.06.018
1064-9689/22/© 2021 Elsevier Inc. All rights reserved.

perineural, intracranial, and orbital involvement from these subsites is less common.[2] High-quality pretreatment and posttreatment baseline imaging is important, because anatomic distortion and evolving posttreatment changes can make it challenging for radiologists to distinguish treatment-induced changes from recurrent disease or complication.[1,3] This article clarifies the rationale for HN cancer surveillance by MR imaging; discusses recommended surveillance protocoling; and reviews treatment approaches, appearance of common posttreatment changes, and pearls for identifying disease recurrence in a subsite-based approach.

SURVEILLANCE INTERVAL AND PROTOCOLING
Surveillance Interval

For neoplasms surveilled by MR imaging, a baseline pretreatment scan helps guide the interpretation of posttreatment imaging, because recurrent neoplasm frequently mimics imaging characteristics of the original disease.[5] Aside from immediate postoperative imaging performed to evaluate for residual disease within the first 6 months, there is no consensus for an appropriate interval for continued imaging surveillance in HN cancer beyond 6 months in asymptomatic patients. The Neck Imaging Reporting and Data System (NI-RADS) has been developed by the American College of Radiology (ACR) to standardize the approach, reporting, and management recommendations of HN cancer surveillance imaging[6] and has shown high reproducibility.[7] Per NI-RADS, standard surveillance imaging for HN squamous cell carcinoma (SCCa) includes baseline imaging 8 to 12 weeks after completion of definitive therapy with follow-up imaging every 6 months for 2 years from the baseline scan.[6]

Magnetic Resonance Imaging Strength and Basic Protocoling

For HN MR imaging, a minimum field strength of 1.5 or 3 T (T) is required. 3-T magnets provide better contrast resolution, although are more prone to susceptibility artifacts, which can limit evaluation of soft tissue/bone/air interfaces in the HN.[8] A head or neck coil may be used depending on the anatomic location of the primary malignancy, and a combination HN coil allows evaluation of cervical lymphadenopathy.[9]

Posttreatment surveillance imaging benefits from a small field of view (FOV) of 18 to 19 cm in multiple planes tailored to the primary malignancy site, with additional coverage of anatomy from the anterior skull base to the thoracic inlet depending on the need for evaluation of lymph nodes. A slice thickness of 2.5 to 5 mm is preferred, except in cases of isotropic volumetric imaging. A conventional anatomic workhorse protocol in the HN include precontrast T1-weighted (T1W), T2-weighted (T2W) with fat suppression (FS), and postcontrast T1W FS (T1FS) sequences in axial and coronal planes. Precontrast T1W sequences should be performed without FS for improved delineation between normal T1-hyperintense fat and neoplasm, which is typically T1 isointense to hypointense. T2W sequences should be performed with FS to increase conspicuity of T2-hyperintense pathologic processes. Postcontrast T1W sequences should be performed with FS to maximize conspicuity of enhancement.[8,10] At the skull base, dedicated precontrast T1 and postcontrast FS volumetric imaging with multiplanar reconstructions may add value in the evaluation of marrow invasion and PNS, especially near cisternal structures and neuroforamina.[11]

Fat-suppression Techniques

FS techniques include spectral or frequency-selective FS; inversion recovery sequences, including short tau inversion recovery (STIR) and turbo inversion recovery magnitude (TIRM), chemical shift-based Dixon methods, and hybrid techniques. STIR/TIRM imaging is limited to noncontrast acquisitions because contrast T1 shortening nulls signal intensity. Dixon methods use simultaneously acquired in-phase and opposed-phase images to produce pure fat and water images,[12] and has shown superior uniformity of FS compared with frequency-selective and inversion recovery techniques in the HN.[13,14]

Diffusion and Perfusion Imaging

Diffusion-weighted imaging (DWI) is routinely used to increase sensitivity for detection of recurrence and nodal metastasis and to differentiate posttherapeutic radiation changes and residual or recurrent disease.[15] At present, most practices use qualitative DWI sequences for clinical applications, although quantitative DWI has shown promise in the evaluation of HN cancers in research.[10,16–18]

Perfusion-weighted MR imaging providing qualitative and/or quantitative analysis of blood delivery to tissues also remains in the research realm. Dynamic contrast enhancement (DCE) is more commonly used than dynamic susceptibility contrast techniques because of the challenges of field inhomogeneity and susceptibility artifact.[8] When used alongside conventional MR imaging, DCE may aid in local recurrence detection in the surgical bed.[9] DCE also shows promise in differentiating enhancing posttreatment change from local recurrence[19] and differentiating benign from malignant salivary gland neoplasms.[20] Arterial spin labeling (ASL), a perfusion technique that requires no administration of contrast, remains predominantly investigational in its HN applications but has shown promise in staging and distinguishing recurrent HN cancer from postradiation changes.[21,22]

magnetic Resonance Imaging Nodal Screening

Regional nodal metastasis is considered the most important prognostic indication in patients with HN SCCa, thus the FOV of T2 FS and T1 postcontrast FS imaging should be increased to cover the neck if there is any suspicion of cervical lymphadenopathy.[23] DWI has been shown to improve detection of small metastatic lymph nodes (4–9 mm) using apparent diffusion coefficient (ADC) values, although this requires quantitative analysis because most normal nodes also show some degree of diffusion abnormality.[24]

SINONASAL MALIGNANCIES
Introduction

There are more than 70 subtypes of sinonasal malignancies, which are broadly subclassified into epithelial or nonepithelial lesions.[25] Epithelial neoplasms include SCCa, adenocarcinoma, and sinonasal undifferentiated carcinoma (SNUC).[26] Nonepithelial malignancies in the sinonasal cavities include sarcoma, lymphoma, and melanoma.[27] Most sinonasal malignancies are diagnosed in advanced stages. Therefore, orbital and intracranial invasion at time of presentation or disease recurrence can directly affect staging and prognosis. The goal of pretreatment imaging is to delineate lesion extent facilitating biopsy and/or surgical resection, and provide a basis for comparison for posttreatment imaging.

Treatment Approach and Posttreatment Changes

The most common treatment approach for sinonasal cancer is complete surgical resection with postoperative radiotherapy.[28] Surgical approaches range from minimally invasive endoscopy to traditional open resections.[29] Open resections require complex regional or free flap reconstructions posing challenges to postoperative image interpretation. Graft material used for anterior skull base resection and/or granulation tissue may mimic disease recurrence in the postoperative setting. Postradiation changes from techniques such as intensity-modulated radiation therapy and proton beam therapy may also confound posttreatment imaging.[28] Inflammatory changes and denervation are expected after surgery and radiation therapy, and these findings may persist for as long as 30 months, complicating posttreatment evaluation.[30]

Magnetic Resonance Imaging Surveillance Pearls

MR imaging is critical for detection of recurrent or progressive disease, which are often asymptomatic and can involve areas not accessible by clinical inspection.[4] Baseline postoperative imaging should be obtained 3 months after the end of definitive treatment.[3] After this point, MR imaging follow-up strategies are variable, but can be performed every 3 to 6 months for the first 2 years, with yearly screening afterward for 5 years for SCCa or SNUC, or 10 years in the case of adenocarcinoma.[4]

MR imaging signal characteristics of recurrent disease are variable, so attention should be focused on the surgical margins and interfaces between native and reconstructed tissue. Familiarity with the fatty appearance, T1-hypointense and T2-hypointense aponeurosis, and striated pattern of muscle in most free flaps can be helpful to define flap edges and differentiate normal postoperative changes from recurrent lesions.[4] Any soft tissue nodule along the edge of a resection or flap bed should be considered suspicious until proved otherwise, especially if it mimics the signal characteristics of pretreated neoplasm[4] (**Fig. 1**). Malignant dural invasion at time of initial treatment places patients at increased risk of dural recurrence, so attention should be paid to the intracranial compartment at time of follow-up (**Fig. 2**). DWI can increase sensitivity for recurrent disease, but susceptibility artifact can limit its power in this region.[31]

PNS presents as enlargement and abnormal enhancement of nerves adjacent to the resection site, possibly with remodeling and destruction of skull base foramina and fissures, and denervation atrophy of innervated muscles.[4] For maxillary and nasal cavity neoplasms, careful evaluation should be directed along the maxillary division of the trigeminal nerve (V2), whereas evaluation of the ophthalmic division (V1) is necessary for frontal sinus neoplasms and those with orbital invasion. PNS is expected to retain abnormal enhancement indefinitely after being fully treated with radiotherapy, so familiarity with pretreatment imaging and the radiotherapy field is necessary to evaluate for any increase in extent of PNS findings.

NASOPHARYNGEAL CARCINOMA
Introduction

Nasopharyngeal carcinoma (NPC), the most common neoplasm of the nasopharyngeal subsite, is

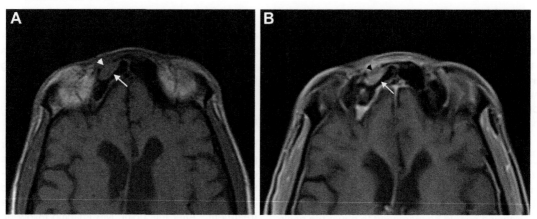

Fig. 1. A 73-year-old man with history of nasal cavity SCCa treated with radiotherapy and endoscopic surgery 2 years prior. Axial precontrast T1W (*A*) and axial postcontrast T1W (*B*) images show an enhancing lesion (*white arrow*) centered in the outer table of the right frontal sinus with aggressive osseous erosion (*black arrowhead*). Pathology confirmed recurrent sinonasal SCCa.

an epithelial carcinoma that arises from the mucosal lining, most commonly in the pharyngeal recess (fossa of Rosenmuller).[32] Primary NPC staging depends on extent of local invasion. Assessment by MR imaging is the gold standard because intracranial extension of disease, prevertebral muscle invasion, and perineural disease spread are common and suboptimally evaluated on CT.

Treatment Approach and Posttreatment Changes

Radiotherapy is the primary method of treatment of nonmetastatic NPC. However, chemotherapy may be used in several treatment scenarios.[32]

For patients with regional failure, neck dissection is the primary salvage method.[33] Treatment of metastatic NPC involves a combination of radiotherapy and/or palliative chemotherapy.[32]

Postradiation findings on MR include skin thickening, ill-defined edema and enhancement within the subcutaneous and deep face spaces, mucositis, and inflammatory changes of the paranasal sinuses. Given its proximity to the fossa of Rosenmuller, eustachian tube dysfunction, and resultant mastoid fluid opacification are common. Sialoadenitis, followed by chronic fatty atrophy, are also encountered because the salivary glands are highly sensitive to radiation. Masticator space denervation myositis can present as linear T2W signal hyperintensity and enhancement in the

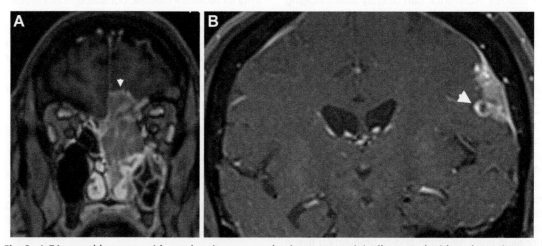

Fig. 2. A 74-year-old woman with nasal cavity neuroendocrine tumor, originally treated with endoscopic resection and chemotherapy, followed by recurrent disease treated by reresection and chemoradiation 1 year later. Coronal postcontrast T1FS image at time of presentation (*A*) shows intracranial invasion by the primary tumor (*arrowhead*). Coronal postcontrast T1FS image of the brain 1.5 years after initial treatment (*B*) shows a new dural-based enhancing mass (*arrowhead*) that shows irregular interfaces with the brain, compatible with dural recurrence.

acute setting and fatty atrophy chronically.[34] In the central skull base bones, radiotherapy causes transformation of red marrow into yellow marrow, leading to fatty marrow replacement presenting as uniform marrow T1 hyperintensity.

Magnetic Resonance Imaging Surveillance Pearls

Highly radiosensitive NPCs often decrease in size within the first 3 months following radiotherapy,[35] although residual treated tissue is expected in the early phases of imaging surveillance. Close imaging follow-up is necessary to exclude persistent viable neoplasm.[36] MR readily differentiates between mature fibrous scar (with signal hypointensity on all pulse sequences), benign nasopharyngeal mucosal thickening or mucositis (with T2 signal hyperintensity and peripheral enhancement), and recurrent neoplasm (with intermediate T2 signal intensity and solid enhancement).[37] Similarly, MR distinguishes postradiation changes from neoplasm recurrence in the deep neck spaces.[36] Despite these capabilities, imaging characteristics of viable neoplasm, treated disease, edema, or immature fibrosis can occasionally overlap.[38] Comparison with pretreatment imaging is helpful to identify new nodular soft tissue that has similar imaging characteristics to the primary neoplasm, a finding highly suspicious for recurrence.[36]

Persistent deossification and marrow signal abnormality are expected in the posttreatment setting in patients with known skull base involvement, and do not immediately indicate treatment failure. However, new or progressive marrow T1 signal hypointensity and enhancement raise suspicion for osseous neoplasm recurrence, osteoradionecrosis, or a combination of the two. MR imaging offers higher sensitivity for progressive osseous involvement, because marrow infiltration can precede cortical erosion detectable on CT, although the two modalities are complementary in delineating the extent of skull base erosion and involvement of skull base neuroforamina and vascular structures.[36]

NPC has a tendency for PNS, often involving the pterygopalatine fossa (PPF) and cranial nerve (CN) V2 branches by direct extension via the sphenopalatine foramen or the palatovaginal canal.[39] PNS may be characterized by nerve thickening and enhancement, loss of fat signal within or around the skull base foramina and the PPF, lateral bowing of the cavernous sinus, and replacement of the cerebrospinal fluid signal within the Meckel caves.[3] Nodal spread of nasopharyngeal carcinoma occurs initially to retropharyngeal or level IIB lymph nodes, necessitating close evaluation of the retropharyngeal spaces[3] (**Fig. 3**).

ORBITAL MALIGNANCIES
Introduction

MR imaging is vital for characterization of retrobulbar extent of orbital, conjunctival, and lacrimal gland malignant neoplasms, because ophthalmologic examination is limited by the fundoscopic FOV.[40] MR imaging surveillance can provide valuable information for local disease recurrence and extension into surrounding structures, PNS, and intracranial extension.

Orbital Lymphoma

The most common malignancy of the orbit, lymphoma, appears moderately hypointense on T1W and T2W MR images, with avid enhancement and low ADC values, distinguishing them from other benign orbital processes.[41] Localized disease is typically treated with radiation therapy, whereas systemic disease is treated with chemotherapy.[42] Surgery has no role in primary ocular lymphoma treatment except for biopsy.[43,44] Expected postradiation findings include edema and enhancement in the treatment site and lacrimal gland. Careful attention should be paid on follow-up imaging to evaluate for progressive orbital/bone invasion and PNS along V1.

Malignant Uveal Melanoma

Malignant uveal melanoma is the most common primary intraocular neoplasm in adults. The diagnosis can typically be made on fundoscopic examination; however cross-sectional imaging may be necessary in the case of opaque lenses or significant subretinal effusion.[41] Melanin contents cause hyperintense T1W and hypointense T2W signal abnormalities, and neoplasms often show restricted diffusion[41,45] (**Fig. 4**). Postcontrast imaging can help differentiate enhancing neoplasm from retinal detachment. Local treatment of uveal melanoma consists of globe-preserving therapies such as radiation, laser therapy, or surgical resection, or more aggressive therapies, including enucleation.[46] However, nearly 50% of patients develop metastatic disease with dismal outcomes because of lack of effective therapies.[46] New research indicates that DWI can be helpful for evaluating response to treatment, because reduction in the mean ADC values between pretreatment MR imaging and the first posttreatment MR imaging may correlate with increased risk of disease progression.[47] In patients treated with brachytherapy, it is important to evaluate the

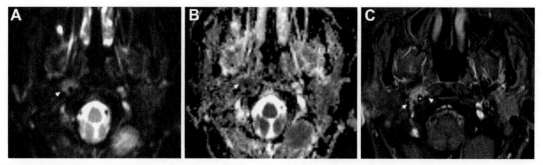

Fig. 3. A 30 woman with history of stage III, T2N2 NPC partially treated with chemoradiation in 2014 stopped prematurely secondary to poor tolerance 5 years prior. Axial DWI (*A*), ADC (*B*), and postcontrast T1FS (*C*) images show enhancing tissue with associated restricted diffusion (*arrowheads*) encasing the proximal right internal carotid artery (*asterisk*) in the retropharyngeal space, compatible with retropharyngeal nodal recurrence of nasopharyngeal carcinoma.

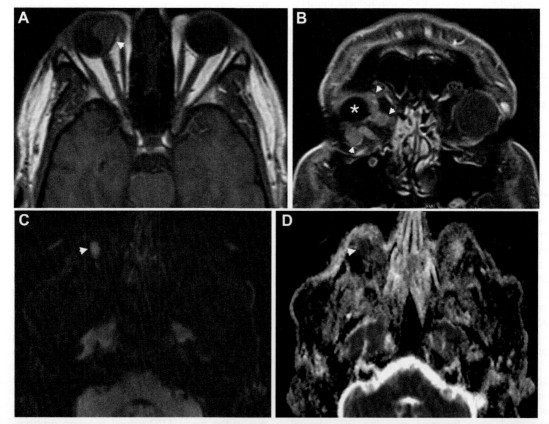

Fig. 4. A 57-year-old man with stage IV uveal melanoma of the right orbit treated with orbital exenteration. Axial precontrast T1W image from the pretreatment scan (*A*) shows a slightly hyperintense right choroidal mass (*arrowhead*). Surveillance examination 1 year later with coronal T1 postcontrast (*B*), axial DWI (*C*), and axial ADC (*D*) shows multifocal enhancing nodularity (*arrowheads*) with restricted diffusion surrounding the globe prosthesis (*white asterisk*) compatible with recurrent disease.

orbital apex and cavernous sinus for early signs of recurrence on coronal precontrast T1W images.

SALIVARY GLAND MALIGNANCIES
Introduction

MR imaging surveillance is most typically performed for treated salivary neoplasms in the parotid glands, the orbits, and the palate given their propensity for perineural spread and intraorbital and intracranial extension. Malignant parotid neoplasms may be categorized into low-grade, intermediate-grade, or high-grade categories.[48] MR imaging is important to characterize the margins of primary parotid neoplasms. Well-circumscribed margins imply benign or low-grade entities, whereas poorly marginated lesions frequently are high-grade malignancies.

Treatment Approach and Posttreatment Changes

Complete surgical excision is the primary treatment modality in the management of benign and malignant salivary gland neoplasms. Total parotidectomy and facial nerve resection are typically required in patients with extensive disease or those with facial nerve involvement.[48] Neck dissection, chemotherapy, and radiotherapy are addition treatment modalities used in some treatment scenarios.[48]

Parotidectomy changes range from partial to total resection of the parotid gland, and could include facial nerve sacrifice and/or resection of adjacent structures, including skin, mastoid, mandible, and muscles of mastication.[49] In the early posttreatment period, inflammatory/infectious changes, including enhancing scar, postoperative fluid collections, hematomas, and abscesses, easily mimic or obscure recurrence, thus treatment history and preoperative imaging are crucial for accurate interpretation. Fibrotic scar typically shows T2 hypointensity without enhancement. Reconstructive changes, including grafts or flaps, may be encountered on postoperative imaging,[50] the imaging appearance of which varies depending on the amount of muscle versus fat in the donor tissue. Over time, denervation often results in muscle volume degeneration and fatty infiltration.[51]

Magnetic Resonance Imaging Surveillance Pearls

Violation of neoplasm margins or spillage at time of original resection predisposes the patient to multifocal recurrence. Baseline imaging is typically recommended 3 months after initial therapy. Surveillance is guided by clinical suspicion for recurrence rather than standard imaging follow-up intervals. Some institutions incorporate standard imaging surveillance intervals, which vary depending on the clinical grade of the initial disorder.[50]

Recurrences generally appear expansile with intermediate T2 signal and moderate enhancement.[50] DWI improves differentiation of posttreatment change and recurrence, and shows restricted diffusion with low ADC values, compatible with hypercellularity.[52] DCE-MR imaging can differentiate recurrence from postoperative changes given different enhancement kinetics.[53]

Facial or trigeminal nerve palsies in the setting of salivary gland malignancies indicate possible PNS.[39] Classically associated with, but not limited to, adenoid cystic carcinoma, PNS may be antegrade or retrograde with contiguous or discontinuous patterns.[54] Attention should be paid to the parotid bed for areas of asymmetric linear enhancement, particularly dorsal to the mandibular ramus, for evidence of PNS along the auriculotemporal nerve, a route of communication between the facial and trigeminal nerves. Attention should also be paid to the fat plane at the stylomastoid foramen to evaluate for PNS along the facial nerve into the skull base (**Fig. 5**). Although the intraosseous segments of the facial nerve could show normal scattered enhancement (particularly within the mastoid, tympanic, and geniculate segments), asymmetry in the intensity and thickness of enhancement and any enhancement in the canalicular and cisternal segments of the nerve indicate the presence of intraosseous or intracranial PNS. The greater superficial petrosal nerve, directed anteromedially from the geniculate ganglion, is a route of potential PNS from the facial nerve to the vidian nerve.[55] The PPF, infratemporal fossa, foramen ovale, and Meckel cave should also be scrutinized to exclude trigeminal nerve involvement.[39]

Within the oral cavity, minor palatal salivary gland cancers may spread to V2 via the PPF by way of the greater and lesser palatine nerves. Once neoplasm has reached the PPF, PNS may continue through the foramen rotundum to the cavernous sinus and Meckel cave intracranially. More rarely, oral mucosal or salivary gland neoplasms of the palate and maxillary sinus may also develop PNS via palatine and superior alveolar branches, respectively.[39]

SKULL BASE MALIGNANCIES
Introduction

The skull base contains multiple foramina, which allow vessels and nerves to pass from the

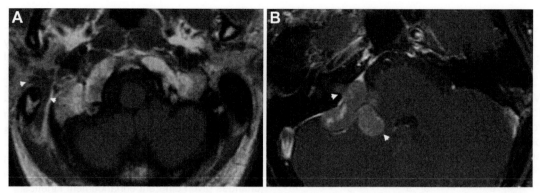

Fig. 5. A 49-year-old man with a history of parotid adenocarcinoma presents with new right facial nerve palsy. Axial precontrast T1W at the skull base (A) shows asymmetric T1-hypointense soft tissue extending toward the right stylomastoid foramen (*arrowheads*). Axial postcontrast T1FS image (B) shows nodular enhancing mass at the porus acusticus and cerebellopontine angle (*arrowheads*). Findings are compatible with PNS along extracranial and intracranial facial nerve.

intracranial cavity to the neck/face, and may form conduits for PNS and intracranial spread in patients with skull base neoplasms. In addition to carcinomas arising from the sinonasal cavities and nasopharynx, which could secondarily involve the skull base, common malignant neoplasms found at the skull base include chondrosarcomas, chordomas, and metastatic disease, which all have a predilection for the petrous apex.

The petrous temporal bone contains or is bordered by several important vascular structures and foramina, including the petrous carotid canal, the internal auditory canal, the jugular bulb, and Meckel cave.[56] On initial imaging, chondrosarcomas and chordomas show low to intermediate T1W signal and very high T2W signal, with variable

degrees of enhancement[57] (**Fig. 6**). Given the similar MR imaging findings between these neoplasms, the location of the initial mass can help differentiate the initial diagnosis. Chondrosarcomas typically arise within the petroclival junction at the petroclival synchondrosis, whereas chordomas are typically central within the clivus.[57,58] DWI can also be used to help differentiate chondrosarcomas from chordomas, because chondrosarcomas are associated with higher ADC values.[59]

Treatment Approach and Magnetic Resonance Imaging Surveillance Pearls

Careful evaluation of preoperative imaging must be performed to accurately describe neoplasm extent, including dural, neuroforaminal, and

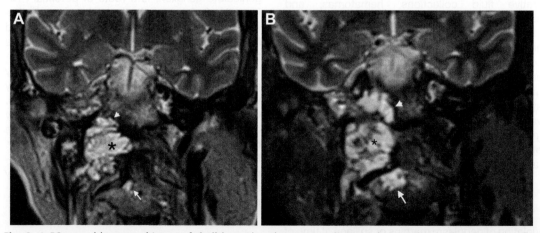

Fig. 6. A 56-year-old woman history of skull base chondrosarcoma diagnosed more than a decade prior, after resection and proton beam radiation at time of initial treatment with multiple additional recurrences and reresections. Coronal precontrast T2W at 14 years postdiagnosis (A) and 15 years postdiagnosis (B) clearly show progression of characteristically T2 hyperintense disease involving the right occiput (*white arrowhead*), lateral mass of C1 (*black asterisk*), and C2 vertebral body (*white arrow*).

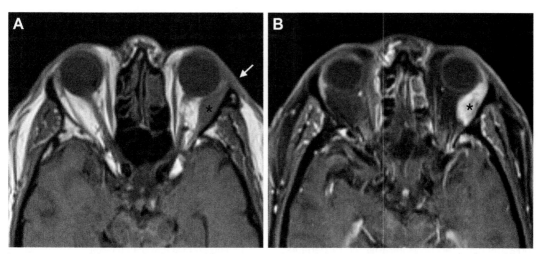

Fig. 7. A 79-year-old man with a history of SCCa resected from left temple. The patient complained of left facial pain, inability to raise left eyebrow, and numbness along left midface 6 months posttreatment. Axial precontrast T1W (*A*) shows postsurgical thickening of the left lateral periorbital skin (*arrow*) and a T1-isointense mass (*asterisk*) in the left superolateral orbit along the lateral rectus muscle, inseparable from the lacrimal gland. Axial postcontrast T1FS (*B*) image shows avid enhancement in the mass (*asterisk*), consistent with recurrent SCCa.

vascular involvement. For chondrosarcoma centered at the petroclival junction, a low subtemporal craniotomy with removal of the petrous apex and clivus provides access to extradural and intradural components.[57] For chordomas centered in the clivus, endonasal endoscopic resections are becoming the preferred method of resection. When the carotid canal is involved, subtotal resection with adjuvant radiotherapy is generally preferred. Alternatively, some investigators recommend carotid resection in the case of complete petrous carotid encasement, particularly in

low-grade malignant neoplasms.[60] Correlation with the extent of surgical resection, as well as baseline postoperative imaging, helps differentiate residual treated neoplasm from viable recurrent disease, which would be expected to show growth across multiple studies (see **Fig. 6**).

CUTANEOUS MALIGNANCIES

Most nonmelanoma skin cancers are managed clinically. However, deeply invasive neoplasms and those showing high-risk and aggressive

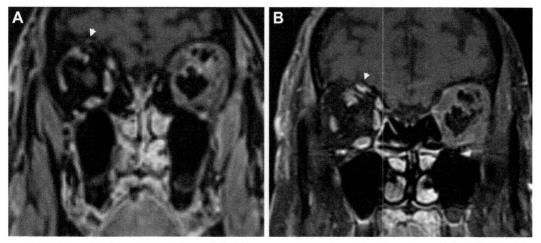

Fig. 8. A 79-year-old man with a history of facial cutaneous SCCa invading left orbit treated with left orbital exenteration and radiotherapy, now with new skin nodule on the right brow. Coronal postcontrast T1FS images from 1.5 years posttreatment (*A*) and 2 years posttreatment (*B*) show new abnormal thickening and enhancement along the right CN V1 division (*arrowhead*) extending from the supraorbital notch to the right cavernous sinus, highly concerning for contralateral PNS.

features on biopsy necessitate imaging for optimal management.[61] Aggressive skin cancers near the orbit may invade by direct extension into the orbital contents or by retrograde perineural spread.[62] Painful, fixed neoplasms involving the orbital rim or medial canthus, a displaced globe, or reduced extraocular muscle range of motion should prompt imaging to assess for orbital invasion[61](Fig. 7). Although CT may provide evaluation of the orbital bony margins, MR imaging is superior at characterizing soft tissue invasion and PNS along the superior orbital wall and the supraorbital notch, the expected location of V1[63] (Fig. 8).

Depending on the location of the primary skin cancer, V2, V3, and the facial nerve may be involved by PNS, especially because occult scalp neoplasms can present as intraparotid or periauricular nodal metastases because of their nodal drainage patterns. As discussed earlier, spread between the facial and trigeminal nerves via communicating nerves may also occur.[64] Thus, careful evaluation for direct and indirect signs of PNS along the expected paths of these nerves is necessary.[65]

SUMMARY

Given its superior soft tissue contrast resolution, MR imaging is best used in the evaluation of recurrent HN cancers, which may involve the orbits, intracranial structures, the skull base, and CNs. Cancers arising from the sinonasal cavities, nasopharynx, orbits, parotid and minor salivary glands, and the skin thus benefit the most from MR imaging surveillance. High-quality pretreatment and baseline posttreatment MR imaging help differentiate posttreatment changes from active residual or recurrent disease on follow-up surveillance. Advanced MR imaging techniques such as DWI and perfusion-weighted imaging have also shown promise in increasing specificity in HN cancer surveillance.

REFERENCES

1. Saito N, Nadgir RN, Nakahira M, et al. Posttreatment CT and MR imaging in head and neck cancer: what the radiologist needs to know. Radiographics 2012; 32(5):1261–82 [discussion: 1282–4].
2. De Felice F, Musio D, Tombolini V. Follow-up in head and neck cancer: a management dilemma. Adv Otolaryngol 2014;2015:1–4.
3. Seeburg DP, Baer AH, Aygun N. Imaging of patients with head and neck cancer: from staging to surveillance. Oral Maxillofacial Surg Clin N Am 2018;30(4): 121 33.
4. Farina D, Borghesi A, Botturi E, et al. Treatment monitoring of paranasal sinus tumors by magnetic resonance imaging. Cancer Imaging 2010;10: 183–93.
5. Glastonbury CM. Head and Neck Squamous Cell Cancer: Approach to Staging and Surveillance. In: Hodler J, Kubik-Huch RA, von Schulthess GK, eds Diseases of the Brain, Head and Neck, Spine 2020-2023: Diagnostic Imaging. Cham (CH): Springer; 2020. p.215-222.
6. Aiken AH, Rath TJ, Anzai Y, et al. ACR Neck Imaging Reporting and Data Systems (NI-RADS): A White Paper of the ACR NI-RADS Committee. J Am Coll Radiol 2018;15(8):1097–108.
7. Abdelaziz TT, Abdel Razk AAK, Ashour MMM, et al. Interreader reproducibility of the Neck Imaging Reporting and Data system (NI-RADS) lexicon for the detection of residual/recurrent disease in treated head and neck squamous cell carcinoma (HNSCC). Cancer Imaging 2020;20(1):61.
8. Junn JC, Soderlund KA, Glastonbury CM. Imaging of Head and Neck Cancer With CT, MRI, and US. Semin Nucl Med 2020;51(1):3–12.
9. Lee JY, Cheng KL, Lee JH, et al. Detection of local recurrence in patients with head and neck squamous cell carcinoma using voxel-based color maps of initial and final area under the curve values derived from DCE-MRI. AJNR Am J Neuroradiol 2019;40(8):1392–401.
10. Tshering Vogel DW, Thoeny HC. Cross-sectional imaging in cancers of the head and neck: how we review and report. Cancer Imaging 2016;16(1):20.
11. Hudgins PA, Baugnon KL. Head and Neck: Skull Base Imaging. Neurosurgery 2018;82(3):255–67.
12. Ma J. Dixon techniques for water and fat imaging. J Magn Reson Imaging 2008;28(3):543–58.
13. Gaddikeri S, Mossa-Basha M, Andre JB, et al. Optimal Fat Suppression in Head and Neck MRI: Comparison of Multipoint Dixon with 2 Different Fat-Suppression Techniques, Spectral Presaturation and Inversion Recovery, and STIR. AJNR Am J Neuroradiol 2018;39(2):362–8.
14. Wendl CM, Eiglsperger J, Dendl LM, et al. Fat suppression in magnetic resonance imaging of the head and neck region: is the two-point DIXON technique superior to spectral fat suppression? Br J Radiol 2018;91(1085):20170078.
15. Thoeny HC, De Keyzer F, King AD. Diffusion-weighted MR imaging in the head and neck. Radiology 2012;263(1):19–32.
16. Abdel Razek AA, Gaballa G, Ashamalla G, et al. Dynamic susceptibility contrast perfusion-weighted magnetic resonance imaging and diffusion-weighted magnetic resonance imaging in differentiating recurrent head and neck cancer from postradiation changes. J Comput Assist Tomogr 2015; 39(6):849–54.

17. Abdel Razek AA, Kandeel AY, Soliman N, et al. Role of diffusion-weighted echo-planar MR imaging in differentiation of residual or recurrent head and neck tumors and posttreatment changes. AJNR Am J Neuroradiol 2007;28(6):1146–52.

18. Abdel Razek AA, Kamal E. Nasopharyngeal carcinoma: correlation of apparent diffusion coefficient value with prognostic parameters. Radiol Med 2013;118(4):534–9.

19. Choi YJ, Lee JH, Sung YS, et al. Value of Dynamic Contrast-Enhanced MRI to Detect Local Tumor Recurrence in Primary Head and Neck Cancer Patients. Medicine (Baltimore) 2016;95(19):e3698.

20. Lam PD, Kuribayashi A, Imaizumi A, et al. Differentiating benign and malignant salivary gland tumours: diagnostic criteria and the accuracy of dynamic contrast-enhanced MRI with high temporal resolution. Br J Radiol 2015;88(1049):20140685.

21. Abdel Razek AAK, Nada N. Arterial spin labeling perfusion-weighted MR imaging: correlation of tumor blood flow with pathological degree of tumor differentiation, clinical stage and nodal metastasis of head and neck squamous cell carcinoma. Eur Arch Otorhinolaryngol 2018;275(5):1301–7.

22. Abdel Razek AAK. Arterial spin labelling and diffusion-weighted magnetic resonance imaging in differentiation of recurrent head and neck cancer from post-radiation changes. J Laryngol Otol 2018; 132(10):923–8.

23. Sadick M, Schoenberg SO, Hoermann K, et al. Current oncologic concepts and emerging techniques for imaging of head and neck squamous cell cancer. GMS Curr Top Otorhinolaryngol Head Neck Surg 2012;11:Doc08.

24. Vandecaveye V, De Keyzer F, Vander Poorten V, et al. Head and neck squamous cell carcinoma: value of diffusion-weighted MR imaging for nodal staging. Radiology 2009;251(1):134–46.

25. Desai DD, Brandon BM, Perkins EL, et al. Staging of Sinonasal and Ventral Skull Base Malignancies. Otolaryngol Clin North Am 2017;50(2):257–71.

26. Virk JS, Chan J, Dimitrov L, et al. Sinonasal cancer: an overview of the emerging subtypes. J Laryngol Otol 2020;134(3):191–6.

27. Dean KE, Shatzkes D, Phillips CD. Imaging Review of New and Emerging Sinonasal Tumors and Tumor-Like Entities from the Fourth Edition of the World Health Organization Classification of Head and Neck Tumors. AJNR Am J Neuroradiol 2019; 40(4):584–90.

28. Llorente JL, Lopez F, Suarez C, et al. Sinonasal carcinoma: clinical, pathological, genetic and therapeutic advances. Nat Rev Clin Oncol 2014;11(8):460–72.

29. Snyderman CH, Carrau RL, Kassam AB, et al. Endoscopic skull base surgery: principles of endonasal oncologic surgery. J Surg Oncol 2008;97(8): 658–64.

30. Raviv J, Downing L, Le QT, et al. Radiographic assessment of the sinuses in patients treated for nasopharyngeal carcinoma. Am J Rhinol 2008; 22(1):64–7.

31. Ailianou A, Mundada P, De Perrot T, et al. MRI with DWI for the Detection of Posttreatment Head and Neck Squamous Cell Carcinoma: Why Morphologic MRI Criteria Matter. AJNR Am J Neuroradiol 2018; 39(4):748–55.

32. Chen YP, Chan ATC, Le QT, et al. Nasopharyngeal carcinoma. Lancet 2019;394(10192):64–80.

33. Liu YP, Li H, You R, et al. Surgery for isolated regional failure in nasopharyngeal carcinoma after radiation: Selective or comprehensive neck dissection. Laryngoscope 2019;129(2):387–95.

34. Becker M, Schroth G, Zbären P, et al. Long-term changes induced by high-dose irradiation of the head and neck region: imaging findings. Radiographics 1997;17(1):5–26.

35. Sham JS, Wei WI, Kwan WH, et al. Nasopharyngeal carcinoma. Pattern of tumor regression after radiotherapy. Cancer 1990;65(2):216–20.

36. Ng SH, Liu HM, Ko SF, et al. Posttreatment imaging of the nasopharynx. Eur J Radiol 2002;44(2):82–95.

37. Ng SH, Wan YL, Ko SF, et al. MRI of nasopharyngeal carcinoma with emphasis on relationship to radiotherapy. J Magn Reson Imaging 1998;8(2):327–36.

38. Chong VF, Fan YF. Detection of recurrent nasopharyngeal carcinoma: MR imaging versus CT. Radiology 1997;202(2):463–70.

39. Badger D, Aygun N. Imaging of Perineural Spread in Head and Neck Cancer. Radiol Clin North Am 2017; 55(1):139–49.

40. Tailor TD, Gupta D, Dalley RW, et al. Orbital neoplasms in adults: clinical, radiologic, and pathologic review. Radiographics 2013;33(6):1739–58.

41. Purohit BS, Vargas MI, Ailianou A, et al. Orbital tumours and tumour-like lesions: exploring the armamentarium of multiparametric imaging. Insights Imaging 2016;7(1):43–68.

42. Eckardt AM, Lemound J, Rana M, et al. Orbital lymphoma: diagnostic approach and treatment outcome. World J Surg Oncol 2013;11:73.

43. Esik O, Ikeda H, Mukai K, et al. A retrospective analysis of different modalities for treatment of primary orbital non-Hodgkin's lymphomas. Radiother Oncol 1996;38(1):13–8.

44. Yadav BS, Sharma SC. Orbital lymphoma: role of radiation. Indian J Ophthalmol 2009;57(2):91–7.

45. Erb-Eigner K, Willerding G, Taupitz M, et al. Diffusion-weighted imaging of ocular melanoma. Invest Radiol 2013;48(10):702–7.

46. Yang J, Manson DK, Marr BP, et al. Treatment of uveal melanoma: where are we now? Ther Adv Med Oncol 2018;10. 1758834018757175.

47. Bitencourt F, Bitencourt AGV, Chojniak MMM, et al. Response Evaluation of Choroidal Melanoma After

Brachytherapy Using Diffusion-Weighted Magnetic Resonance Imaging (DW-MRI): Preliminary Findings. Front Oncol 2020;10:825.

48. Lewis AG, Tong T, Maghami E. Diagnosis and Management of Malignant Salivary Gland Tumors of the Parotid Gland. Otolaryngol Clin North Am 2016; 49(2):343–80.

49. Quer M, Guntinas-Lichius O, Marchal F, et al. Classification of parotidectomies: a proposal of the European Salivary Gland Society. Eur Arch Oto-Rhino-Laryngology 2016;273(10):3307–12.

50. Abdel Razek AAK, Mukherji SK. Imaging of post-treatment salivary gland tumors. Neuroimaging Clin N Am 2018;28(2):199–208.

51. Syed F, Spector ME, Cornelius R, et al. Head and neck reconstructive surgery: what the radiologist needs to know. Eur Radiol 2016;26(10):3345–52.

52. Razek AA, Megahed AS, Denewer A, et al. Role of diffusion-weighted magnetic resonance imaging in differentiation between the viable and necrotic parts of head and neck tumors. Acta Radiol 2008;49(3): 364–70.

53. Samir S, El-Adalany MA, Hamed EE. Value of dynamic contrast enhanced magnetic resonance imaging in the differentiation between post-treatment changes and recurrent salivary gland tumors. Egypt J Radiol Nucl Med 2016;47(2):477–86.

54. Panizza B, Warren TA, Solares CA, et al. Histopathological features of clinical perineural invasion of cutaneous squamous cell carcinoma of the head and neck and the potential implications for treatment. Head Neck 2014;36(11):1611–8.

55. Sommerville J, Gandhi M. Postoperative Imaging and Surveillance in Large Nerve Perineural Spread. J Neurol Surg B Skull Base 2016;77(2):182–92.

56. Schmalfuss IM. Petrous apex. Neuroimaging Clin N Am 2009;19(3):367–91.

57. Oghalai JS, Buxbaum JL, Jackler RK, et al. Skull base chondrosarcoma originating from the petroclival junction. Otol Neurotol 2005;26(5):1052–60.

58. Brown RV, Sage MR, Brophy BP. CT and MR findings in patients with chordomas of the petrous apex. AJNR Am J Neuroradiol 1990;11(1):121–4.

59. Yeom KW, Lober RM, Mobley BC, et al. Diffusion-weighted MRI: distinction of skull base chordoma from chondrosarcoma. AJNR Am J Neuroradiol 2013;34(5):1056–61. S1051.

60. Tzortzidis F, Elahi F, Wright DC, et al. Patient outcome at long-term follow-up after aggressive microsurgical resection of cranial base chondrosarcomas. Neurosurgery 2006;58(6):1090–8 [discussion: 1090–8].

61. Humphreys TR, Shah K, Wysong A, et al. The role of imaging in the management of patients with nonmelanoma skin cancer: When is imaging necessary? J Am Acad Dermatol 2017;76(4):591–607.

62. Veness MJ, Biankin S. Perineural spread leading to orbital invasion from skin cancer. Australas Radiol 2000;44(3):296–302.

63. Turkmen A, Temel M, Gokce A, et al. Orbital exenteration for the treatment of advanced periocular skin cancer. Eur J Plast Surg 2013;36(2):69–74.

64. Galloway TJ, Morris CG, Mancuso AA, et al. Impact of radiographic findings on prognosis for skin carcinoma with clinical perineural invasion. Cancer 2005; 103(6):1254–7.

65. Mendenhall WM, Amdur RJ, Hinerman RW, et al. Skin cancer of the head and neck with perineural invasion. Am J Clin Oncol 2007;30(1):93–6.

Preimaging and Postimaging of Graft and Flap in Head and Neck Reconstruction

Ahmed Abdel Khalek Abdel Razek, MD[a,†], Gehad A. Saleh, MD[a],
Adel T. Denever, MD[b], Suresh K. Mukherji, MD, MBA, FACR[c,*]

KEYWORDS

• MR imaging • Flap • Head and neck

KEY POINTS

• Free flaps are the gold standard in head and neck reconstructive surgery.
• Increased radiologist's knowledge and familiarity with the predictable postoperative normal imaging of the flap of the head and neck.
• MR imaging appearance of a flap imitates its composition and the denervation sequelae.
• Most tumor recurrence occurs at the borders of the flap; recurrence could be a challenge to determine due to the altered anatomy.
• Imaging helps to discriminate recurrence from posttreatment changes and monitoring patients after flap reconstruction.

INTRODUCTION

Head and neck reconstructive surgery is now frequently performed after surgical resection of a sizable tumor. The altered neck anatomy after reconstructive surgery causes complexity to the imaging, so it is a must for the radiologist to gain this knowledge for accurate interpretation. Tissue transfer from one site to another includes both grafts and flaps. Precise preoperative planning and evaluation of the vascular supply is critical to improving surgical outcomes.[1,2] Postoperative imaging is mandatory for the evaluation of serious complications that threaten flap viability such as vascular thrombosis and monitoring patient for detection of tumor recurrence that was difficult by clinical examination due to postoperative and postradiation fibrosis.[3–7]

BASIC BACKGROUND
Definition of Flaps and Grafts

Graft

Grafts do not carry their own blood supply and depend on angiogenesis. Grafts are transferred from the donor site and typically, must lie within 1 to 2 mm of the recipient blood supply, limiting the type and amount of the harvested tissue. Graft types are autograft (from a patient), allograft (from a donor), or alloplastic (synthetic). Grafts are suitable for skin and subcutaneous defects, but frequently do not match to the natural skin, and finally may contract. Grafts are mainly performed as a brief coverage of the defect for future settlement of a flap or to cover donor-site defects in reconstructive surgery.[7,8]

[a] Faculty of Medicine, Department of Diagnostic Radiology, Mansoura University, Elgomhoria Street, Mansoura 35512, Egypt; [b] Faculty of Medicine, Department of Surgery, Mansoura University, Elgomhoria Street, Mansoura 35512, Egypt; [c] Marian University, Head and Neck Radiology, ProScan Imaging, Carmel, IN, USA
[†] Deceased
* Corresponding author.
E-mail address: sureshmukherji@hotmail.com

Magn Reson Imaging Clin N Am 30 (2022) 121–133
https://doi.org/10.1016/j.mric.2021.07.004
1064-9689/22/© 2021 Elsevier Inc. All rights reserved.

Flaps

Flaps are the gold standard in head and neck reconstruction and are more commonly performed for maxillofacial reconstructions, as flaps carry their own blood supply and are safely moved and transfer large amounts of tissue compared with the grafts. The radiographic appearance of donor sites and types of tissue depend on the individual components of the flap which may contain skin, fat, muscle and/or bone.[5–9]

Types of Head and Neck Flaps

Flaps are classified according to defect proximity as local, regional, or free flaps. **Table 1** shows the types of commonly used head and neck flaps and their vascular pedicles.[10,11]

Local flaps

Local flaps are frequently used to reconstruct small surgical defects with good outcomes, such as V-Y flaps or rhomboid flaps. Local flaps are favored for defects including the eyelids, nose, and lips.[10]

Pedicled regional flaps

Pedicle flaps are used to close the primary surgical defect. These flaps preserve the native vascular pedicle. The pectoralis major pedicle flap is the most frequently used pedicle flap in the head and neck reconstruction owing to its admirable vascular supply and is characteristically favored for postradiation necks. Pedicle flap reconstruction is an easier technique to accomplish than free flap and can be achieved in patients with prior radiation therapy. Also, pedicle flaps are used if free tissue transfer is contraindicated or failed. These flaps are technically limited by the pedicle length and associated with more donor site morbidity than a free flap.[8]

Free flaps (microvascular free tissue transfer)

Free flaps are the principal reconstructive technique for complex surgical defects, especially younger patients. The vascularized tissue is harvested from the donor site to reconstruct the surgical defect with microvascular anastomosis of the native vessels to the local regional blood supply. Free flaps have improved outcomes and enhance the cosmetic appearance. There is also less donor site morbidity. Free flaps can be of several tissue types depending on the recipient site requirements. The anterolateral thigh (ALT) flap, rectus abdominis flaps, and the osteocutaneous fibula flaps are the most frequently performed flaps in head and neck reconstruction, as they permit the transfer of several components with a reliable long pedicle.[8–10]

Tissue Composition of Head and Neck Flaps

Flaps are classified according to tissue composition into simple and composite flaps. The simple

Table 1 Types of head and neck flaps and their vascular pedicles	
Locoregional Flaps	**Vascular Pedicle**
Nasoseptal flap	Nasoseptal branch of sphenopalatine a.
Pericranial or galeal-pericranial flap	Supratrochlear and supraorbital a.
Temporalis muscle	Deep temporal a.
Temporoparietal fascia	Superficial temporal a.
Pectoralis muscle	Pectoral branch of thoracoacromial a.
Latissimus dorsi muscle	Thoracodorsal a.
Free Flaps	
Rectus abdominis	Deep inferior epigastric a. and v.
Latissimus dorsi	Thoracodorsal a. and v.
Radial forearm	Radial a. and cephalic v. or venae comitantes
Anterolateral thigh	Descending branch of lateral circumflex femoral a. and venae comitantes
Fibular	Peroneal a. and venae comitantes
Radius	Radial a. and venae comitantes
Iliac crest	Deep circumflex a. and v.
Scapular	Circumflex scapular a. and v.
Jejunum	Superior mesenteric a. and v.

Abbreviations: a, artery; v, vein

flap contains a single tissue type, and the complex flap involves more than one tissue. The tissue composition of the flap may be myocutaneous, fascial, osseous, or visceral. **Table 2** shows the tissue composition of the head and neck flap.[9–12]

Myocutaneous flaps

Myocutaneous flaps contain muscle, skin, vessels, and fascia. Common flaps include rectus abdominus and latissimus dorsi and are often used for skull base reconstruction.

Rectus abdominis free flaps Rectus flaps comprise one of the paired anterior abdominal muscles that are particularly beneficial due to the flexible flap design. The long pedicle (up to 10–15 cm) permits the insertion of rectus free flaps into distant defects, even those on the opposite side. Rectus free flaps are often used to reconstruct large surgical defect because of the bulkiness.[10,11]

Latissimus dorsi free flaps Latissimus dorsi free flaps are the largest muscular flaps. The cutaneous component can be positioned externally or internally to replace the lost skin or mucosa, allowing latissimus flaps to be used to reconstruct large floor of mouth or skull base surgical defects. Myocutaneous flaps display a varied range of enhancement that does not predict flap failure.[7,12]

Fascial flaps

Fascial free flaps are almost completely fasciocutaneous and contain a skin paddle, fascia, vessels, and subcutaneous tissue. Common fascial flaps include ALT and radial forearm free (RFF) flaps.

ALT flaps provide a longer vascular pedicle (up to 15 cm) and satisfactory tissue bulk and are often used for reconstruction following total glossectomy and orbital exenteration. The ALT flap is transferred from the proximal part of the lower limb with relatively minor morbidity at the donor site.[7]

RFF flaps have a thin pliable flap with a long pedicle and a substantial caliber, making it perfect for small-to-medium defects such as partial glossectomy and maxillectomy defects. This graft can also be rolled into a tube graft to reconstruct a pharyngeal defect. The RFF flap is picked from the volar side of the forearm and comprises the radial artery. Preoperative Allen test is critical to confirm a satisfactory collateral blood supply of the hand through the ulnar artery to avoid postoperative hand ischemia.

Osseous flaps

Osseous flaps are composite flaps permitting concurrent replacement of bone and soft tissue. Osteocutaneous free flaps have become a favorite technique for maxillary and mandibular defects, as long segments of bone could be fashioned using plate sand screws.[8]

Fibula osteocutaneous flaps are the preferred vascularized bone flap, as it provides the longest and strongest bone stock. The merits of the fibular flaps are the characteristic satisfactory length of its vascular pedicle (peroneal artery and its venae comitantes), excellent bone quality, tolerating several segmental osteotomies for proper contouring, and appropriate thickness for dental implantation. Preoperative angiographic assessment is necessary to confirm that the peroneal artery is not supplying the foot, as it may cause foot ischemia if transferred.[13–15]

Scapular osteocutaneous flaps are more commonly used for complex midface (hard palate or orbital) reconstructions owing to its long and large vessel diameters up to14 cm and 3 to 4.5 mm, respectively. One or two skin paddles can be gained and be totally separated from the osseous element.

Table 2
Tissue composition of head and neck flaps

Type	Donor Site	Surgical Defect
Myocutaneous	Rectus abdominus	Skull base and orbit
	Latissimus dorsi	Skull
Fascial	Radial forearm	Oral cavity, tongue, palate, nose, face, lip, pharynx, larynx
	Anterolateral thigh	Oral cavity, tongue, pharynx, larynx, cervical esophagus
Osseous	Fibula	Mandible
	Scapula, radius, and iliac crest	Mandible and midface
Visceral	Jejunal and ileal flaps	Pharynx and esophagus

Visceral flaps

Jejunum free flaps are performed for the reconstruction of pharyngoesophageal defects. This flap is technically challenging and relies on the jejunal artery that is vulnerable to ischemia. When successful, jejunal flaps allow for the quick return of swallowing, due to its exceptional motility, and lower incidence of stricture and fistula formation.[16]

PREOPERATIVE IMAGING WORKUP

Potential flap candidates should undergo preoperative imaging within 12 months of the surgical procedural.[13]

Preoperative cross-sectional imaging with computed tomography (CT) and MR for assessing the extent of the tumor, planning of the resection margin, and determining the type and size of the flap.

Preoperative ascular mapping should be performed of the donor site for all potential free flap candidates.

Imaging aids the surgeon to select the appropriate vessels by idenfying vessels greater than 3 mm that can be used for anastomosis to the local blood supply.[17] The most commonly used arteries for microvascular anastomosis are the facial, superior thyroid, and lingual arteries and all branches of the external carotid artery, whereas the internal and external jugular veins are frequently used for venous anastomoses.[8]

Method of Examinations

Accurate preoperative vascular mapping is important for preoperative planning for microvascular free tissue transfer.

Color Duplex Sonography

Color duplex sonography (CDS) provides both anatomic information along with quantitative analysis of the dominant perforator, helping to identify the most favorable anastomotic vessels. However, CDS does not create a 2-dimensional (2D) or 3D image and has a limited mapping of the subfascial and intramuscular course of the perforators.[18,19]

Computed Tomography Angiography

CT angiography (CTA) is the method of choice for preoperative vascular mapping, as it offers a global vascular map beside evaluation of the intraflap soft tissue and recognition of small perforators (3 mm), reducing operative time with improving accuracy. The disadvantages of CTA are its radiation exposure. Dual-phase CTA obtains a delayed set of images to highlight venous vasculature and

decreases the intraoperative multiple vessel explorations.[17,20]

Magnetic Resonance Angiography

There are several advantages of magnetic resonance angiography (MRA) over CTA, as it has no radiation exposure or potentially nephrotoxic iodinated contrast agents. MRA also can be achieved without contrast injection. The main disadvantages of MRA are the high cost and the less precise detection of smaller perforators, compared with CTA (vessels up to 1.0 mm in MRA vs 0.3 mm in CTA). MRA has been used in the preoperative planning of the fibular free flap and anterolateral thigh flaps.[21–25]

Digital Subtraction Angiography

Digital subtraction angiography is the gold standard for evaluation of perforators. However, it is an invasive procedure, with radiation exposure and vasoconstricting effect limiting precise measurement of small vessels.[26]

POSTOPERATIVE IMAGING
Postoperative Surveillance Imaging

The main role of postoperative surveillance imaging is early detection of complication or recurrence. CT and PET-CT are suitable for assessing the postoperative neck in most cases, whereas MR imaging is favored in complex cases near the skull base with perineural spread. The suggested time of baseline postoperative imaging is at 2 to 3 months, and surveillance varies from case to case.[8–11]

Normal Imaging Appearance of Flap

The CT or MR imaging appearance of the free flap reconstruction imitates the flap components. The normal imaging appearance of flaps of head and neck is listed in **Table 3**. The familiarity of normal changes over time is critical to avoid misreading the expected postoperative changes of the flap as recurrence. Also, the knowledge of altered surgical bed anatomy is principal for precise imaging assessment; therefore, it is vital to obtain the appropriate operative details.[27]

Nasoseptal flaps

The nasoseptal flaps are isointense on T1 and T2 images. They have variable enhancement with a characteristic C-shaped configuration in coronal and sagittal images. The distinctive imaging appearance of the vascular pedicle is best shown on contiguous axial images, which helps recognize the flap.[28–30]

Table 3
Normal postoperative imaging appearance of head and neck flaps

Flap	Normal Imaging Appearance
Pedicled regional flap	Loss of muscle bulk at donor site; the rotated vascular pedicle is typically identified
Nasoseptal flap	C-shaped enhancing flap at the skull base defect with its vascular pedicle rising from the sphenopalatine foramen
Fasciocutaneous flap	Unevenness of soft tissue volume and altered fascial planes; feeding vessels are larger with different course than normal vasculature
Myocutaneous flap	Early the flaps preserve muscle bulk with soft tissue attenuation On MR imaging, neither T2-hyperintensity nor the variable or absent enhancement of the muscular component is a dependable indicator of flap failure. A critical sign of benignity is the piercing clear borders between the flap and the adjacent natural recipient bed. Then gradually volume loss and fatty denervation atrophic changes are detected
Osteocutaneous flap	Bone segment fashioned to close the defect using many osteotomies and saved with plates and screws
Jejunal flap	Jejunal folds could be detected on imaging

Fasciocutaneous flaps

Fasciocutaneous flaps are detected on CT as mild asymmetry of soft tissue and altered fascial planes; the feeding vessels are larger with aberrant course compared with the normal vasculature (**Fig. 1**). On MR, fasciocutaneous flaps commonly reveal persistent non-masslike enhancement and T2 hyperintensity; the flap becomes smaller overtime.[31]

Myocutaneous flaps

Myocutaneous flap may show postoperative swelling and edema in first few weeks following the procedures. Over months to years, myocutaneous flaps often under muscle atrophy and fat infiltration. The muscular component may reveal persistent and variable enhancement for many months. Early postoperative CT shows a bulky flap with soft-tissue attenuation. MR imaging shows the flap to be isointense to muscle with characteristic muscle striations. The enhancement pattern is variable. The muscle component tends to show denervation atropy over time[7,16,31] (**Fig. 2**).

Osseous flaps

Bone grafts are often cut into smaller sections to reconstruct curved contours of mandible. Grafts are usually secured using plates and screws. The soft tissues attached to bone flaps are useful for providing bulk to large surgical defects. The osteomyocutaneous iliac crest free flap is a reconstructive option for segmental mandibular resection.[32] Panorex and reconstructed 3D CT images can be used to assess the bony component of the flap (**Fig. 3**).

Visceral flaps

On imaging and barium studies, jejunal, rugal folds, and haustra can be identified with jejunal, gastric, and colon interposition, respectively[16] (**Fig. 4**).

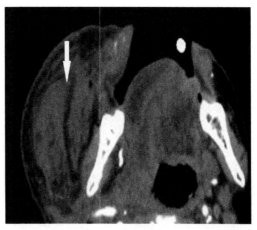

Fig. 1. Normal fasciocutaneous flaps. Axial postcontrast CT scan shows heterogeneous soft tissue thickening (*arrow*) is seen involving the flap in right mandibular region with prominent larger feeding vessels.

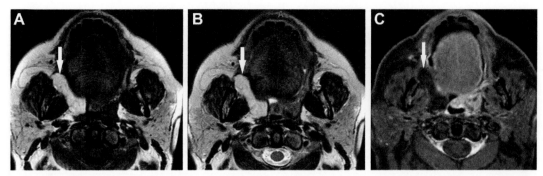

Fig. 2. Normal myocutaneous flap after oral retromolar trigone cancer. (*A*) Axial T1WI shows hyperintense flap (*arrow*) in the right retromolar region with fine linear hyointense striation within flap. (*B*) Axial T2WI shows less hyperintensity of the flap (*arrow*). (*C*) Fat-suppressed contrast T1WI shows hypointensity by signal drop of the fat (*arrow*).

Site-specific Head and Neck Flaps

Lateral skull base and infratemporal fossa
For lateral skull base reconstruction, the nearby temporalis muscle is the best choice for rotated flaps based off the deep temporal arteries. The transferred flap is easily recognized by the attached temporalis muscle to the mandibular coronoid process, the absent muscle bulk in the temporal fossa, as well as the osteotomy of the zygomatic arch.[30–32]

Anterior skull base reconstruction
The nasoseptal flap is used to close small endoscopically formed skull base defects, whereas pericranial flaps are used for open skull base defects. Free-tissue transfers such as ALT or rectus abdominis are reserved for large defects.[32–34]

Orbit and midface reconstruction
The midface defect is reconstructed with flaps that contain both bony and soft tissue components. The large defect often requires a bulky flap, such as arectus abdominis flap, whereas the bony reconstruction of the orbital is usually performed with RFF. Virtual planning and 3D printed models permit a better position of the RFF and improve the efficacy[35] (**Fig. 5**).

Hard palate and maxilla reconstruction
Maxillary reconstructive surgeries aim to separate the oral cavity from the nasal cavity and improve cosmesis by reestablishing facial contour. Based on the defect, the reconstruction may be accomplished with soft tissue or a complex osteocutaneous flap.[5,10]

Oral cavity and oropharynx reconstruction
RFF are commonly used after partial glossectomies to allow the residual normal tongue movement, as the flexible skin paddle can be fashioned to renovate the complex relationships of the tongue base. Large resections requiring segmental mandibulectomies are often reconstructed with fibular free flap to improve both function and cosmesis.[8,10]

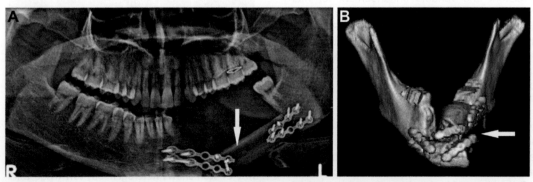

Fig. 3. Normal bone graft and flap after cancer mandible. (*A*) Panorama shows mandibular reconstruction with fibular graft (*arrow*) fixed by plates. (*B*) 3D reconstructed CT image shows satisfactory flap (*arrow*) reconstruction of the mandible.

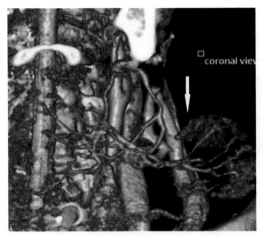

Fig. 4. Normal visceral flap after pharyngectomy. CTA shows adequate vascularity of the free jejunal flap (*arrow*) (jejunal branches from superior mesenteric artery).

Hypopharynx and laryngeal reconstruction

Laryngectomies are reconstructed with pectoralis major flap, whereas complete laryngopharyngectomy is rebuilt with RFF or ALT. There is a distinguishing appearance of pharyngeal reconstruction with pectoralis major, as the flap has a rolled appearance with reversed tissue plane and the skin making the inner pseudomucosal coat of the neopharynx. Also, the absent pectoralis muscle in its normal position and the rotated pedicles have a distinctive imaging finding[7,10] (**Fig. 6**).

Mandibular reconstruction

Mandibular reconstructive surgery aims to rebuild mandibular continuity and maintain function. Bone grafts are performed for small defects, whereas free tissue transfers are used in large composite defects; the most used are the fibular, iliac crest, and scapular flaps. Fibular free flaps are the gold standard for mandibular reconstructions principally in defects with more than one osteotomy

because of its long pedicle, segmental perforators tolerating many osteotomies, and better facial contouring. The scapular osteocutaneous flap may be used in cases with significant peripheral vascular disease[10,32] (see **Fig. 3**).

POSTOPERATIVE COMPLICATIONS
Classification of Complication

Postoperative complications can be categorized as an early or late complication; most of them occur early after surgery, frequently related to the surgical technique. Early complications such as vascular occlusion and fluid collection are frequently clinically observed and seldom necessitate cross-sectional imaging. More frequently imaged complications arise later and comprise fistulas, flap necrosis, and recurrence.[7]

Flap Vascularity and Viability

Vascular occlusion is the main cause for flap loss; venous thrombosis is more common. The use of interposition vein graft and previous radiotherapy increase the risk. Nonthrombotic vascular complications include vasospasm, stenosis, and external compression of the pedicle by hematoma or hardware.[36] Flap ischemia is best assessed clinically and hardly acquired cross-sectional imaging. Management comprises reexploration with probable thrombectomy and anastomosis revision with a rescue rate of 50% to 75%.[7,37]

Early detection of a deteriorating flap and fast intervention is critical for flap salvage. Doppler is helpful to assess both the arterial and venous outfow. MR imaging is not routinely performed to assess flap viability.[10] The normal postoperative appearance of flaps is very variable and ranges from almost no enhancement to diffuse strong enhancement. Therefore, postoperative MR enhancement is not reliable to predict flap necrosis.[38,39]

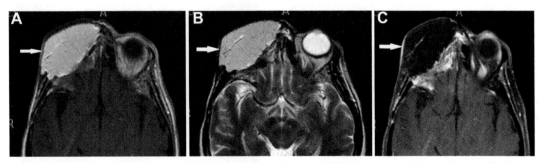

Fig. 5. Normal pericranial flap after orbital exenteration. (*A*) Axial T1WI shows sizable hyperintense flap (*arrow*) with striated appearance. (*B*) T2WI shows less hyperintensity of the flap. (*C*) Fat-suppressed contrast T1WI shows flap hypointensity by signal drop of the fat (*arrow*). T1WI, T1-weighted imaging; T2W1, T2-weighted imaging.

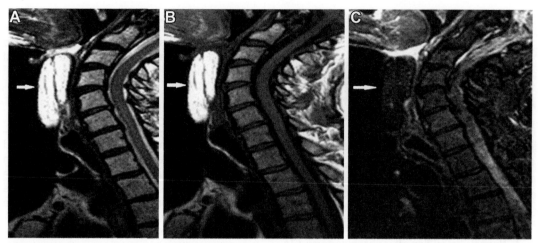

Fig. 6. Normal myocutaneous flap after laryngoectomy. (*A*) T1WI shows hyperintense flap (*arrow*) with linear hypointense striations within flap. (*B*) T2WI shows less hyperitnesity of the flap (*arrow*). (*C*) Fat-suppressed contrast T1WI shows hypointense of the fat (*arrow*).

Fluid Collection

Seroma or hematoma

Seroma or hematoma may occur instantly after reconstruction and gradually resolve; sporadically ultrasound may be requested to detect a quickly expanding hematoma, which may necessitate evacuation (**Fig. 7**).

Abscess

Postoperative abscess may occasionally occur. Patients are usually fever and pain. CT and MR imaging show peripheral enhancement (**Fig. 8**), which may differentiate between tumor recurrence and other collections.[10]

Leakage

Pharyngocutaneous fistula

Pharyngocutaneous fistula occurs early postoperative period. Delayed occurrence suggests local recurrence and warrants evaluation with MR imaging or CT. The fistulous tract and/or strictures are best evaluated by swallowing studies. On CT or MR imaging, fistula is suggested by detecting a skin defect, subcutaneous gas at late postoperative period, or gas inside the flap with distorted anatomy.[40,41]

Cerebrospinal fluid leakage

CT or MR imaging can detect the location of the skull base defect. The prevalence of cerebrospinal fluid leak is less with skull base reconstructive surgery using free flaps rather than locoregional flaps.[8]

Tumor Recurrence

Clinical assessment for recurrence is limited by the flap bulkiness. Therefore, the radiologist plays a crucial role in the recognition of the recurrence

The primary site of recurrence mostly occurs at the anastomotic site, which must be assessed carefully. The imaging features of recurrent tumors are an enlarging mass, nodal recurrence, or perineural spread.[39,42]

Recurrent tumors reveal a variable enhancement pattern and may cause bone erosion or encasement of vital structures. CT provides better evaluation of cortical bony abnormalities. The presence of new low-density areas, soft tissue nodule, and/or loss of fat within a flap is considered recurrence until proved otherwise[43–45] (**Figs. 9 and 10**). Dual-energy CT (DECT): DECT-derived iodine content and overlay are significantly lower in metastatic cervical lymph nodes (LNs) compared with the inflammatory LNs.[46] On CT perfusion, the recurrent tumors had significantly

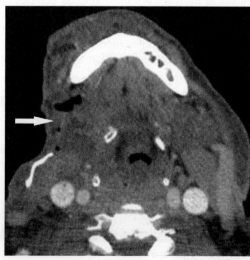

Fig. 7. Postflap seroma. Axial CT scan shows postoperative fluid collection (*arrow*), no enhancing soft issue.

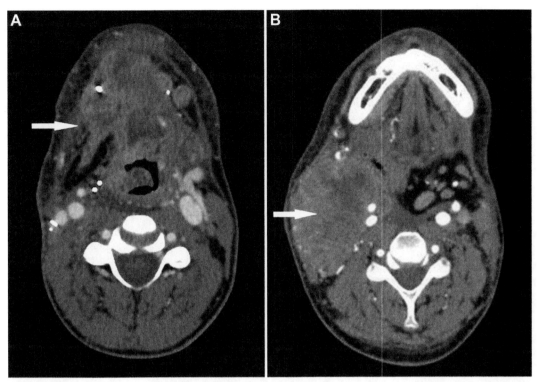

Fig. 8. Postflap recurrence. (*A*) Axial postcontrast CT scan shows heterogeneous soft tissue mass (*arrow*) is seen involving the flap in the right mandibular region. (*B*) Axial postcontrast CT scan in another patient shows large right-sided metastatic necrotic cervical lymph nodes (*arrow*).

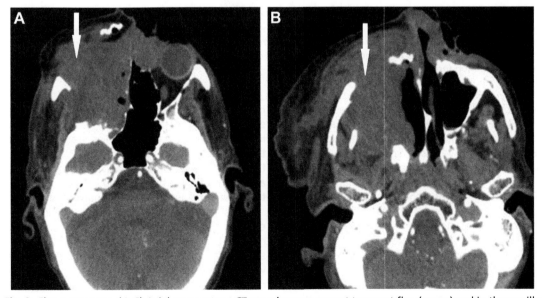

Fig. 9. Flap recurrence. (*A*, *B*) Axial postcontrast CT scan shows recurrent tumor at flap (*arrow*) and in the maxilla and right check after 1 year of surgery.

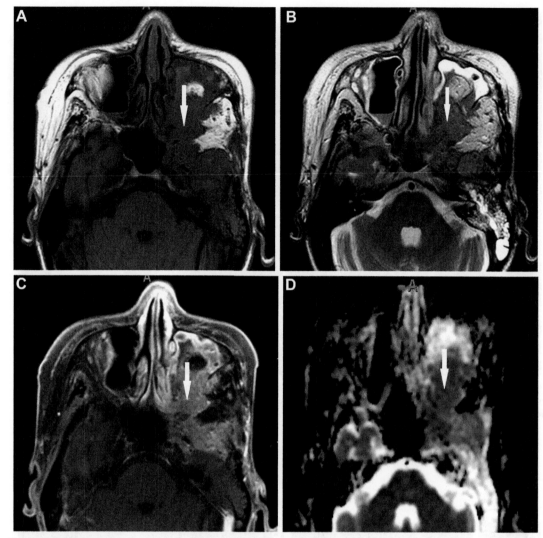

Fig. 10. Postflap marginal recurrence after maxillary reconstruction. (*A*) Axial T1WI shows hypointense lesion is seen along the margin of the flap (*arrow*). (*B*) Axial T2WI shows the hypointensity of the lesion (*arrow*). (*C*) Axial contrast T1WI shows intense heterogenous enhancement of the recurrent tumor (*arrow*). (*D*) ADC map shows restricted diffusion (*arrow*).

higher blood flow, blood volume, and permeability surface area product with decreased mean transit time compared with posttherapeutic changes.[47,48] PET with fludeoxyglucose *scan* revealed higher diagnostic accuracy for local and overall recurrence compared with contrast-enhanced CT. PET/CT better not be achieved before 2 months after the accomplishment of treatment to prevent false-positive results by persistent local inflammation; in general, 12 weeks interval is advised.[49]

MR imaging is superior to CT owing to its excellent tissue delineation and contrast resolution. Unenhanced T2-weighted and STIR sequences help to differentiate recurrence from radiation fibrosis, as the latter displays hypointensity. Tumor recurrence enhancement is better defined on fat-saturated postcontrast T1-weighted images and indicated by a new focal soft tissue thickening at the surgical margin. Postoperative chronic scar tissue is hypointense on T1 and T2 images, scars, and granulation tissue and shows retraction over time, but neoplastic tissue continues to grow.[50,51]

Diffusion-weighted imaging is valuable in differentiating benign posttreatment changes from recurrence, as the latter revealed true diffusion restriction and lower apparent diffusion coefficient values.[52–55] Diffusion tensor imaging parameters revealed significantly lower mean diffusivity and higher fractional anisotropy values compared with postradiation changes.[56,57] Intravoxel incoherent motion (IVIM) offers quantitative parameters reflecting diffusion and perfusion characteristics. IVIM parameters (D, D*, and f) can discriminate recurrence from postchemoradiation fibrosis.[58,59] Dynamic susceptibility contrast T2*-weighted perfusion-weighted MR imaging helps in the detection of recurrent tumors, as it exhibits a higher mean dynamic susceptibility contrast percentage (DSC%) than posttherapeutic changes.[60,61] Arterial spin labeling The tumor blood flow for recurrent masses is higher than in postradiation changes.[62–64] MR spectroscopy evidenced higher choline/creatine ratios in recurrent tumor and metastatic LNs compared with posttreatment changes and inflammatory LNs.[65]

Dehiscence

Dehiscence of flap covering surgical hardware may cause hardware exposure and extrusion, frequently perceived with constant tobacco use.[66]

SUMMARY

Understanding the imaging appearances of the postoperative grafts and flaps is important due to continuing advances in surgical reconstructive techniques. Postoperative head and neck follow-up is challenging, so to deliver accurate imaging, radiologists must gain a basic knowledge of the surgical choices, ranging from skin grafts to variable types of flaps and skill to differentiate between normal enhancing flaps and recurrent tumors, particularly because recurrences could be missed by clinical examination.

CLINICS CARE POINTS

- Knowledge of the normal appearance of flaps helps prevent misdiagnosing recurrent tumor from normal flap.
- Radiographic appearance of donor sites and types of tissue depend on the individual components of the flap which may contain skin, fat, muscle and/or bone.

REFERENCES

1. Eid IN, Arosarena OA. Reconstruction of cutaneous cancer defects of the head and neck. Otolaryngol Clin North Am 2021;54:379–95.
2. Kim HS, Chung CH, Chang YJ. Free-flap reconstruction in recurrent head and neck cancer: a retrospective review of 124 cases. Arch Craniofac Surg 2020;21:27–34.
3. Prince ADP, Broderick MT, Neal MEH, et al. Head and neck reconstruction in the vessel depleted neck. Front Oral Maxillofac Med 2020;2:13.
4. Lim X, Rajagopal R, Silva P, et al. A systematic review on outcomes of anterior skull base reconstruction. J Plast Reconstr Aesthet Surg 2020;73:1940–50.
5. Kanatas AN, Lowe D, Rogers SN. Free flap donor site during early review consultations: is it really an issue? Br J Oral Maxillofac Surg 2020;58:e115–8.
6. Pichardo P, Purdy N, Haugen T. Implantation of squamous cell carcinoma in a free flap donor site. Ann Otol Rhinol Laryngol 2020;129:935–40.
7. McCarty JL, Corey AS, El-Deiry MW, et al. Imaging of surgical free flaps in head and neck reconstruction. AJNR Am J Neuroradiol 2019;40:5–13.
8. Syed F, Spector ME, Cornelius R, et al. Head and neck reconstructive surgery: what the radiologist needs to know. Eur Radiol 2016;26:3345–52.
9. Chang EI, Chu CK, Chang EI. Advancements in imaging technology for microvascular free tissue transfer. J Surg Oncol 2018;118:729–35.
10. Learned K, Malloy K, Loevner L. Myocutaneous flaps and other vascularized grafts in head and neck reconstruction for cancer treatment. Magn Reson Imaging Clin North Am 2012;20:495–513.
11. Hudgins P. Flap reconstruction in the head and neck: expected appearance, complications, and recurrent disease. Eur J Radiol 2002;44:130–8.
12. Pinel-Giroux FM, El Khoury MM, Trop I, et al. Breast reconstruction: review of surgical methods and spectrum of imaging findings. Radiographics 2013;33:435–53.
13. Abou-Foul AK, Fasanmade A, Prabhu S, et al. Anatomy of the vasculature of the lower leg and harvest of a fibular flap: a systematic review. Br J Oral Maxillofac Surg 2017;55:904–10.
14. Abou-Foul AK, Borumandi F. Anatomical variants of lower limb vasculature and implications for free fibula flap: systematic review and critical analysis. Microsurgery 2016;36:165–72.
15. Gryseleyn R, Schlund M, Pigache P, et al. Influence of preoperative imaging on fibula free flap harvesting. J Stomatol Oral Maxillofac Surg 2017;118:265–70.
16. Welkoborsky H-J, Deichmüller C, Bauer L, et al. Reconstruction of large pharyngeal defects with microvascular free flaps and myocutaneous pedicled flaps. Curr Opin Otolaryngol Head Neck Surg 2013;21:318–27.
17. Chen Y-W, Yen J-H, Chen W-H, et al. Preoperative computed tomography angiography for evaluation of feasibility of free flaps in difficult reconstruction of head and neck. Ann Plast Surg 2016;76:S19–24.
18. Huang JW, Huang CS, Shih YC, et al. Comparison of perioperative outcomes between endoscope-

assisted technique and handheld acoustic Doppler for perforator identification in fasciocutaneous flaps. Medicine 2018;97:e10849.

19. Paydar KZ, Hansen SL, Chang DS, et al. Implantable venous Doppler monitoring in head and neck free flap reconstruction increases the salvage rate. Plast Reconstr Surg 2010;125:1129–34.

20. Avraham T, Franco P, Brecht LE, et al. Functional outcomes of virtually planned free fibula flap reconstruction of the mandible. Plast Reconstr Surg 2014; 134:628e–34e.

21. Schuderer JG, Meier JK, Klingelhöffer C, et al. Magnetic resonance angiography for free fibula harvest: anatomy and perforator mapping. Int J Oral Maxillofac Surg 2020;49:176–82.

22. Razek AA, Saad E, Soliman N, et al. Assessment of vascular disorders of the upper extremity with contrast-enhanced magnetic resonance angiography: pictorial review. Jpn J Radiol 2010;28:87–94.

23. Lohan DG, Tomasian A, Krishnam M, et al. MR angiography of lower extremities at 3T: presurgical planning of fibular free flap transfer for facial reconstruction. Am J Roentgenol 2008;190:770e6.

24. Razek AA, Gaballa G, Megahed AS, et al. Time resolved imaging of contrast kinetics (TRICKS) MR angiography of arteriovenous malformations of head and neck. Eur J Radiol 2013;82:1885–91.

25. Fukaya E, Grossman RF, Saloner D, et al. Magnetic resonance angiography for free fibula flap transfer. J Reconstr Microsurg 2007;23:205–11.

26. Alolabi N, Dickson L, Coroneos CJ, et al. Preoperative angiography for free fibula flap harvest: a meta-analysis. J Reconstr Microsurg 2019;35:362–71.

27. Chong J, Chan LL, Langstein HN, et al. MR imaging of the muscular component of myocutaneous flaps in the head and neck. AJNR Am J Neuroradiol 2001;22:170–4.

28. Learned KO, Adappa ND, Lee JY, et al. MR imaging evolution of endoscopic cranial defect reconstructions using nasoseptal flaps and their distinction from neoplasm. AJNR Am J Neuroradiol 2014;35: 1182–9.

29. Learned KO, Adappa ND, Loevner LA, et al. MR imaging evaluation of endoscopic cranial base reconstruction with pedicled nasoseptal flap following endoscopic endonasal skull base surgery. Eur J Radiol 2013;82:544–51.

30. Kang MD, Escott E, Thomas AJ, et al. The MR imaging appearance of the vascular pedicle nasoseptal flap. Am J Neuroradiol 2009;30:781–6.

31. Sedrak P, Lee PS, Guha-Thakurta N, et al. MRI findings of myocutaneous and fasciocutaneous flaps used for reconstruction of orbital exenteration defects. Ophthalmic Plast Reconstr Surg 2014;30: 328–36.

32. Sandler ML, Griffin M, Xing MH, et al. Postoperative imaging appearance of Iliac crest free flaps used for

33. Xu X, Lwin S, Ting E, et al. Magnetic resonance imaging study of the pericranial flap and its local effects following endoscopic craniofacial resection. Laryngoscope 2021;131:E90–7.

34. Kim CS, Patel U, Pastena G, et al. The magnetic resonance imaging appearance of endoscopic endonasal skull base defect reconstruction using free mucosal graft. World Neurosurg 2019;126:e165–72.

35. Fu K, Liu Y, Gao N, et al. Reconstruction of maxillary and orbital floor defect with free fibula flap and whole individualized titanium mesh assisted by computer techniques. J Oral Maxillofac Surg 2017;75: 1791.e1.

36. Seres L, Makula E, Morvay Z, et al. Color Doppler ultrasound for monitoring free flaps in the head and neck region. J Craniofac Surg 2002;13:75–8.

37. Abdel Razek AA, Denewer AT, Hegazy MA, et al. Role of computed tomography angiography in the diagnosis of vascular stenosis in head and neck microvascular free flap reconstruction. Int J Oral Maxillofac Surg 2014;43:811–5.

38. Saito N, Nadgir RN, Nakahira M, et al. Posttreatment CT and MR imaging in head and neck cancer: what the radiologist needs to know. Radiographics 2012; 32:1261–82.

39. Gillespie J. Imaging of the post-treatment neck. Clin Radiol 2020;75. 794.e7–794.e17.

40. ingh R, Karantanis W, Fadhil M, et al. Meta-analysis on the rate of pharyngocutaneous fistula in early oral feeding in laryngectomy patients. Am J Otolaryngol 2021;42:102748.

41. Khoo MJW, Ooi ASH. Management of postreconstructive head and neck salivary fistulae: a review of current practices. J Plast Reconstr Aesthet Surg 2021;10: S1748–6815.

42. González Moreno IM, Torres Del Río S, Vázquez Olmos C. Follow-up in head and neck cancer. What the radiologist must know. Radiologia 2020; 62:13–27.

43. Abdel Razek AAA, Abdelaziz TT. Neck imaging reporting and data system: what does radiologist want to know? J Comput Assist Tomogr 2020;44:527–32.

44. Abdel Razek AAK, Mukherji SK. Imaging of posttreatment salivary gland tumors. Neuroimaging Clin North Am 2018;28:199–208.

45. Jacobson A, Cohen O. Review of flap monitoring technology in 2020. Facial Plast Surg 2020;36:722–6.

46. Tawfik AM, Razek AA, Kerl JM, et al. Comparison of dual-energy CT-derived iodine content and iodine overlay of normal, inflammatory and metastatic squamous cell carcinoma cervical lymph nodes. Eur Radiol 2014;24:574–80.

47. Razek AA, Tawfik AM, Elsorogy LG, et al. Perfusion CT of head and neck cancer. Eur J Radiol 2014;83: 537–44.

48. Tawfik AM, Razek AA, Elsorogy LG, et al. Perfusion CT of head and neck cancer: effect of arterial input selection. AJR Am J Roentgenol 2011;196:1374–80.

49. Suenaga Y, Kitajima K, Ishihara T, et al. FDG-PET/contrast-enhanced CT as a post-treatment tool in head and neck squamous cell carcinoma: comparison with FDG-PET/non-contrast-enhanced CT and contrast-enhanced CT. Eur Radiol 2016;26:1018–30.

50. Ishiyama M, Richards T, Parvathaneni U, et al. Dynamic contrast-enhanced magnetic resonance imaging in head and neck cancer: differentiation of new H&N cancer, recurrent disease, and benign post-treatment changes. Clin Imaging 2015;39:566–70.

51. Abdel Razek AAK. Routine and advanced diffusion imaging modules of the salivary glands. Neuroimaging Clin North Am 2018;28:245–54.

52. Abdel Razek A, Mossad A, Ghonim M. Role of diffusion-weighted MR imaging in assessing malignant versus benign skull-base lesions. Radiol Med 2011;116:125–32.

53. Abdel Razek AA, Kamal E. Nasopharyngeal carcinoma: correlation of apparent diffusion coefficient value with prognostic parameters. Radiol Med 2013;118:534–9.

54. Abdel Razek AA, Kandeel AY, Soliman N, et al. Role of diffusion-weighted echo-planar MR imaging in differentiation of residual or recurrent head and neck tumors and posttreatment changes. AJNR Am J Neuroradiol 2007;28:1146–52.

55. Abdel Razek AA, Elkhamary S, Al-Mesfer S, et al. Correlation of apparent diffusion coefficient at 3T with prognostic parameters of retinoblastoma. AJNR Am J Neuroradiol 2012;33:944–8.

56. Razek AAKA. Diffusion tensor imaging in differentiation of residual head and neck squamous cell carcinoma from post-radiation changes. Magn Reson Imaging 2018;54:84–9.

57. Khalek Abdel Razek AA. Characterization of salivary gland tumours with diffusion tensor imaging. Dentomaxillofac Radiol 2018;47:20170343.

58. Liang L, Luo X, Lian Z, et al. Lymph node metastasis in head and neck squamous carcinoma: efficacy of intravoxel incoherent motion magnetic resonance imaging for the differential diagnosis. Eur J Radiol 2017;90:159–65.

59. Noij DP, Martens RM, Marcus JT, et al. Intravoxel incoherent motion magnetic resonance imaging in head and neck cancer: a systematic review of the diagnostic and prognostic value. Oral Oncol 2017; 68:81–91.

60. Abdel Razek AA, Gaballa G. Role of perfusion magnetic resonance imaging in cervical lymphadenopathy. J Comput Assist Tomogr 2011;35:21–5.

61. Abdel Razek AA, Gaballa G, Ashamalla G, et al. Dynamic susceptibility contrast perfusion-weighted magnetic resonance imaging and diffusion-weighted magnetic resonance imaging in differentiating recurrent head and neck cancer from postradiation changes. J Comput Assist Tomogr 2015;39:849–54.

62. Abdel Razek AAK, Talaat M, El-Serougy L, et al. Clinical applications of arterial spin labeling in brain tumors. J Comput Assist Tomogr 2019;43:525–32.

63. Abdel Razek AAK. Arterial spin labelling and diffusion-weighted magnetic resonance imaging in differentiation of recurrent head and neck cancer from post-radiation changes. J Laryngol Otol 2018; 132:923–8.

64. Razek AAKA. Multi-parametric MR imaging using pseudo-continuous arterial-spin labeling and diffusion-weighted MR imaging in differentiating subtypes of parotid tumors. Magn Reson Imaging 2019;63:55–9.

65. Razek AA, Nada N. Correlation of choline/creatine and apparent diffusion coefficient values with the prognostic parameters of head and neck squamous cell carcinoma. NMR Biomed 2016;29:483–9.

66. Day KE, Desmond R, Magnuson JS, et al. Hardware removal after osseous free flap reconstruction. Otolaryngol Neck Surg 2014;150:40–6.

MR Imaging of Salivary Gland Tumors

Elliott Friedman, MD[a],*, Maria Olga Patino, MD[a], Ahmed Abdel Khalek Abdel Razek, MD[b],[†]

KEYWORDS

- Salivary • Parotid • MR imaging • Benign • Malignant • Perfusion • Staging

KEY POINTS

- Contrast-enhanced MR imaging is the best imaging modality to evaluate salivary gland neoplasms.
- Irregular margins, extraglandular spread, low T2 signal, low apparent diffusion coefficient, cervical lymphadenopathy, and perineural spread are imaging features suggestive of malignancy.
- Overlap exists between the appearance of benign and malignant tumors.
- Multiparametric advanced MR imaging combining diffusion-weighted imaging and perfusion MR imaging helps to distinguish between pleomorphic adenoma, Warthin tumor, and malignancy.

INTRODUCTION

Salivary gland tumors (SGT) are among the most histopathologically heterogeneous groups of tumors in humans. Salivary malignancies are uncommon, with approximately 1 malignancy per 100,000 population in the United States.[1] Unlike other head and neck malignancies, which are overwhelmingly squamous cell carcinoma, salivary gland malignancies constitute a variety of histologies with a classification system that continues to change over time.[2] The 2017 World Health Organization classification for SGTs lists more than 30 different benign and malignant salivary epithelial tumors.[3]

Benign and malignant SGTs most commonly present as painless, enlarging salivary masses, and may also overlap in clinical presentation with nonneoplastic entities.[4] The proportion of benign to malignant neoplasms varies by the gland involved, with the risk of malignancy in adults increasing as gland size decreases for the major salivary glands. The majority of parotid gland tumors in adults are benign (roughly 80% benign to 20% malignant), but given that it is the most common location for neoplasms to occur, most malignancies occur in the parotid gland. More than one-half of submandibular gland neoplasms are benign, and the overwhelming majority of sublingual gland tumors are malignant, to the point, that regardless of appearance, sublingual masses should be considered malignant until proven otherwise.[5] Minor SGTs are more likely to be malignant; however, the proportion of benign to malignant varies by subsite[5,6] (**Fig. 1**). SGTs are much less common in children than adults and differ in some key respects. A greater proportion of SGTs in children occur in the parotid gland, and there is a higher frequency of nonepithelial tumors and a greater chance of malignancy in epithelial tumors, especially in younger children.[7]

STAGING OF SALIVARY GLAND TUMORS

The primary role of imaging in salivary gland masses is to define the extent of tumor, and in the case of malignancies, to characterize features that allow appropriate staging by American Joint Committee on Cancer TNM criteria.[8] Reporting criteria should include local extension with specific regard to criteria that affect T staging, and the presence of any perineural spread, metastasis to lymph nodes and distant sites (brain, bone, and

None of the authors have commercial or financial conflicts to disclose.
[a] Department of Neuroradiology, University of Texas Health Science Center at Houston, 6431 Fannin Street, MSB 2.130B, Houston, TX 77030, USA; [b] Department of Diagnostic Radiology, Faculty of Medicine, Mansoura University, Elgomhoria Street, Mansoura 35512, Egypt
[†] Deceased
* Corresponding author.
E-mail address: efried77@gmail.com

Magn Reson Imaging Clin N Am 30 (2022) 135–149
https://doi.org/10.1016/j.mric.2021.07.006

mri.theclinics.com

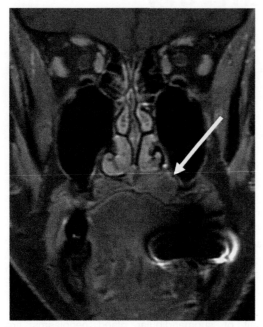

Fig. 1. Coronal fast spin T1-weighted image with contrast shows a mildly enhancing mass in the left palate, which turned out to be an adenoid cystic carcinoma.

lungs) (**Box 1**). Minor SGTs are staged according to their site of origin.

MR IMAGING PROTOCOLS AND TECHNIQUES

MR imaging is the preferred imaging modality to evaluate soft tissue masses, including SGTs. MR imaging provides better tissue characterization than a computed tomography (CT) scan, and is the optimal modality to define the local extent of disease and, in the case of malignancy, to assess for perineural spread of disease. Regardless of the modality used, imaging is usually not reliable to determine a histopathologic diagnosis and ultimately biopsy or excision is necessary to provide a specific diagnosis. Even definitively distinguishing benign from malignant disease is not always possible by imaging. Certain MR imaging characteristics and advanced imaging techniques can be used to suggest that a mass is more or less likely to be malignant, as discussed elsewhere in this article. This distinction has important management implications, because benign parotid tumors are often treated by local excision or superficial parotidectomy and malignancies are treated by total parotidectomy with or without facial nerve sacrifice.

A general face protocol should be used for evaluation of major SGTs and minor salivary gland neoplasms of the oral cavity. Ideally, both precontrast and postcontrast imaging should be

---

Box 1
Reporting of salivary gland masses

Local extent (T staging)

   T1: Tumor <2 cm without extraparenchymal extension

   T2: Tumor 2 to 4 cm without extraparenchymal extension

   T3: Tumor greater than 4 cm or extraparenchymal extension

   T4a: Invasion of skin, mandible, external auditory canal, or facial nerve

   T4b: Invasion of skull base or pterygoid plates or encases the internal carotid artery

Nodal involvement—Size of largest node (<3 cm, 3–6 cm, or >6 cm), single or multiple pathologic nodes, ipsilateral or bilateral/contralateral involvement, or extranodal extension

Metastatic disease—bones, lung, brain, and other sites

---

performed, with a field of view no larger than 250 × 250 mm. At our institution, imaging sequences include axial, coronal, and sagittal T1 without fat saturation, axial T2 without fat saturation, coronal T2 short T1 inversion recovery or Dixon, and postcontrast axial and coronal T1 with fat saturation, at a 3-mm slice thickness. Axial diffusion-weighted imaging (DWI) is also performed; however, in the case of oral cavity and palate masses, coronal plane DWI is used. Postcontrast fat-saturated 3-dimensional (3D) T1-weighted imaging is helpful for high resolution assessment for perineural spread. Either MR imaging or CT scan of the neck is adequate to screen for metastatic lymphadenopathy.

Appropriate presurgical planning requires that the location of the mass superficial or deep to the facial nerve be determined to plan the appropriate operative approach and to minimize the risk of intraoperative facial nerve injury. The facial nerve is not identified directly on conventional cross-sectional imaging, and several indirect methods have been proposed to estimate its intraparotid course with varying levels of accuracy.[9] In recent years, techniques with increased spatial and contrast resolution including high resolution 3D steady state imaging techniques (Fast Imaging Employing Steady-state Acquisition imaging sequence in magnetic resonance imaging, constructive interference in steady state, 3D DWI reversed fast imaging with steady state precession) and diffusion tensor imaging have been shown to be reliable for delineation of the main trunk and cervicofacial and temporofacial divisions of the facial nerve in the parotid gland.[10–13]

DISTINGUISHING BENIGN FROM MALIGNANT

Differentiating benign from malignant neoplasms is important for preoperative treatment planning. Clinically, the presence of cranial neuropathies, such as facial weakness or numbness, is highly suggestive of malignancy. Certain imaging characteristics on conventional imaging can suggest that a mass is more likely to be malignant; however, benign and malignant salivary neoplasms demonstrate a considerable amount of overlap in their imaging appearance as well as with some nonneoplastic lesions. Ill-defined tumor margins and extraglandular invasion of tumor are suggestive of malignancy, although infectious or inflammatory disease also characteristically has poorly defined margins and benign tumors may be complicated by a sialadenitis. Some low-grade malignancies, like mucoepidermoid carcinoma, may have well-defined margins (**Fig. 2**).

T2 hypointensity, which is present in highly cellular tumors, is suggestive of malignancy but can also be seen in some granulomatous or chronic inflammatory diseases. A Warthin tumor (WT) can also have internal areas of low T2 signal. A mass with well-defined borders and T2 hyperintensity that is located in the superficial lobe is more likely to be benign[14] (**Fig. 3**).

Intratumoral cystic changes can be seen in both benign and malignant neoplasms; however, central cystic changes are much more commonly seen in malignancies.[15] The degree of tumor enhancement and the speed of growth are not reliable indicators of malignancy. Rapid growth, which is often associated with higher grade malignancies, can be seen with infectious or other inflammatory disease.

Conversely, adenoid cystic carcinoma, is a notoriously slow growing malignancy.

Even cervical lymphadenopathy is not without its exceptions in predicting malignancy. WT can rarely arise in cervical lymph nodes and infectious and other inflammatory diseases can mimic metastatic lymphadenopathy.

PERINEURAL SPREAD

Perineural invasion, a finding highly correlated with more aggressive malignancies, is best assessed by MR imaging. Involved nerves include branches of the trigeminal (V) or facial (VII) nerves, or the auriculotemporal nerve, a small branch of the mandibular division of the trigeminal nerve that courses posterior to the mandibular condyle and enters the parotid gland to join with branches of the facial nerve. It represents an important route of perineural spread from the parotid gland intracranially through the foramen ovale[16] (**Fig. 4**).

DIFFUSION-WEIGHTED IMAGING AND DIFFUSION TENSOR IMAGING

DWI of the salivary glands can be performed using either single or multishot echo planar imaging, or non–echo planar imaging. DWI is now a routine part of most face and neck MR imaging protocols in the workup of inflammatory and neoplastic masses and post-treatment follow-up. As a generalization, malignant tumors of the neck without cystic or necrotic components are more likely to have a lower mean apparent diffusion coefficient (ADC) value than benign tumors, presumably owing to their more densely packed cellularity and higher nucleus to cytoplasm ratio.[17] Multiple studies evaluating ADC thresholds have shown that there is a considerable overlap and lack of significant difference in ADC values for distinguishing

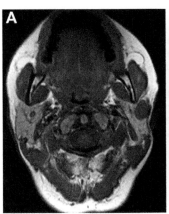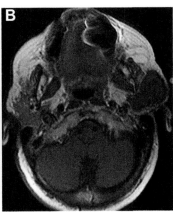

Fig. 2. Axial T1-weighted imaging shows superficial lobe left parotid masses in 2 patients. (*A*) Pleomorphic adenoma has well-defined margins and (*B*) carcinoma ex pleomorphic adenoma has ill-defined margins.

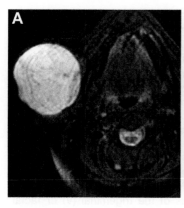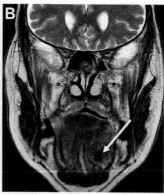

Fig. 3. (*A*) Axial T2-weighted imaging shows a lesion brighter than cerebrospinal fluid, found to be pleomorphic adenoma. (*B*) Coronal T2-weighted imaging shows a mass with low T2 signal in the floor of mouth, pathologically proven clear cell carcinoma.

benign from malignant salivary neoplasms. In particular, WT, a benign parotid mass, typically has ADC values as low or lower than malignant neoplasms, with ranges overlapping with malignant lesions. Only pleomorphic adenoma (PA), was distinguishable from all other parotid masses, with the exception of myoepithelioma, based on its facilitated diffusion[18] (**Fig. 5**).

Lower ADC values have been correlated with higher tumor grade and tumor T stage, and tumor T stage has been inversely correlated with overall prognosis.[19] Fractional anisotropy, a common metric of diffusion tensor imaging, has been shown in multiple studies to be significantly higher in malignant compared with benign SGTs.[20,21] DWI can also be used to monitor patients after treatment, with restricted diffusion and low ADC value concerning for recurrent tumor and a high ADC value more suggestive of treatment-related changes.[22]

MR PERFUSION

Multiple techniques exist for perfusion imaging. Malignant tumors tend to have higher angiogenesis which is associated with increased tumor

blood volume, arteriovenous shunt formation, altered capillary transit time, and increased capillary permeability. Dynamic susceptibility contrast MR perfusion, follows the first pass of gadolinium-based contrast agents through the brain measuring T2 or T2* signal changes. The susceptibility effects of the paramagnetic contrast agent are used to generate a contrast concentration time curve from which cerebral blood flow and cerebral blood volume maps can be created. Malignant tumors can be distinguished from benign tumors, both PA and WT, based on a higher dynamic susceptibility contrast percent signal loss. Dynamic contrast-enhanced MR perfusion, also known as permeability imaging, measures the T1 signal before, during, and after contrast administration and a time–intensity curve is generated and a transfer constant can be calculated. Four distinct time–intensity curve patterns have been described based on wash-in, washout, and time to peak contrast enhancement. Type A curves with progressive enhancement are typical of PA. Type B curves with early enhancement (<150 s) and high washout (>30%) are characteristic of WT and lymphoma. Malignancies most commonly show a type C curve with early

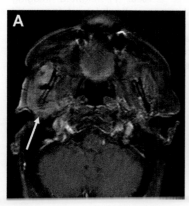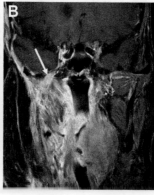

Fig. 4. Adenoid cystic carcinoma. Fast spin T1-weighted image with contrast axial (*A*) and coronal (*B*) images show thickened enhancement posterior to the mandibular condyle secondary to perineural spread along the auriculotemporal nerve (*A*) and perineural extension along the mandibular nerve to the foramen ovale (*B*).

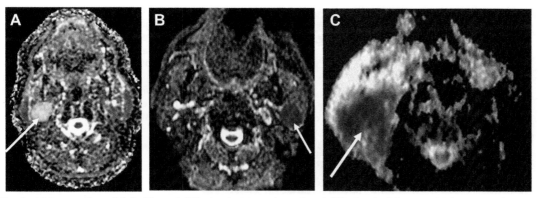

Fig. 5. ADC maps show (*A*) facilitated diffusion in PA, and restricted diffusion in (*B*) WT and (*C*) mucoepidermoid carcinoma.

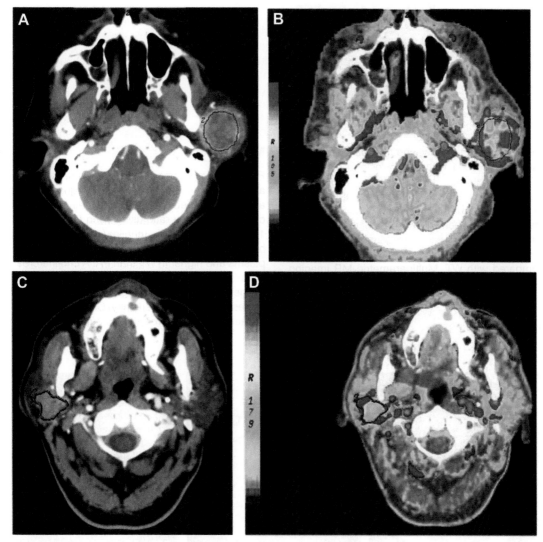

Fig. 6. Postcontrast CT scan and blood flow maps from PA (*A*, *B*) and parotid carcinoma (*C*, *D*) show increased blood flow in both tumors; however, there is significantly higher blood flow in the PA (210 mL/100 g/min) than carcinoma (76 mL/100 g/min).

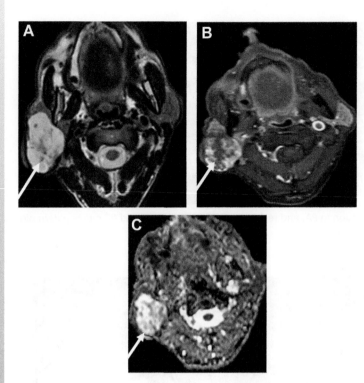

Fig. 7. PA in the superficial lobe of the right parotid gland. Axial T2-weighted imaging (*A*), fast spin T1-weighted image with contrast (*B*) and ADC map (*C*) show a T2 hyperintense, heterogeneously enhancing mass with facilitated diffusion. Note the extension through and widening of the stylomandibular tunnel.

enhancement and low washout. Type D curves are flat and are seen with cystic lesions and some WTs. Arterial spin labeling uses magnetically labeled blood as an endogenous contrast agent to calculate the tumor blood flow (TBF). The mean TBF has been shown to be higher in benign tumors compared with malignancies; however, this difference is more pronounced with PA compared with WT. Multiparametric MR imaging combining DWI and quantitative ADC with perfusion MR imaging has been shown to improve distinction of PA, WT, and salivary malignancies[23–26] (**Fig. 6**).

MR SPECTROSCOPY

Proton MR spectroscopy has been shown to be able to distinguish benign from malignant tumors as well as between PA and WT based on choline/creatinine ratio using echo times of either 136 or 272 ms. The choline/creatinine ratio is higher in benign than malignant salivary neoplasms and higher in WT than PA. A choline/creatinine threshold of more than 2.4 has been suggested to have a high positive predictive values for predicting benignity. Choline is a marker of membrane turnover and is found in malignant

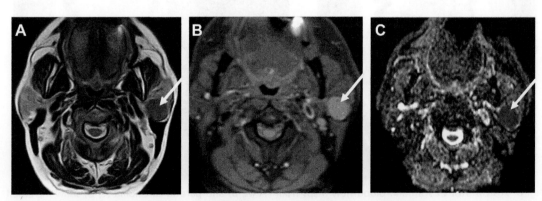

Fig. 8. Superficial lobe left parotid WT. Axial T2-weighted imaging (*A*), fast spin T1-weighted image with contrast (*B*), and ADC map (*C*) show a low T2 signal enhancing mass with low ADC values.

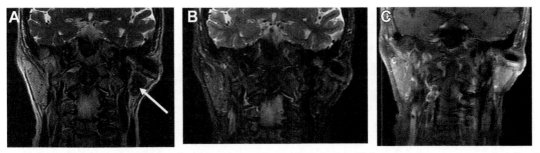

Fig. 9. Oncocytoma. Coronal T2-weighted imaging without (*A*) and with (*B*) fat saturation shows a well-defined mass in the left parotid gland (*A*) that disappears on fat-saturated imaging (*B*). The mass is also inconspicuous on T1 postcontrast imaging (*C*).

tumors as well as in hypercellular benign tumors and inflammatory processes.[27]

HISTOLOGIC CLASSIFICATION OF TUMORS
Benign Neoplastic Tumors

Pleomorphic adenoma
PA, also known as benign mixed tumor, is the most common neoplasm of the salivary glands, accounting for 70% to 80% of all benign major

SGTs. PA most commonly occur in the parotid gland, with up to 90% arising in the superficial lobe, and usually solitary.[28] Recurrent lesions are most commonly multifocal subcutaneous or parotid space masses, estimated to occur in 1% to 4% of cases based on current surgical techniques of facial nerve preservation with wide local excision or lateral lobectomy. Most recurrences occur within 10 years of surgery, but rarely have been reported decades later.[29]

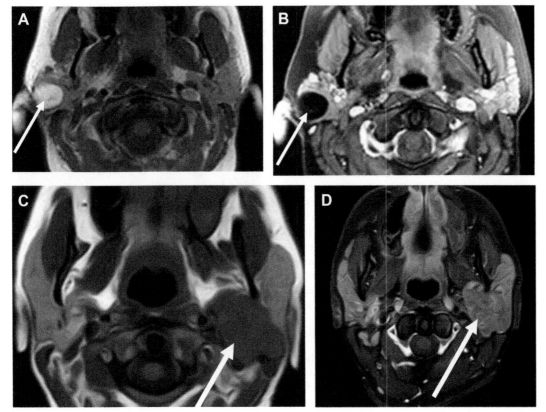

Fig. 10. Axial T1 (*A, C*) and fast spin T1-weighted image with contrast (*B, D*) images show a lipoma of the right parotid gland with T1 bright fat signal (*A*), which suppresses with fat saturation (*B*). Schwannoma of the left parotid appears as a well-defined mass (*C*) with swirled enhancement (*D*).

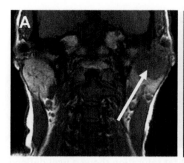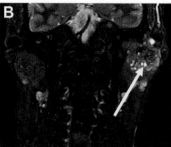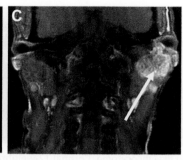

Fig. 11. Intermediate grade mucoepidermoid carcinoma. Coronal T1 (*A*), fast spin T2 (*B*) and fast spin T1+C (*C*) shows a heterogeneously enhancing left parotid mass with areas of low T2 signal and microcystic changes.

PA are composed of a variable amount of epithelial, myoepithelial, and stromal cellular elements, and the myxoid stroma is responsible for the characteristic high T2 signal of these tumors. A T2 signal greater than cerebrospinal fluid is specific for PA.[30] PA are usually well-defined masses with smaller tumors demonstrating homogenous T2 hyperintensity and enhancement. Larger PAs may have heterogeneous signal owing to areas of necrosis, hemorrhage, and/or dystrophic calcifications.[31] PA can be distinguished from other salivary tumors, except myoepithelioma by its facilitated diffusion on DWI or diffusion tensor imaging.[20] PA most commonly show a progressive time–intensity curve on dynamic contrast-enhanced MR perfusion[24] (**Fig. 7**).

Although percentages vary by study, PA have a risk of malignant degeneration into carcinoma ex PA, reported to be 9.5% in PA left untreated for 15 years.[32]

Myoepithelioma

Formerly considered a variant of PA was recognized by the World Health Organization as a distinct entity in 1991. They are benign tumors mostly made of myoepithelial cells that account for 1.5% of all SGTs and most commonly arise in the parotid glands. The peak incidence is in the third decade. Myoepitheliomas can undergo malignant transformation. They are less prone to recur than PA.[33–35] Imaging is nonspecific; however, it is generally well-defined masses with intermediate to high T2 signal and homogeneous enhancement.[36] The ADC values are elevated and not significantly differentiated from PA.[18]

Warthin tumor

WT, also known as papillary cystadenoma lymphomatosum, are slow growing tumors that arise almost exclusively in the parotid gland, most commonly at the tail, but can uncommonly develop in periparotid or cervical lymph nodes. WT is the second most common parotid gland tumor, most commonly arising in the sixth to eighth

decades, induced by smoking, and likely with a more equal sex distribution than has been reported in older literature. Histologically, these tumors are monomorphic adenomas composed of oncogenic epithelium and lymphoid stroma. Tumors are multicentric in 12% to 20% and bilateral in 5% to 14% of cases.[37,38] Malignant transformation is extremely rare.

WT are typically well-defined masses with intermediate to high T2 signal, although foci of hypointense T2 signal may be present. WT have average ADC values that are typically lower than malignancies, and most commonly with a type B time–intensity curve.[39] Adjunct techniques can support the diagnosis with increased uptake on FDG PET and on technetium 99m pertechnetate scans (**Fig. 8**).

Oncocytoma

Oncoytomas are rare tumors representing less than 1% of SGTs. Oncocytomas are slow growing

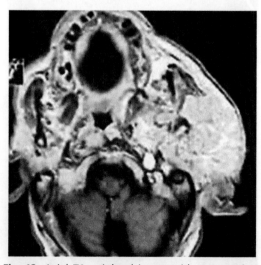

Fig. 12. Axial T1-weighted image with contrast in a patient with adenoid cystic carcinoma shows an aggressive left parotid mass with spread to the masticator and parapharyngeal spaces

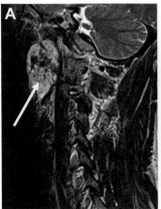 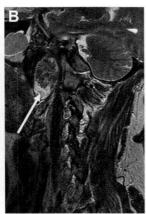 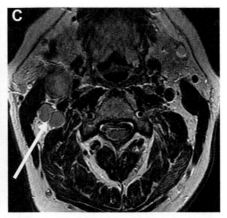

Fig. 13. Sagittal T2-weighted imaging obtained 9 years apart show a PA (*A*) that subsequently transformed into carcinoma ex PA (*B*). Note the increased amount of low T2 signal in (*B*). Axial T2-weighted imaging (*C*) shows metastatic lymphadenopathy associated with the carcinoma ex PA.

tumors most commonly arising in the parotid gland in the sixth to eighth decades, and may be unilateral or bilateral. They are composed of oncocytes, which are mitochondrial rich epithelial cells. Oncocytomas have been called the vanishing tumor owing to their isointense to parotid signal on fat-saturated T2 and postcontrast T1-weighted imaging (**Fig. 9**). Similar to WT, oncocytomas demonstrate uptake on PET and technetium 99m scans.[40]

Mesenchymal tumors

Mesenchymal tumors account for 1.5% to 5.0% of major SGTs, and are predominantly benign neoplasms, including schwannoma, neurofibroma, lipoma, hemangioma, solitary fibrous tumor, dermatofibrosarcoma protuberans, and desmoid tumor.[41] Some of these tumors can have very specific imaging features, such as lipomas, with a diffuse fat signal, and peripheral nerve sheath tumors with the target and fascicular signs. The target sign is central hypointense and peripheral hyperintense T2 signal and the fascicular sign describes multiple T2 hypointense ring-like structures within a T2 hyperintense mass[42] (**Fig. 10**).

Malignant Tumors

Mucoepidermoid carcinoma

Mucoepidermoid carcinomas are the most common salivary malignancy in both children and adults. They account for 3% to 15% of all SGTs and represent about 30% of all salivary gland malignancies. They can occur in any major salivary gland, with more than 80% arising in the parotid, especially the superficial lobe, or in the minor salivary glands. Radiation exposure is a risk factor.[28] Histologically, mucoepidermoid

carcinomas can be classified into 3 grades (low, intermediate, and high), and this grading has shown to correlate with the clinical behavior of the tumor, and propensity to infiltrate, metastasize, and recur.[43–45]

Mucoepidermoid carcinoma can have an incredibly diverse imaging appearance, which varies by tumor grade. Low-grade lesions tend to be well-defined, often with T2 hyperintense cystic areas, and can mimic PA. Even low-grade tumors can have ill-defined margins owing to peritumoral inflammatory changes. Higher grade lesions tend to have fewer cystic areas and a lower T2 signal, poorly defined margins, and metastasis, most commonly to the parotid or cervical lymph nodes, (**Fig. 11**). Perineural spread and distant metastases may also occur.[46]

Adenoid cystic carcinoma

Adenoid cystic carcinoma is a slow growing, infiltrative epithelial malignancy with a very high propensity for perineural spread. It is the second most common primary parotid malignancy in adults, with a slight female predominance. Histologically, it is characterized by a tubular, cribriform, or solid growth pattern, with solid components associated with more aggressive behavior, a poorer prognosis, and lymph node metastasis. Minor salivary glands, particularly along the palate, are involved more frequently than all the major salivary glands combined. Metastasis is most common to the lungs, with lymph node metastasis occurring less frequently. There is a tendency for recurrence, which may occur years after surgery.[47,48]

Imaging is nonspecific. As with other malignancies, higher grade lesions tend to have lower T2 and ADC signal with infiltrative margins. Attention

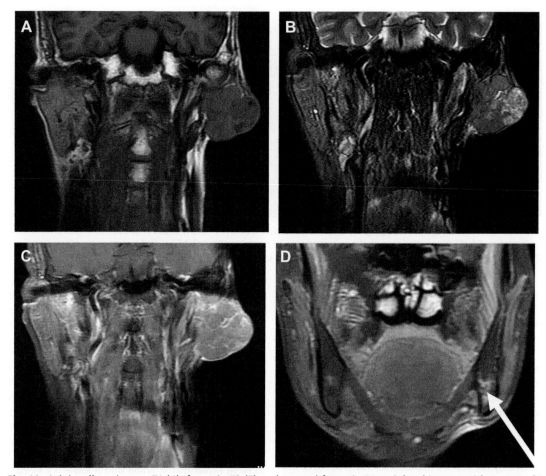

Fig. 14. Acinic cell carcinoma. T1 (*A*), fast spin T2 (*B*) and coronal fast spin T1-weighted images with contrast (*C, D*) show a mildly enhancing mass with predominantly hypointense T2 signal in the left parotid. (*D*) Perineural spread along the inferior alveolar nerve.

should be paid for perineural spread (facial, auriculo-temporal, or mandibular nerves for parotid tumors and inferior alveolar and palatine nerves for oral cavity lesions). These slow growing tumors may not demonstrate FDG avidity on PET[49] (**Fig. 12**).

Carcinoma ex pleomorphic adenoma
Carcinoma ex PA, also called malignant mixed tumor, is a malignancy arising within a PA and has shown an increased incidence over the past decade. The rate of malignant transformation is variably reported in the literature, estimated to be up to 15%, although increasing with a longer duration of preexisting PA. Clinically, rapid growth or new facial pain or paralysis in a preexisting salivary mass is concerning for malignant degeneration. On imaging, areas of low T2 and low ADC signal, irregular margins, metastatic lymphadenopathy, and perineural spread are concerning for development of carcinoma ex PA.[50–52] Tumor size larger

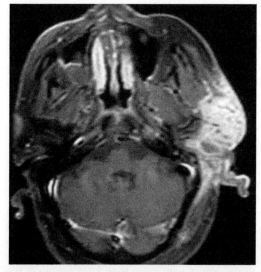

Fig. 15. Lymphoma. Axial fast spin T1-weighted image with contrast shows poorly defined enhancing mass in the left parotid gland with extraglandular extension into adjacent soft tissues.

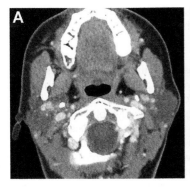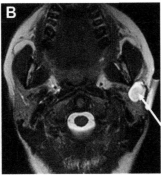

Fig. 16. Axial postcontrast CT scan (*A*) and T2-weighted imaging (*B*) show a discrete T2 hyperintense mass in the left parotid gland, found to be PA, which is inconspicuous on a CT scan.

than 4 cm, lymphadenopathy, and distant metastatic disease indicate a poorer prognosis[53] (**Fig. 13**).

Acinic cell carcinoma

Acinic cell carcinomas are generally slow-growing, low-grade malignancies and are the third most common salivary malignancy in adults and second most common in children, with a mild female predilection. Of these tumors, 80% to 90% occur in the parotid glands. Acinic cell carcinoma is the most common parotid epithelial malignancy to present bilaterally. Risk factors include radiation exposure and familial predisposition. There is a tendency for local recurrence, which may occur many years after treatment. Metastases are most common to lymph nodes, lungs, and bone.[54,55] Imaging finds are nonspecific and may simulate a benign appearance (**Fig. 14**).

Mammary analog secretory carcinoma

Mammary analog secretory carcinoma was a new addition to the 2017 World Health Organization classification and pathologically resembles secretory carcinoma of the breast. First described in 2010, it is a rare malignancy, usually low grade, and most commonly found in the parotid glands, however, with a potential for high-grade transformation. There are no distinctive clinical or radiologic criteria; however, most commonly mammary analog secretory carcinoma appears as a small, well-defined parotid mass.[56]

Lymphoma

Lymphoma of the salivary glands is rare, mostly occurring in the parotids, and accounting for less than 5% of all lymphomas and approximately 2% of salivary tumors. Parotid lymphoma can be secondary to systemic disease or primary nodal or

---

Box 2
Potential pitfalls in MR imaging interpretation

Interpretation	Pitfall
T2 hyperintensity does not mean a mass is cystic	Administer contrast to distinguish solid and cystic masses
	PA is characteristically a T2 hyperintense mass
Well-defined tumor margins mean a mass is benign	Low-grade malignancies may have well-defined margins
Ill-defined margins suggest malignancy	Infectious/inflammatory disease has ill-defined margins
	Sialoadenitis may complicate benign tumors
Low ADC values are concerning for malignancy	WT has ADC values, which tend to be lower than malignancies
Perineural spread of tumor is seen with aggressive malignancy	Perineural disease may appear noncontiguous on MR imaging
Abnormal lymph nodes are concerning for metastatic disease	Infectious/inflammatory disease can mimic metastatic lymphadenopathy
Heterogeneous enhancement with or without cystic postoperative changes signify recurrent tumor disease	Postoperative changes can mimic residual or recurrent tumor disease

parenchymal (mucosa-associated lymphoid tissue associated), typically B-cell, lymphoma. The incidence of mucosa-associated lymphoid tissue lymphoma is markedly increased in patients with autoimmune disorders, particularly Sjögren syndrome. High tumor cellularity characteristically results in restricted diffusion. Primary lymphoma may present as single or multiple distinct masses or diffuse involvement with well-demarcated or ill-defined margins. Mucosa-associated lymphoid tissue-associated lymphomas are more likely to have cystic changes. Secondary lymphoma presents as discrete nodules or diffuse gland involvement. Bilateral involvement may be present and there may be associated periparotid and cervical lymphadenopathy[57,58] (**Fig. 15**).

Metastasis

Metastatic disease to the salivary glands most frequently involves the parotid gland, which is the exclusive site for lymphatic spread as it is the only salivary gland with lymph nodes. Most commonly, the primary tumor in these cases is from cutaneous malignancies of the scalp, face, or external ear, which drain to parotid and periparotid nodes. Distant metastases are reported to occur most commonly from the kidney, lung, and breast. Imaging is nonspecific and may feature

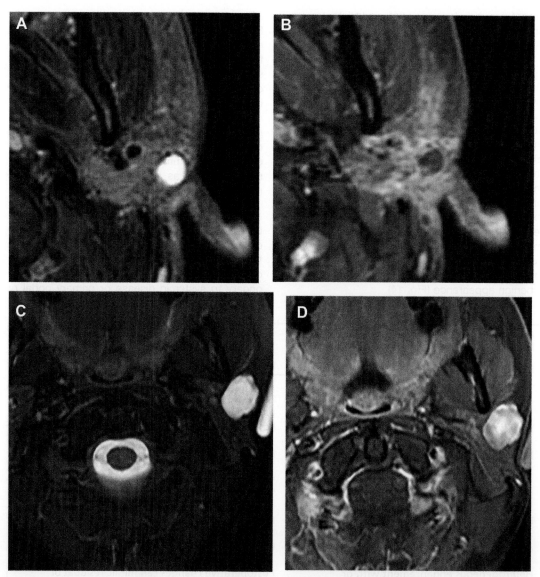

Fig. 17. Axial fast spin T2-weighted imaging (*A, C*) show 2 similar appearing well-defined T2 hyperintense lesions in the left parotid space. Fast spin T1-weighted image with contrast distinguishes the postoperative sialocele (*B*) from the PA (*D*). Not all T2 bright lesions are cystic.

only a solitary mass. Metastases can have well or ill-defined margins.[59,60]

MR IMAGING PITFALLS

Some glandular masses are inconspicuous from surrounding salivary gland tissue by CT scan, and consequently MR imaging, with its superior tissue characterization, is the preferred imaging modality to assess noninflammatory masses of the salivary glands (**Fig. 16**). Although certain MR imaging findings can be used to suggest that a mass is more likely to be benign or low-grade malignant versus as a high-grade malignancy, interpreting radiologists should be aware of potential imaging pitfalls that may confound interpretation (**Box 2, Fig. 17**).

SUMMARY

MR imaging findings are usually not specific for a particular histopathologic diagnosis and ultimately biopsy or excision is required for definitive diagnosis. We can use certain conventional MR Imaging features to suggest that a mass is more likely to be a benign or low-grade malignancy versus high-grade, and adding advanced MR techniques (DWI/diffusion tensor imaging, perfusion, spectroscopy) can aid in this distinction. It is important to be cognizant of potential pitfalls when interpreting imaging, and keep in mind that the smaller the gland, the higher the likelihood of malignancy, such that sublingual masses should be considered malignant regardless of appearance until proven otherwise.

REFERENCES

1. American Cancer Society online statistics. 2017. Available at: cancer.org. Accessed July 15, 2020.

2. Boukheris H, Curtis RE, Land CE, et al. Incidence of carcinoma of the major salivary glands according to the WHO classification, 1992-2006: a population-based study in the United States. Cancer Epidemiol Biomarkers Prev 2009;18(11):2899–906.

3. El-Naggar AK, Chan JKC, Grandis JR, et al. WHO classification of head and neck tumors. 4th edition. Lyon (France): WHO; 2017.

4. Lee W, Tseng T, Hsu H, et al. Salivary gland tumors: a 20-year review of clinical diagnostic accuracy at a single center. Oncol Lett 2014;7:583–7.

5. Bradley P. Frequency and histopathology by site, major pathologies, symptoms and signs of salivary gland neoplasms. Adv Otorhinolaryngol 2016;78:9–16.

6. Sreenivasa P, V Bhosale R. Frequency and distribution pattern of minor salivary gland tumors: a clinico-pathological retrospective study. Int J Contemp Med Surg Radiol 2018;3:84–6.

7. Luna MA, Batsakis JG, El-Naggar A. Salivary gland tumors in children. Ann Otol Rhinol Laryngol 1991; 100:869–71.

8. Amin MB, Edge SB, Greene FL, et al, editors. AJCC cancer staging manual. 8th edition. Chicago: Springer; 2017.

9. Kim JY, Yang HC, Lee S, et al. Effectiveness of anatomic criteria for predicting parotid tumour location. Clin Otolaryngol 2016;41:154–9.

10. Chu J, Zhou Z, Hong G, et al. High-resolution MRI of the intraparotid facial nerve based on a microsurface coil and a 3D reversed fast imaging with steady-state precession DWI sequence at 3T. AJNR Am J Neuroradiol 2013;34:1643–8.

11. Li C, Li Y, Zhang D, et al. 3D-FIESTA at 3 T demonstrating branches of the intraparotid facial nerve, parotid ducts, and relation with benign parotid tomours. Clin Radiol 2012;67:1078–82.

12. Guenette JP, Ben-Shlomo N, Jayender J, et al. MR Imaging of the extracranial facial nerve with the CISS sequence. AJNR Am J Neuroradiol 2019;40: 1954–9.

13. Rouchy R, Attye A, Medici M, et al. Facial nerve tractography: a new tool for detection of perineural spread in parotid cancers. Eur Radiol 2018;28: 3861–71.

14. Christe A, Waldherr C, Hallett R, et al. MR Imaging of parotid tumors: typical lesion characteristics in MR Imaging improve discrimination between benign and malignant disease. AJNR Am J Neuroradiol 2011;32:1202–7.

15. Kato H, Kanematsu M, Watanabe H, et al. Salivary gland tumors of the parotid gland: CT and MR imaging findings with emphasis on intratumoral cystic components. Neuroradiol 2014;56:789–95.

16. Schmalfuss IM, Tart RP, Mukherji S, et al. Perineural tumor spread along the auriculotemporal nerve. AJNR Am J Neuroradiol 2002;23:303–11.

17. Thoeny HC, De Keyzer F, King AD. Diffusion-weighted MR Imaging in the Head and Neck. Radiol 2012;263:19–32.

18. Habermann CR, Arndt C, Graessner J, et al. Diffusion-weighted echo-planar MR Imaging of primary parotid gland tumors: is a prediction of different histologic subtypes possible? AJNR Am J Neuroradiol 2009;30:591–6.

19. Razek AA, Elkhamary SM, Nada N. Correlation of apparent diffusion coefficient with histopathological parameters of salivary gland cancer. J Oral Maxillofac Surg 2019;48:995–1000.

20. Takumi K, Fukukura Y, Hakamada H, et al. Value of diffusion tensor imaging in differentiating malignant from benign parotid gland tumors. Eur J Radiol 2017;95:249–56.

21. Razek AA. Characterization of salivary gland tumors with diffusion tensor imaging. Dentomaxillofac Radiol 2018;47:20170343.

22. Razek AA, Mukherji SK. Imaging of posttreatment salivary gland tumors. Neuroimag Clin North Am 2018;28:199–208.

23. Essig M, Shiroishi MS, Nguyen TB, et al. Perfusion MRI: the five most frequently asked technical questions. AJR Am J Roentgenol 2013;200:24–34.

24. Lam PD, Kuribayashi A, Imaizumi A, et al. Differentiating benign and malignant salivary gland tumors: diagnostic criteria and the accuracy of dynamic-contrast enhanced MRI with high temporal resolution. Br J Radiol 2015;88:20140685.

25. Razek AA. Multi-parametric MR Imaging using pseudo-continuous arterial-spin labeling and diffusion-weighted MR Imaging in differentiating subtypes of parotid tumors. Magn Reson Imaging 2019;63:55–9.

26. Razek AA, Samir S, Ashmalla GA. Characterization of parotid tumors with dynamic susceptibility contrast perfusion-weighted Magnetic Resonance Imaging and diffusion-weighted imaging. J Comput Assist Tomogr 2017;41:131–6.

27. King AD, Yeung DK, Ahuja AT, et al. Salivary gland tumors at in vivo Proton MR Spectroscopy. Radiol 2005;237:563–9.

28. Som PM, Brandwein-Genslet MS. Anatomy and pathology of the salivary glands. In: Som PM, Curtin HD, editors. Head and neck imaging. 5th edition. St Louis (MO): Mosby; 2011. p. 2449–609.

29. Moonis G, Patel P, Koshkareva Y, et al. Imaging characteristics of recurrent pleomorphic adenoma of the parotid gland. AJNR Am J Neuroradiol 2007;28:1532–6.

30. Tsushima Y, Matsumoto M, Endo K, et al. Characteristic bright signal of parotid pleomorphic adenomas on T2-weighted MR images with pathologic correlation. Clin Radiol 1994;49:485–9.

31. Yerli H, Aydin E, Coskun M, et al. Dynamic multislice computed tomography findings for parotid gland tumors. Comput Assist Tomogr 2007;31:309–16.

32. Seifert G. Histopathology of malignant salivary gland tumours. Oral Oncol Eur J Cancer 1992;28B:49–56.

33. Barca I, Novembre D, Cordaro R, et al. Myoepithelioma of the parotid gland: a case report with review of the literature. Oral Maxillofac Surg Cases 2020;6:100131.

34. Ellis GL, Auclair PL. Tumors of the salivary glands. In: AFIP Atlas of Tumor Pathology, Series 4. Washington, DC: American Registry of Pathology; 2008.

35. Alos I, Cardesa A, Bombi JA, et al. Myoepithelial tumors of salivary glands: a clinicopathological, immunohistochemical, ultrastructural and flow cytometric study. Sem Diagn Pathol 1996;13:138–47.

36. Sciubba JJ, Brannon RB. Myoepithelioma of salivary glands: report of 23 cases. Cancer 1982;49:562–72.

37. Raghu AR, Shweta R, Kundendu, et al. Warthin's tumor: a case report and review of Pathogenesis and its histological subtypes. J Clin Diagn Res 2014;8:37–40.

38. Tunc O, Gonuldas B, Arslanhan Y, et al. Changes in Warthin's tumor incidence: a 20-year joinpoint trend analysis. Eur Arch Otorhinol 2020;277:3431–4.

39. Ikeda M, Motoori K, Hanazawa T, et al. Warthin tumor of the parotid gland: diagnostic value of MR imaging with histopathologic correlation. AJNR Am J Neuroradiol 2004;25:1256–62.

40. Patel ND, Zante AV, Eisele DW, et al. Oncocytoma: the vanishing parotid mass. AJNR Am J Neuroradiol 2011;32:1703–6.

41. Cho KJ, Ro J, Choi J, et al. Mesenchymal neoplasms of the major salivary glands: clinicopathological features of 18 cases. Eur Arch Otorhinolaryngol 2007;265:47–56.

42. Shimizu K, Iwai H, Ikeda K, et al. Intraparotid facial nerve schwannoma: a report of five cases and an analysis of MR imaging results. AJNR Am J Neuroradiol 2005;26:1328–30.

43. Goode RK, Auclair PL, Ellis GL. Mucoepidermoid carcinoma of the major salivary glands: clinical and histological analysis of 234 cases with evaluation of grading criteria. Cancer 1998;82:1217–24.

44. Brandwein MS, Ivanov K, Wallace DI, et al. Mucoepidermoid carcinoma. A clinicopathologic study of 80 patients with special reference to histological grading. Am J Surg Pathol 2001;25:835–45.

45. Nance AM, Seethala RR, Wang Y, et al. Treatment and survival outcomes based on histological grading in patients with head and neck mucoepidermoid carcinoma. Cancer 2008;113:2082–9.

46. Kashiwagi N, Dote K, Kawano K, et al. MRI findings of mucoepidermoid carcinoma of the parotid gland: correlation with pathologic features. Br J Radiol 2012;85:709–13.

47. Min R, Siyi L, Wenjun Y, et al. Salivary gland adenoid cystic carcinoma with cervical lymph node metastasis: a preliminary study of 62 cases. Int J Oral Maxillofac Surg 2012;41:952–7.

48. Histopathological grading of adenoid cystic carcinoma of the head and neck: analysis of currently used grading systems and proposal for simplified grading scheme. Oral Oncol 2015;51:71–6.

49. Purohit BS, Ailianou A, Dulguerov N, et al. FDG-PET/CT pitfalls in oncological head and neck imaging. Insights Imag 2014;5:585–602.

50. Andreasen S, Therkildsen M, Bjorndal K, et al. Pleomorphic adenoma of the parotid gland 1985-2010: a Danish nationwide study of incidence, recurrent rate, and malignant transformation. Head Neck 2016;38(Supp 1):E1364–9.

51. Kato H, Kanematsu M, Mizuta K, et al. Carcinoma ex pleomorphic adenoma of the parotid gland: radiologic-pathologic correlation with MR imaging including diffusion-weighted imaging. AJNR Am J Neuroradiol 2008;29:865–7.

52. Seifert G, Sobin LH. Histological typing of salivary gland tumors. In: World Health Organization International histological classification of tumors. 2nd edition. Berlin: Springer-Verlag; 1991. p. 20–1.

53. Gupta A, Koochakzadeh S, Neskey DM, et al. Carcinoma ex pleomorphic adenoma: a review of incidence, demographics, risk factors, and survival. Am J Otolaryngol 2019;40:102279.

54. Durand N, Mourrain-Langlois E, LeClair F, et al. Synchronous bilateral acinic cell carcinoma of the parotid: when a tumor reveals another one. Eur Ann Otorhinolaryngol Head Neck Dis 2013;130:22–5.

55. Al-Zaher N, Obeid A, Al-Salam S, et al. Acinic cell carcinoma of the salivary glands: a literature review. Hematol Oncol Stem Cell Ther 2009;2:259–64.

56. Bissinger O, Götz C, Kolk A, et al. Mammary analogue secretory carcinoma of salivary glands: diagnostic pitfall with distinct immunohistochemical profile and molecular features. Rare Tumors 2017; 9:89–92.

57. Kato H, Kanematsu M, Goto H, et al. Mucosa-associated lymphoid tissue lymphoma of the salivary glands: MR imaging findings including diffusion-weighted imaging. Eur J Radiol 2012;81:e612–7.

58. Zhu L, Wang P, Yang J, et al. Non-Hodgkin lymphoma involving the parotid gland: CT and MR imaging findings. Dentomaxillofac Radiol 2013;42: 20130046.

59. Seifert G, Hennings K, Caselitz J, et al. Metastatic tumors to the parotid and submandibular glands—analysis and differential diagnosis of 108 cases. Pathol Res Pract 1986;181:684–92.

60. Kashiwagi N, Murakami T, Toguchi M, et al. Metastases to the parotid nodes: CT and MR imaging findings. Dentomaxillofac Radiol 2016;45: 20160201.

Update on MR Imaging of Soft Tissue Tumors of Head and Neck

Justin D. Rodriguez, MD[a], A. Morgan Selleck, MD[b],
Ahmed Abdel Khalek Abdel Razek, MD[c,†], Benjamin Y. Huang, MD, MPH[d,*]

KEYWORDS

- Soft tissue tumors • MR imaging • Lipoma • Sarcoma • Head and neck • WHO, fifth edition
- Rhabdomyosarcoma

KEY POINTS

- The recently published fifth edition of the *WHO Classification of Bone and Soft Tissue Tumours* includes several new entities and further incorporates genetic information into tumor classification.
- Imaging features of most soft tissue tumors in the head and neck frequently are nonspecific, and narrowing the differential diagnosis requires consideration of location, patient demographics, and clinical presentation.
- Advanced imaging techniques, such as diffusion-weighted and dynamic contrast-enhanced MR imaging, can be helpful in distinguishing some malignant and benign tumors.

INTRODUCTION

Soft tissue tumors represent a heterogeneous collection of benign and malignant lesions that develop from various nonepithelial and extraskeletal elements, including adipose tissue, smooth and skeletal muscle, tendon, cartilage, fibrous tissue, blood vessels, and lymphatics. These tumors are formally cataloged in the *WHO Classification of Soft Tissue and Bone Tumours*, which was updated in 2020 with the publication of the fifth edition.[1] The newest update introduced several recently described tumor types, summarized new prognostic information for existing entities, and further incorporated newly discovered genetic data into the current classification of soft tissue tumors. Currently, the World Health Organization (WHO) classification delineates 11 different groups of soft tissue tumors based on their presumed histologic origin. The categories include adipocytic, fibroblastic/myofibroblastic, so-called fibrohistiocytic, vascular, pericytic, smooth muscle, skeletal muscle, gastrointestinal stromal, chondro-osseous, peripheral nerve sheath, and tumors of uncertain differentiation (**Box 1**). In addition, the fifth edition adds a new category, "Undifferentiated small round cell sarcomas of bone and soft tissue," which includes Ewing sarcoma and several more recently described Ewing-like sarcomas characterized by specific genetic alterations.[1]

Compared with epithelial neoplasms, which make up greater than 90% of cancers in the head and neck, tumors arising from the soft tissues of this region are relatively infrequent. The estimated annual incidence of head and neck soft tissue neoplasms is approximately only 300 per 100,000 individuals.[2] These tumors can be categorized further based on their biologic potential into benign, intermediate

[a] Department of Radiology, Duke University, 2301 Erwin Rd, Durham, NC 27705, USA; [b] Department of Otolaryngology/Head and Neck Surgery, University of North Carolina Hospitals, 170 Manning Drive, CB 7070, Physicians Office Building, Rm G190A, Chapel Hill, NC 27599, USA; [c] Department of Radiology, Mansoura University, Elgomheryia Street, Mansoura 35512, Egypt; [d] Department of Radiology, UNC School of Medicine, 101 Manning Drive, CB#7510, Chapel Hill, NC 27599, USA
[†] Deceased
* Corresponding author.
E-mail address: bhuang@med.unc.edu

Magn Reson Imaging Clin N Am 30 (2022) 151–198
https://doi.org/10.1016/j.mric.2021.06.019

Box 1
Selected soft tissue tumors of the head and neck in the *WHO Classification of Bone and Soft Tissue Tumours*, fifth edition

Adipocytic tumors

  Benign

    Lipoma (including angiolipoma, myolipoma, chondroid lipoma, and spindle cell/pleomorphic lipoma)

    Lipomatosis

    Lipoblastoma and lipoblastomatosis

    Hibernoma

    ASLT[a]

  Intermediate—locally aggressive

    Atypical lipomatous tumor/well-differentiated liposarcoma

  Malignant

    Liposarcoma (dedifferentiated, myxoid, pleomorphic, and myxoid pleomorphic[a])

Fibroblastic and myofibroblastic tumors

  Benign

    Nodular fasciitis

    MO

    Fibromatosis colli

    EWSR1-SMAD3–positive fibroblastic tumor (emerging)[a]

    Angiofibroma of soft tissue[a]

  Intermediate—locally aggressive

    Desmoid fibromatosis

  Intermediate—rarely metastasizing

    DFSP

    SFT[b]

    IMT

    Superficial CD34-positive fibroblastic tumor[a]

  Malignant

    Infantile fibrosarcoma

    Adult fibrosarcoma

    MFS

    LGMS

So-called fibrohistiocytic tumors

  Benign

    TGCT

    Deep fibrous histiocytoma

  Intermediate—rarely metastasizing

    Plexiform fibrohistiocytic tumor

    GCT-ST

  Malignant

    Malignant TGCT

Pericytic (perivascular) tumors

  Benign and intermediate

    Glomus tumor

    Myopericytoma, including myofibroma

    Angioleiomyoma

  Malignant

    Malignant glomus tumor

Smooth muscle tumors

  Benign

    Leiomyoma

  Intermediate

    EBV-associated smooth muscle tumor[a]

  Malignant

    Inflammatory LMS[a]

    LMS

Skeletal muscle tumors

  Benign

    Rhabdomyoma

  Malignant

    ERMS

    ARMS

    Pleomorphic RMS

    Spindle cell/sclerosing RMS

    Ectomesenchymoma[c]

GIST

  GIST

Chondro-osseous tumors

  Benign

    Soft tissue chondroma

  Malignant

    Extraskeletal osteosarcoma

    Mesenchymal chondrosarcoma

Peripheral nerve sheath tumors

  Benign

    Schwannoma

    Neurofibroma

    Perineurioma

Granular cell tumor

BTT/neuromuscular choristoma

Malignant

MPNST

MMNST[a]

Tumors of uncertain differentiation

Benign

Intramuscular myxoma

Juxta-articular myxoma

Malignant

NTRK-rearranged spindle cell neoplasm (emerging)[a]

Synovial sarcoma

ASPS

Undifferentiated soft tissue sarcoma[a] (including spindle cell, pleomorphic, and round cell subtypes)

Undifferentiated small round cell sarcomas of soft tissue[d]

Malignant

Ewing sarcoma

Round cell sarcoma with EWSR1–non-ETS fusions[a]

CIC-rearranged sarcoma[a]

Sarcoma with BCOR genetic alterations[a]

Other tumors (described in the WHO Classification of Head and Neck Tumours)

BSNS

Nasopharyngeal angiofibroma

Sinonasal glomangiopericytoma

[a]New entity in the fifth edition of the WHO Classification of Head and Neck Tumours.[b]Benign and malignant forms also exist.[c]Previously in the peripheral nerve sheath tumor category.[d]Previously described in the category of tumors of unknown differentiation.

(locally aggressive), intermediate (rarely metastasizing), and malignant neoplasms. A large majority of soft tissue tumors are benign, with malignant tumors accounting for less than 1% overall.[1,2] Among soft tissue sarcomas, approximately 5% to 15% arise in the head and neck, although it is notable that in children, approximately a third of soft tissue sarcomas arise in this region.[3–5]

Virtually any tumor of soft tissue origin can be found in the head and neck; however, a relatively small subset is encountered with any degree of frequency, with the most common benign tumors occurring in the region being lipomas. Among

head and neck sarcomas, approximately 80% arise from the soft tissues. In adults, the specific topographic area determines the types of sarcomas that are most likely to be encountered. In the region of the neck, including the pharynx and larynx, liposarcoma, synovial sarcoma, and malignant peripheral nerve sheath tumor (MPNST) predominate; in the skin of the scalp and face, angiosarcoma and dermatofibrosarcoma protuberans (DFSP) are the most common; in the sinonasal tract, MPNST is encountered most frequently, followed by myxofibrosarcoma (MFS); and, in the oral cavity, leiomyosarcoma (LMS) and rhabdomyosarcoma (RMS) are most prevalent.[3] In children and adolescents, RMS is by far the most common soft tissue malignancy, followed by Ewing sarcoma.[3,5,6]

Soft tissue tumors that appear commonly in the head and neck region also are included in the separately published WHO Classification of Head and Neck Tumours,[7] the fourth edition of which was published in 2017. This volume describes tumors based on site of occurrence, which include the nasal cavity, paranasal sinuses, and skull base; nasopharynx; hypopharynx, larynx, trachea and parapharyngeal space; oral cavity and mobile tongue; oropharynx; neck and lymph nodes; and salivary glands.[7] For the most part, the entries in the head and neck tumor classification overlap those in the soft tissue and bone tumor classification; however, a few entities, including nasopharyngeal angiofibroma, sinonasal glomangiopericytoma, and biphenotypic sinonasal sarcoma (BSNS), are unique to the former publication.

Soft tissue tumors in the head and neck often present a clinical diagnostic challenge, because they frequently present with a nonspecific history and physical examination findings—usually consisting of a painless, enlarging subcutaneous or submucosal mass. Imaging remains an important diagnostic adjunct, with ultrasonography (US), computed tomography (CT), or MR imaging all potentially having roles in lesion characterization or patient management. Although US or CT might be performed initially and frequently is used for biopsy guidance, MR imaging is the ideal imaging modality for these tumors, given its superior contrast resolution and ability to better characterize the lesion location, extension, and involvement of nearby structures in the setting of the highly complex anatomy of the head and neck. In many instances, however, a specific tissue diagnosis is not possible with imaging alone. The literature on the accuracy of MR imaging of soft tissue neoplasms, although not head and neck specific, has demonstrated a wide variability. Some studies have reported the accuracy of imaging to differentiate malignant from benign soft tissue tumors as high as 85% to 90%,[8,9] but other studies have demonstrated an accuracies as low as 50%.[10–12] The ability to noninvasively diagnose specific tumor type has proved even more challenging, with studies reporting accuracies as low as 16% for diagnosing soft tissue tumors.[10,11] Nevertheless, even when a specific diagnosis cannot be made noninvasively, imaging often plays an essential role in the evaluation and management of patients with soft tissue tumors, because it can aid in tumor staging, planning of biopsies or surgical resections, evaluating response to treatment, and detecting tumor recurrences.

This article reviews the most recent update to the WHO classification of soft tissue tumors, introduces entities new to the classification, and discusses the clinical and MR imaging characteristics of several soft tissue tumors in the head and neck. Although a comprehensive review of every entity in the classification is beyond the scope of this text, this article attempts to highlight tumors that arise with greater frequency in the head and neck or that are new or have distinctive characteristics. Where possible, the focus is on differentiating clinical and MR imaging features that may allow diagnosing specific tumors or to narrow the imaging differential diagnosis.

CLINICAL AND IMAGING FEATURES THAT MAY AID IN DIFFERENTIATING SOFT TISSUE TUMORS

Differentiating types of soft tissue tumors, or even differentiating benign from malignant tumors, is difficult and frequently impossible by imaging alone. Whenever possible, clinical features, including age of the patient, duration and rapidity of onset of the mass, presence of pain, concomitant medical conditions or genetic syndromes, and history of trauma or prior irradiation should be taken into consideration. Multiplicity, location of the mass, and certain characteristic imaging features including calcification, MR imaging signal intensity, and vascularity of a lesion, also can be helpful in paring the list of potential differential diagnoses.

Patient Demographics and Clinical History

Imaging always should be correlated with clinical and demographic data when interpreting studies. Patient age can be an important discriminator in constructing a differential, because several entities, such as RMSs, infantile hemangiomas, lipoblastoma, fibromatosis colli, and myofibroma, occur primarily in younger children. Hibernomas, desmoid-type fibromatoses, synovial sarcomas, and Ewing sarcomas occur primarily in adolescents and young adults, whereas lesions, such as liposarcoma, angiosarcoma, and undifferentiated pleomorphic sarcoma, occur primarily in older adults.

A patient's clinical presentation may also further improve specificity in diagnosis. Painless, slow-growing, and long-standing masses are more likely to represent benign lesions, whereas the presence of pain or a rapid increase in the size of a mass is worrisome for malignancy.[13] Past medical history also can provide clues to diagnosis. For instance, a calcified mass arising in an area of previous trauma to the area may suggest a diagnosis of MO. Alternatively, a history of prior irradiation to the site of a tumor should invoke the possibility of a radiation-induced sarcoma, particularly if the mass arises years after completion of radiation therapy. The median latency period between radiation exposure and sarcoma development has been estimated at approximately 9 years to 11 years, with a range of 3 years to 36 years.[14,15] Numerous types of sarcomas are reported in the postradiation setting, with common histologies including LMS, fibrosarcoma, undifferentiated pleomorphic sarcoma, angiosarcoma, and osteosarcoma.

In some cases, history of a predisposing condition or syndrome or the presence of concomitant lesions may be helpful in making diagnoses. For example, desmoid-type fibromatosis is seen in association with Gardner syndrome, cutaneous myxomas can be seen in in patients with Carney complex,[16] and intramuscular myxomas are seen in association with fibrous dysplasia in patients with Mazabraud syndrome.[17]

Lesion Morphology and MR imaging Signal Characteristics

A higher likelihood of malignancy is suggested by the presence of certain conventional imaging features, including larger lesion volume; extracompartmental spread; presence of poorly defined margins; a broad interface with adjacent fascia; heterogeneous signal intensity on all MR imaging pulse sequences; high signal intensity on T2-weighted images; invasion of bone or neurovascular structures; intratumoral hemorrhage or necrosis; or marked primarily peripheral enhancement.[18] Although the relative sensitivity and specificity of any individual sign is quite low, the probability of malignancy increases with the number of suspicious features present. In general, size more than 5 cm and location beneath the deep fascia are signs associated more frequently with malignancy. Size smaller than 3 cm, lobulated or smooth well-defined margins, and superficial location are more suggestive of a benign lesion.

Signal intensity on MR imaging and contrast enhancement features on either CT or MR imaging occasionally can be helpful. Very low signal intensity on T2-weighted images may indicate the presence of hemosiderin, calcification, or fibrous tissue. For example, identification of a low signal lesion in the region of the temporomandibular joint (TMJ) is highly suggestive of a tenosynovial giant cell tumor (TGCT), which is characterized by intratumoral hemosiderin deposition (**Fig. 1**). Similarly, tumors containing calcification, such as chondrosarcomas, osteosarcomas, and MO, typically demonstrate areas of signal void on T2-weighted images. Tumors containing fibrous tissue, such as desmoid-type fibromatoses, LMS, and fibrosarcoma, also can demonstrate T2-weighted hypointensity relative to muscle, although this is not universally true of all fibrous tumors.[19]

A myxoid tumor can be suspected if a lesion is extremely bright on T2-weighted sequences and hypointense with T1-weighting—presumedly due to the high water content of myxoid tissue—and enhances on MR imaging (distinguishing the mass from a cyst)[20] (**Fig. 2**). On the other hand, the presence of macroscopic fat signal intensity within a lesion (high signal on T1-weighted images that drops out with fat suppression techniques) should narrow the differential to tumors in the adipocytic family of tumors, whereas the presence of multiple signal void regions and/or intense contrast enhancement leads to considering highly vascularized tumors, such as giant cell angiofibroma, hemangiopericytoma, sinonasal glomus tumors, and members of the vascular soft tissue tumor family. Certain other tumors, including angiofibromas, desmoid-type fibromatosis, angioleiomyomas, and hemangiopericytomas, also tend to demonstrate marked enhancement.

Generally speaking, malignant lesions tend to show greater enhancement and a greater rate of enhancement than benign tumors (discussed later). In addition, heterogeneous enhancement, particularly in association with areas of necrosis, suggests malignancy.[18,19] In most cases, however, enhancement alone cannot be used to distinguish benign from malignant lesions reliably.

Lesion Location and Number

Certain tumors more commonly affect specific regions in the head and neck. For instance, fibromatosis colli exclusively involves the sternocleidomastoid muscle, whereas TGCT involves the TMJ. Lesions frequently affecting the orbits include inflammatory pseudotumor and RMS. Soft tissue tumors that more commonly arise in the sinonasal cavities include many sarcomas (fibrosarcoma,

RMS, and LMS), solitary fibrous tumors (SFTs), BSNS, and sinonasal glomangiopericytoma. Some tumors have predilections for certain anatomic compartments, such as skin (DFSP), subcutaneous tissues (lipoma and nodular fasciitis), intermuscular regions (synovial sarcoma, lipoma, and MO), intramuscular compartment (lipoma, liposarcoma, and RMS), and meninges (SFT).[21]

In addition, the presence of multiple lesions may suggest an underlying syndrome, such as neurofibromas in the setting of neurofibromatosis type 1 (NF1), multiple myofibromas in infantile myofibromatosis, desmoid tumors in the setting of Gardner syndrome, or intramuscular myxomas in a patient with Mazabraud syndrome. Finally, infiltrative, transpatial lesions may be seen in patients with sarcomas, lipomas, hemangiomas, and lymphangiomas.

Calcification

The presence of calcification in a lesion occasionally can help establish a tissue diagnosis. Mineralization of the soft tissue may be due to matrix calcification or ossification, which should lead to focusing on chondro-osseous–type tumors. Linear spiculated calcification or amorphous central calcifications are seen in osteosarcoma, whereas stippled and curvilinear calcifications are typical of cartilaginous tumors, such as soft tissue chondroma and chondrosarcoma. Peripheral calcification can be seen in myositis ossificans (MO) and ossifying fibromyxoid tumors. Other tumors that can calcify include lipomas, liposarcoma, undifferentiated sarcoma, synovial sarcoma, and RMS.

Advanced Imaging Techniques

In addition to conventional MR imaging, there are several specialized MR imaging techniques that may complement standard MR imaging pulse sequences. These include diffusion-weighted imaging (DWI) and diffusion tensor imaging (DTI), MR imaging perfusion techniques (including dynamic contrast-enhanced [DCE] imaging), and proton MR imaging spectroscopy, all of which have been employed in the evaluation of musculoskeletal tumors.[22–24] These sequences enable additional in-depth tumor evaluation assessing tumor physiology at a molecular level. Although often not required to make a diagnosis in cases of frankly aggressive lesions, these sequences may be helpful problem-solving tools for evaluating indeterminate soft tissue lesions. A comprehensive review of these techniques is beyond the scope of this article; however, some of the more

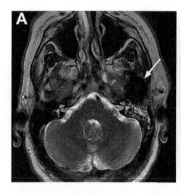
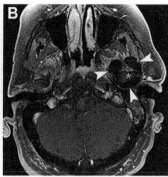

Fig. 1. TGCT in a middle-aged man with gradually changing bite. (*A*) Axial T2-weighted image demonstrates a markedly hypointense mass (*arrow*) centered along the roof of the left TMJ, and possibly extending into the floor of the middle cranial fossa. (*B*) Axial postcontrast, fat-suppressed, T1-weighted image slightly inferior to (*A*) demonstrates a hypointense lesion (*arrowheads*) wrapping around the posterior, medial and lateral aspects of the left mandibular condyle (*asterisk*). The low signal intensity is due to the presence of hemosiderin and is characteristic of TGCTs, which usually occur in the TMJ when they arise in the head and neck.

commonly employed techniques are briefly discussed later.

Diffusion-weighted imaging

DWI is perhaps the most widely incorporated of these advanced MR imaging techniques, having been studied now for several decades with multiple modality subsets developed for further assessment and specificity. In its most basic form, the concept of diffusion imaging is based on the measurement of the free movement of water molecules, and changes and abnormalities in water molecule diffusivity can be used to investigate specific tissue properties. Numerous studies investigating both epithelial and soft tissue tumors have shown that quantitative apparent diffusion coefficient (ADC) assessment may be useful for differentiating between cystic and solid lesions and between benign and malignant neoplasms.[23,25–28]

Although large-scale studies reporting on the use of DWI in characterizing soft tissue tumors in the head and neck region specifically are lacking, inferences can be drawn from literature from soft tissue tumors of other regions of the body. DWI has been shown to have utility in distinguishing between tumoral and normal tissues and in improving specificity for assessing tumor margin infiltration.[29] Still other studies have demonstrated the utility of DWI for differentiating between myxoid and nonmyxoid tumor types and between benign and malignant soft tissue tumors, with most finding that ADC or true diffusion coefficient values are significantly higher in benign mesenchymal tumors compared with malignant ones[23,26–28,30–36] (**Fig. 3**). Various other studies also have shown a negative correlation between

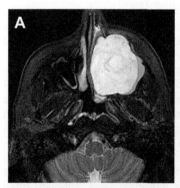
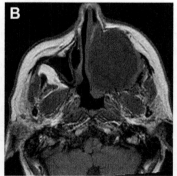
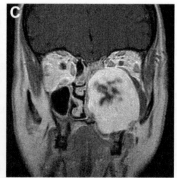

Fig. 2. Low-grade MFS of the left maxillary sinus in a middle-aged woman with left cheek swelling. (*A*) Axial T2-weighted MR image demonstrates an expansile mass centered in the left maxillary sinus, which shows marked hyperintensity, with signal similar to that of CSF. High fluid-like signal intensity on T2-weighted sequences is characteristic of tumors with a high myxoid content. (*B*) On T1-weighted images, the mass is heterogeneously hypointense compared with muscle but is slightly higher in signal than CSF. (*C*) Coronal contrast-enhanced, T1-weighted image shows diffuse enhancement with a few smaller nonenhancing regions centrally, confirming the solid rather than cystic nature of the lesion.

ADC and tumor cellularity in soft tissue tumors[37,38] and at least 1 study noted significantly lower mean ADC values in high-grade malignancies than in low-grade malignant tumors.[35]

Among tumors with myxoid features, mean ADC may not be helpful to distinguish between benign and malignant histologies, but among nonmyxoid histologies, benign tumors appear to show significantly higher ADC values on average than malignant tumors, although these values still appear to overlap substantially.[26,27] Subgroup analyses have revealed interesting trends, however. Teixeira and colleagues[27] reported that in a subset of tumors whose solid components were hyperintense compared with muscle on T2-weighted imaging, the specificity of DWI for differentiating benign and malignant tumors improved substantially. At an ADC cutoff of 1.19, DWI was able to distinguish benign from malignant soft tissue tumors with a sensitivity of 53.3% and a specificity of 65.2%. When the same cutoff was applied to only T2 hyperintense tumors, the specificity increased to 92.9% whereas the sensitivity remained unchanged. When a higher ADC cutoff of 1.68 was used for all tumors, DWI differentiated benign from malignant tumors with a sensitivity of 96.7% and a specificity of 30.4%, but when applied only to tumors, which were T2 hyperintense, the same higher ADC cutoff increased the specificity to 50% while maintaining the same high sensitivity. It also was notable that among their study population, the investigators found that all tumors that demonstrated T2-weighted signal intensities lower than muscle were benign, even though their mean ADC values were not significantly different from those of malignant tumors. They posited that tissue fibrosis might explain the finding of lower ADC values in the T2 hypointense tumors, because fibrotic tissue tends to produce lower signal intensity on T2-weighted images and probably influences ADC values in a negative direction.[27]

Several investigators also have examined the utility of DWI in monitoring treatment response and detecting early recurrences in patients with soft tissue tumors, with multiple studies reporting that tumor ADC values increase relative to pretreatment values following chemotherapy or radiotherapy, even in tumors that appear stable after treatment by size criteria alone,[31,39–42] presumably reflecting the effects of tumor necrosis on ADC. Ithas been suggested , therefore, that change in ADC may be a useful biomarker of response during early treatment before changes in tumor size occur.[43] DWI also has been shown useful in differentiating soft tissue sarcoma recurrence from benign post-treatment changes, with recurrent tumors demonstrating significantly lower diffusion values.[44]

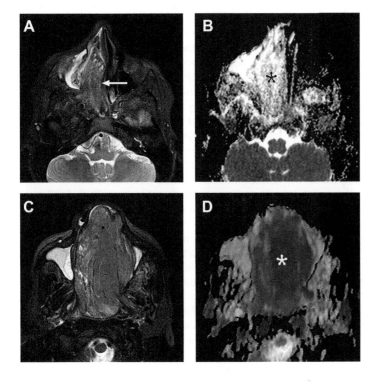

Fig. 3. Relative differences in ADC between benign and malignant tumors. (A) Axial T2-weighted image and (B) axial ADC map in a patient with a nasopharyngeal angiofibroma demonstrates a large heterogeneous and mildly T2 hyperintense mass with scattered low-density foci centered in the right nasal cavity (arrow [A]), which shows high signal intensity on the ADC map (black asterisk [B]), suggestive of facilitated water diffusion. In contradistinction, in a patient with an undifferentiated pleomorphic sarcoma filling both nasal cavities (C, D), although the signal characteristics of the tumor on T2-weighted imaging (C) are similar to those of the angiofibroma in (A), the ADC map (D) demonstrates diffusely low signal (white asterisk), indicating restricted water diffusion, a finding that should raise concern for a more malignant process.

DTI also has been investigated in patients with soft tissue tumors. Historically, this technique has predominantly been utilized in brain imaging; however, more recently it has been applied to the evaluation of cranial nerve tracts as well as peripheral nerves.[45] The anatomic pathway of nerves in the neck has a significant impact on surgical approach and outcomes, so DTI tractography might allow for more accurate preoperative counseling and surgical planning. Akter and colleagues[46] examined 5 patients with head and neck tumors, including vagal nerve schwannoma, thyroid carcinoma, and various salivary gland tumors, with DTI technique and found that 80% of the cases demonstrated agreement in neural pathway between imaging and intraoperative findings. DTI also has been utilized to differentiate between residual squamous cell carcinoma and post radiation changes in an irradiated tumor.[47]

More recently, Gersing and colleagues[48] reported that DTI and tractography can be used to differentiate between schwannomas and neurofibromas accurately and to describe tumor location in relation to nerve fascicles for preoperative planning. In this study, the investigators found that peripheral nerve schwannomas were significantly more likely to be located eccentrically to the nerve than neurofibromas (94.8% vs 0%, respectively; $P<.01$) and that nerve fascicles were more often continuous in schwannomas than in neurofibromas (87.5% vs 0%, respectively; $P = .014$).

More recently, newer DWI techniques have begun use in the head and neck tumor imaging. These techniques included intravoxel incoherent imaging (IVIM) and diffusion kurtosis and are acquired using multiple b-values,[25] a discussion of which is beyond the scope of this article.

Dynamic contrast-enhanced MR imaging

Tissue perfusion in the brain and head and neck can also be assessed via various noninvasive MR imaging techniques, including several employing exogenous contrast agents, such as DCE and dynamic susceptibility contrast MR imaging perfusion imaging or endogenous labeling of arterial blood water as in arterial spin-labeled MR imaging. DCE–MR imaging is perhaps the most widely studied of these techniques for soft tissue tumors. This technique provides information about the vascularity of tissues and their surrounding environments, and quantitative parameters derived from the images can describe the pharmacokinetics of a given region of interest.[49] DCE–MR imaging sequences in turn can be analyzed using both qualitative and quantitative methods. Qualitative analysis relies on visual assessment of time-intensity curves (TICs) to determine the rate of tissue contrast enhancement and washout. In general, malignant tumors tend to demonstrate early and more rapid enhancement with washout compared with benign lesions.[23,49] From these curves, semiquantitative metrics, including initial area under the curve (iAUC), maximum enhancement, time to peak enhancement (TTP), and rate of enhancement can be calculated.

More in-depth pharmacokinetic contrast enhancement modeling allows quantification of blood flow, microvasculature, and capillary permeability of tumors. Commonly used DCE–MR imaging pharmacokinetic metrics include the volume transfer constant (K^{trans}), which characterizes the degree of transfer of contrast from the plasma to the tissue extravascular extracellular space; the extracellular extravascular space volume (V_e); and the transfer rate constant (K_{ep}), which describes the transfer of contrast from the extravascular extracellular compartment into the plasma compartment and is equal to the ratio of K^{trans} and V_e (that is, $K_{ep} = K^{trans}/V_e$). Together, these parameters can be used to describe the vascular profile of a tumor.[49]

Benign lesions tend to have a larger interstitial space and delayed perfusion, which can be reflected as slow continuous enhancement on TICs, whereas malignant tumors, in contrast, tend to have a smaller interstitial space, high vascularity, and increased capillary permeability, leading to early arterial enhancement and higher peak contrast enhancement.[50,51] Using quantitative pharmacokinetic metrics, it also has been shown that malignant soft tissue tumors have significantly higher mean K^{trans} and K_{ep} compared with benign soft tissue tumors.[30] In addition, high-grade soft tissue sarcomas tend to show higher iAUC, shorter TTP, higher K^{trans}, and higher K_{ep} compared with their lower-grade counterparts.[52] DCE–MR imaging also has been shown to help in the assessment of treatment response and the degree of viable residual malignant tumor following neoadjuvant chemotherapy or radiation in soft tissue malignancies[41] and in detecting residual or recurrent tumor after surgical resection.[53]

Moreover, in combination with DWI, DCE has proved in several studies to help differentiate tumor types and monitor treatment response.[41] Sumi and colleagues[54] created tumor profiles based on TICs from DCE–MR imaging in combination with IVIM, which were distinct enough to differentiate squamous cell carcinoma, lymphoma, malignant salivary gland tumors, Warthin tumor, pleomorphic adenoma, and schwannoma. The study also showed that combining IVIM and DCE allowed for a 97% accuracy in differentiating benign and malignant tumors and 89% accuracy for differentiating specific types.

SPECIFIC SOFT TISSUE TUMOR CATEGORIES
Adipocytic Tumors

Adipocytic tumors are mesenchymal tumors that originate from lipocytes (also known as adipocytes). This category of tumors includes lipoma, lipoblastoma, and lipoblastomatosis among its benign entities, and liposarcoma and its numerous variants on the malignant end of the spectrum. New to the fifth edition of the WHO classification are the atypical spindle cell/pleomorphic lipomatous tumor (ASLT) and myxoid pleomorphic liposarcoma (MPL),[1] discussed in further detail later.

Lipomas are the most common mesenchymal tumors, making up approximately 16% of soft tissue tumors, with an annual incidence of 1 in 1000 individuals.[55] Histologically, these tumors are composed of lobules of mature adipocytes and scant connective tissue stroma. Although benign, they may be treated with surgical excision for cosmesis or functional impairment and recur at a rate of less than 5% if superficially located.[1] Anywhere from 17% to 25% of all lipomas occur in the head and neck region.[56,57] These tumors most often are present in the posterior neck, but also they can be found in the parotid, infratemporal fossa, sternocleidomastoid muscle, pharynx, larynx, oral cavity, or retropharyngeal space.[56,58,59] They typically present asymptomatically as soft, well-circumscribed masses in the subcutaneous tissues with slow growth over time.

Most lipomas are well-defined encapsulated masses found subcutaneously or between muscles and other connective tissue structures. They classically demonstrate density and signal characteristics matching that of subcutaneous fat, including high signal intensity on both T1-weighted and T2-weighted images. With fat suppression techniques, the signal within a lipoma drops out completely (**Fig. 4**). Thin septations occasionally may be seen within lipomas, but simple lipomas rarely present a diagnostic challenge.[60–62]

Although conventional lipoma is the most common benign adipocytic tumor, there are several other benign variants, including angiolipoma, chondroid lipoma, myolipoma of soft tissue, spindle cell/pleomorphic lipoma, and hibernoma, which feature adipose tissue intermixed with other tissue types or, in the case of hibernoma, adipose tissue showing brown fat differentiation.[1] These variants may differ from the classic lipomas in regard to both clinical presentation and microscopic appearance. They frequently are characterized by atypical features, such as septae thicker than 2 mm, septal nodularity, soft tissue components, which may be similar in density or signal intensity to muscle or fibrous tissue, enhancement, hemorrhage, or calcification.[60–62] If any of these nonadipocytic elements is present, it may be impossible on imaging to distinguish one of these variants from a liposarcoma. In general, any areas of soft tissue signal or enhancement should be viewed with suspicion and should warrant consideration of biopsy.

When a lesion with the signal characteristics suggesting an adipocytic tumor is seen in a young child, lipoblastoma should be considered. Lipoblastomas arise from embryonal fat cells and thus are diagnosed primarily in the pediatric population, usually in children younger than 3 years of age.[63] These tumors typically exhibit structural gene alterations targeting the PLAG1 gene.[64] Imaging features of lipoblastomas can mimic those of lipomas and low-grade liposarcomas (**Fig. 5**); however, liposarcomas are exceedingly uncommon in children under the age of 5.[65–67]

Lipomatosis and lipoblastomatosis refer to conditions in which there is diffuse overgrowth of mature or immature adipose tissue. In the head and neck, lipomatosis can occur as part of a syndrome (eg, Madelung disease, familial multiple lipomatosis, or congenital infiltrating lipomatosis of the face), and depending on location both lipomatosis and lipoblastomatosis can present with

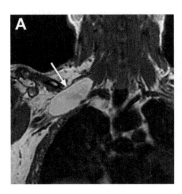
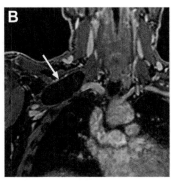

Fig. 4. Lipoma in a 57-year-old man with a right neck mass. (*A*) Coronal unenhanced, T1-weighted and (*B*) coronal contrast-enhanced, fat-suppressed, T1-weighted images through the right neck demonstrate a well-circumscribed, encapsulated mass (*arrows*), which is essentially homogeneously isointense to fat on (*A*) and suppresses completely without internal enhancement on (*B*), which allows confidently making the diagnosis of lipoma.

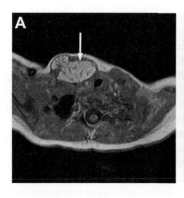
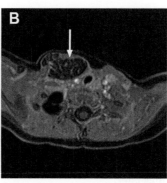

Fig. 5. Lipoblastoma in an 11-month-old boy presenting with a painless right neck mass. (*A*) Axial T1-weighted image demonstrates a bilobed circumscribed mass insinuating within the right sternocleido-mastoid muscle, which is predominantly isointense to subcutaneous fat (*arrow*) with internal strands of more intermediate signal intensity. (*B*) Contrast-enhanced, fat-suppressed, axial T1-weighted image demonstrates drop out of most of the signal within the tumor (*arrow*) confirming its adipocytic nature, with enhancement of the thin internal soft tissue septations. Although the tumor is radiographically indistinguishable from lipoma and low-grade forms of liposarcoma, the patient's very young age favors a diagnosis of lipoblastoma.

significant and sometimes life-threatening complications, including severe functional limitations of breathing and swallowing.[68,69]

An entity new to the fifth edition in the spectrum of benign adipocytic tumors is the ASLT (**Fig. 6**), which is a tumor characterized histologically by ill-defined margins and the presence of variable proportions of mildly to moderately atypical spindle cells, adipocytes, lipoblasts, pleomorphic cells, multinucleated giant cells, and a myxoid or collagenous extracellular matrix. A substantial subset of these tumors demonstrates deletions or losses of 13q14, including RB1 and its flanking genes RCBTB2, DLEU1, and ITM2B.[70] Although they may appear histologically similar to well-differentiated or dedifferentiated liposarcomas, ASLTs do not demonstrate amplification of MDM2 or CDK4. Furthermore, unlike conventional atypical lipomatous tumors, there is no risk for dedifferentiation, although these tumors do have a low tendency for local recurrence if incompletely excised. They have a male predilection (approximately 1.5:1 male:female ratio) and a mean age of presentation in the 50s, although a wide age

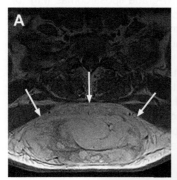
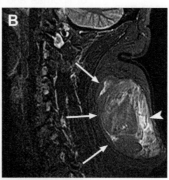
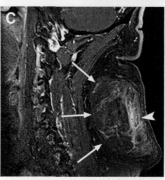

Fig. 6. ASLT in a 50-year-old man presenting with a large posterior neck mass, which had been slowly enlarging over the past decade. (*A*) Axial T1-weighted and (*B*) sagittal STIR images demonstrate a slightly lobulated mass (*arrows*) in the posterior neck, which is predominantly isointense to fat on T1-weighted images and slightly hyperintense to fat on STIR imaging, with internal areas of lower T1-weighted signal and high STIR signal, particularly posteriorly (*arrowhead* [*B*]). (*C*) On a contrast-enhanced, fat-suppressed sequence, the signal in the mass mostly suppresses, but the regions of hyperintensity seen on STIR show corresponding contrast enhancement (*arrowhead*).

range is reported. ASLTs predominantly arise in the limbs and limb girdle; however, they have been reported in a wide distribution of anatomic sites, including in the head, face, and neck, where approximately 10% to 25% are found.[70–72] Occurrence in the larynx and trachea also has been reported. The imaging features of these tumors has not been well described, and they likely are indistinguishable from other benign and malignant adipocytic lesions.

Clinically, adipocytic tumors larger than 5 cm or deep in location are more likely to be malignant.[55–57] Malignant adipocytic tumors include liposarcoma and its variants: atypical lipomatous tumor/well-differentiated, liposarcoma, dedifferentiated liposarcoma, myxoid liposarcoma, pleomorphic liposarcoma, and MPL. Factors thought to contribute to the development of liposarcoma include certain genetic predispositions (eg, neurofibromatosis and familial cancer syndromes), trauma, and previous radiation.[73] The most common variant of liposarcoma in the head and neck is myxoid liposarcoma, which also is the most common subtype in children and young adults and is characterized by translocations producing FUS-DDIT3 or rarely EWSR1-DDIT3 fusion transcripts.[1,67] The neck is the subsite of head and neck liposarcomas involved most frequently, but this tumor also can present at various sites, including the scalp, cheek, hard palate, lip, and thyroid.[73] MR imaging findings of liposarcoma vary depending on the amount of adipose tissue in the lesion with lower-grade lesions having imaging characteristics similar to simple lipomas. Findings suggestive of malignant transformation include the presence of thick septa, enhancement of portions of the tumor, or invasion of adjacent structures (**Fig. 7**). Higher-grade lesions frequently have lower fat content and are more similar to other sarcomas.

MPL is the other new tumor described in the adipocytic tumor category in the fifth edition classification of soft tissue tumors. These tumors show histologic features of both conventional myxoid liposarcoma and pleomorphic sarcoma and lack the gene fusions and amplifications commonly seen in other intermediate and high-grade adipocytic tumors. It is considered a high-grade lesion, which is clinically aggressive with frequent local recurrences, distant metastases, and low overall survival rates.[74] These tumors occur almost exclusively in children and are associated with hereditary tumor syndromes like Li-Fraumeni syndrome. They most frequently involve the mediastinum but also have been reported in the head and neck.[75] There is scant literature on the imaging appearance of MPL, with case reports describing low-attenuation, mildly rim-enhancing complex cystic subcutaneous soft tissue lesions on CT[76] and T2 hyperintense and avidly enhancing soft tissue lesions.[75]

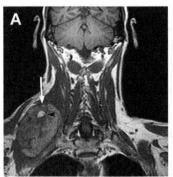
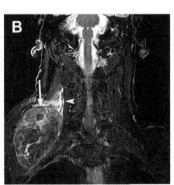
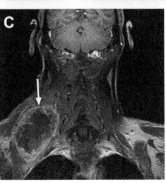

Fig. 7. Pleomorphic liposarcoma in a 59-year-old man with an enlarging right neck mass. (*A*) Coronal T1-weighted, (*B*) STIR, and (*C*) contrast-enhanced, fat-suppressed, T1-weighted images demonstrate a heterogeneous mass (*arrows*) at the base of the right neck. The mass is mostly hyperintense relative to muscle but less intense than subcutaneous fat on the unenhanced T1-weighted image (*A*) but contains at least 1 discrete area that appears iso-intense to fat (*black arrowhead*). On the STIR image (*B*), the lesion suppresses partially, including the aforementioned hyperintense nodule (*A*), suggesting some adipocytic content. Note, however, the edema of the soft tissues adjacent to the superior margin of the tumor (*white arrowhead*), which is not a typical feature seen with benign lipomas. On the contrast-enhanced, T1-weighted sequence (*C*), the mass shows irregular, predominantly peripheral enhancement, a finding not typically seen in benign adipocytic tumors.

Fibroblastic/Myofibroblastic Tumors

Fibroblastic/myofibroblastic tumors make up the largest group of mesenchymal tumors by number and are characterized by a proliferation of fibroblasts and/or myofibroblasts. Demonstrating a wide spectrum of clinical and pathologic features, approximately 76% are regarded as benign, based on biologic potential, 13% as intermediate, and 11% as malignant.[56] Fibroblastic and myofibroblastic tumors are relatively common in children and make up approximately 12% of pediatric soft tissue tumors, with approximately 50% of cases diagnosed within the first year of life and 71% occurring in the first decade. Approximately 25% of these tumors arise in the head and neck region.[19,77–79]

The 2020 WHO update introduced 3 new tumors to the fibroblastic/myofibroblastic tumor category: angiofibroma of soft tissue (a benign tumor occurring primarily in the extremities near large joints),[80] superficial CD34-positive fibroblastic tumor (a low-grade neoplasm of the skin and subcutis with a predilection for the lower extremities),[81] and EWSR1-SMAD3–positive fibroblastic tumor (a benign tumor primarily mainly arising in dermal and subcutaneous locations in the hands and feet).[82] The 2 former tumors have been reported to occur in the neck very rarely,[80,81,83,84] but only scattered reports describing nonspecific MR imaging features of these new tumors exist.[85,86]

Among the more common benign entities in the fibroblastic/myofibroblastic tumor category are fibromatosis colli, nodular fasciitis, and MO. Tumors with intermediate biologic potential include desmoid fibromatosis, DFSP, SFT, and inflammatory myofibroblastic tumor (IMT). Malignant tumors in this category include adult and infantile fibrosarcoma and low-grade fibromyxoid sarcoma (LGMS). In general, the imaging features of most of the entities that comprise this group of tumors are nonspecific; however, patient demographics and tumor location can be useful in narrowing the differential, and certain entities, such as fibromatosis colli, arise in characteristic locations and patient populations.

Fibromatosis colli, also referred to as sternocleidomastoid pseudotumor of infancy, is a self-limited benign fibrous proliferation occurring in the sternocleidomastoid muscle in infants and is the most common cause of a neck mass in the perinatal period. Affected infants typically present within the first 4 weeks to 8 weeks of life (usually in the first 2–4 weeks) with a firm anterior neck mass, usually unilateral with a slight right-sided predilection, and associated torticollis.[1,78] The mass typically increases in size over the course of several weeks and subsequently regresses, with 90% of cases resolving spontaneously during the next 4 months to 8 months. The cause of fibromatosis colli is uncertain, but there often is a history of abnormal intrauterine positioning or birth trauma, leading some to hypothesize it may represent a compartment syndrome due to injury to the sternocleidomastoid during birth or due to intrauterine position.[87] There also may be a genetic component, because 11% of affected children have a family history of the condition.[88]

Pathologic evaluation of fibromatosis colli demonstrates a paucicellular scarlike fibroblastic proliferation with entrapped skeletal muscle.[89] US usually is the diagnostic imaging modality of choice, demonstrating well-defined, unilateral, fusiform expansion of the sternocleidomastoid muscle.[90] On MR imaging, these pseudotumors are isointense to muscle on T1-weighted images, with variable enhancement and hyperintense on T2-weighted images (**Fig. 8**), with occasional subtle patchy and linear areas of decreased signal intensity.[90,91]

Nodular fasciitis is a self-limiting neoplasm usually occurring in the subcutaneous tissues, most commonly seen in second to fourth decades of life. Head and neck involvement occurs in 15% to 20% of patients.[92] The process is characterized histologically by plump, uniform fibroblastic/myofibroblastic cells displaying a tissue culture–like architectural pattern.[1] Recurrent USP6 gene rearrangements have been reported in cases of nodular fasciitis, suggesting it represents a benign neoplasm rather than a reactive tumefactive process, as previously thought. Clinically, nodular fasciitis typically shows rapid growth, with most cases having only a pre-resection duration of less than 2 months to 3 months.[1] Cases occur in all age groups but more often in young adults. Cranial fasciitis, a subtype of the tumor involving the outer table of the skull and contiguous soft tissues of the scalp, develops predominantly in infants with a median age at presentation of 2 years.[93] Some patients report a history of trauma to the site, but most do not. Three subtypes are described: subcutaneous, intramuscular, and intermuscular (fascial) types. The subcutaneous type occurs 3 times to 10 times more commonly than the other subtypes. The intramuscular type typically is larger in size and deeper in location. The intermuscular type generally is less well circumscribed and grows along fascial planes.[92] More superficial lesions have well-defined margins, whereas deeper lesions tend to be infiltrative.

On imaging, nodular fasciitis presents as a mass, often with a broad fascial interface and in some cases demonstrating a tail of tissue

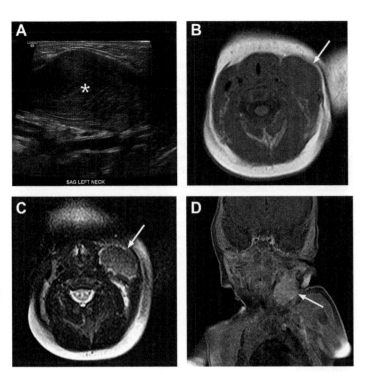

Fig. 8. Fibromatosis colli in a 20-day old man presenting with torticollis and a left neck mass. (*A*) Longitudinal B-mode US image of the left neck demonstrates diffuse, fusiform enlargement of the sternocleidomastoid muscle (*asterisk*). (*B*) Axial T1-weighted and (*C*) axial T2-weighted images demonstrate a mass in the sternocleidomastoid muscle (*arrows*), which is isointense to muscle (*A*) and hyperintense on (*B*). (*D*) Coronal contrast-enhanced, fat-suppressed, T1-weighted image demonstrated diffuse enhancement of the mass (*arrow*). Notice the leftward tilt of the head due to the child's torticollis.

extending along the fascia (fascial tail sign), although this is not a finding specific to nodular fasciitis.[78] Larger lesions can have an aggressive appearance, causing erosion of the adjacent osseous structures. These tumors are heterogeneous on MR imaging and may be solid or partially cystic. The solid components usually are isointense to slightly hyperintense to muscle on T1-weighted images and T2-weighted images, whereas cystic components may demonstrate signal that is hyperintense relative to cerebrospinal fluid (CSF) on T1-weighted images and isointense on T2-weighted images. Variable degrees of enhancement may be seen[92,94] (**Fig. 9**).

MO is a benign, self-limited neoplasm composed of spindle cells and osteoblasts as mesenchymal response to soft tissue injury, which produces metaplastic bone formation in muscles, tendons, and subcutaneous fat.[78] MO can occur at any age but is most common during the second and third decades, and up to 75% of cases occur after trauma.[95] Nontraumatic cases of MO occur more commonly in adults and commonly are seen in association with burns or paralysis.[78] In the head and neck, MO has been reported in the temporalis, masseter, buccinator, myelohyoid, medial pterygoid, scalene, sternocleiodomastoid, and paraspinous muscles.[96–98] As these lesions mature, they typically shrink, with approximately 30% of cases resolving entirely.[78,91,99]

The imaging appearance evolves with maturation of the lesion. Initially, during the early proliferative phase, which occurs up to 3 weeks after the initial trauma, the MR imaging characteristics are nonspecific and are similar to those of other soft tissue tumors, making diagnosis challenging. Three weeks to 7 weeks after trauma, an intermediate calcification and ossification phase occurs. At this stage, a hypointense bony rim gradually develops and is considered diagnostic. During this stage, the muscles surrounding the lesion often are markedly edematous, a finding seen less frequently with soft tissue sarcomas.[78] In the final mature ossification phase, which develops by 6 weeks to 8 weeks, MO demonstrates signal characteristics of bone, with a well-defined, hypointense rim and trabeculae, dense fibrosis, and central adipose tissue. CT demonstrates a well-defined geometric hypodense mass with peripheral calcification in the earlier phases; mature lesions demonstrate dense calcification.[78,91,99]

Desmoid-type fibromatosis, also referred to as desmoid tumor, is a locally aggressive, frequently recurring but nonmetastasizing fibroblastic neoplasm characterized by a proliferation of bland-appearing, spindle-shaped cells arranged in long sweeping fascicles set in a collagenous stroma and irregularly infiltrating through adjacent adipose tissue or muscle.[100] It appears most commonly in the second and third decades but

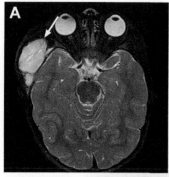
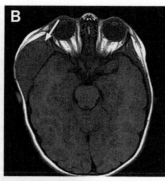
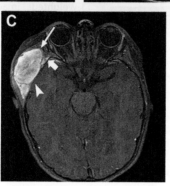

Fig. 9. Cranial fasciitis in a 2-year-old girl with a 6-month history of a slowly enlarging, nontender right temporal mass. (*A*) Axial T2-weighted and (*B*) axial T1-weighted images demonstrate a mass which is hyperintense to muscle on the T2-weighted image and isointense on the T1-weighted image (*long arrows*). (*C*) Contrast-enhanced, axial fat-suppressed, T1-weighted image demonstrates diffuse, avid enhancement of the mass (*long arrow*) with an enhancing fascial tail anteromedially (*short thick arrow*). The normally low signal intensity cortex of the underlying calvarium is not well visualized, which suggests possible erosion by the mass (*arrowhead*).

can be seen at any age. Desmoid tumors occur in the head and neck in up to 15% of cases and in a greater percentage of cases in children. The most common sites of involvement in the head and neck are the supraclavicular and neck regions, followed by the face. Approximately 10% of patients report previous trauma to the region and there also is an association with Gardner syndrome, with up to a third of patients with the syndrome developing desmoid tumors.[21] Desmoids associated with Gardner syndrome are associated with germline *APC* mutations, whereas most sporadic desmoid tumors result from point mutations of the gene that encodes β-catenin (*CTNNB1*).[1] Up to 30% of these tumors recur following resection, and these lesions tend to behave more aggressively in children than in adults.[100]

The MR imaging appearance of desmoid tumor is variable, dependent in part on the cellularity and the amount of collagen and myxoid material that is present. Desmoids usually are ovoid in shape, often with a lobulated or irregular contour. They typically are isointense to slightly hyperintense to muscle on T1-weighted images and of intermediate or variably increased signal intensity on T2-weighted images. Linear and curvilinear strands of decreased signal on T1-weighted and T2-weighted sequences may represent collagen and if extensive should suggest the diagnosis. Furthermore, linear extension of the lesion can be seen

along fascial planes, similar to the fascial tail of nodular fasciitis. Intense enhancement is a common feature of these tumors[101,102] (**Fig. 10**).

DFSP is a locally aggressive cutaneous neoplasm most often arising in young to middle-aged adults, usually presenting as a slow-growing, painless, multinodular, or polypoid cutaneous mass or plaque, which may occur in healthy skin or in an area of repeated trauma. Between 5% and 15% of these tumors occur in the head and neck, with the scalp the most common location involved, followed by the cheek.[3,100] DSFP is infiltrative and lesions in the scalp may invade the periosteum and calvarium or even extend intracranially. It has a high likelihood of local recurrence but almost never metastasizes.[1] On MR imaging, DFSP appears as a cutaneous or subcutaneous mass, which is isointense to muscle on T1-weighted imaging with homogeneous or heterogeneous contrast enhancement. On T2-weighted images, the lesions usually are hyperintense but occasionally may be isokintense or hypointense compared with muscle[103] (**Fig. 11**).

SFT is fibroblastic tumor first described in the pleura but since documented to occur in virtually any anatomic site and organ.[104] Histologically, these tumors have a characteristic appearance composed of bland ovoid or spindled fibroblastic cells with a pattern-less architectural arrangement

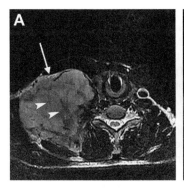
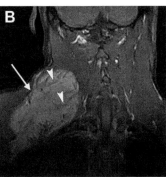

Fig. 10. Desmoid-type fibromatosis in a 19-year-old man with a 1-year history of a slow growing mass in the right neck. (*A*) Axial T2-weighted image demonstrates a hyperintense mass with slightly irregular borders (*arrow*) in the right neck. (*B*) Coronal contrast-enhanced, fat-suppressed, T1-weighted image demonstrates homogeneous, intense enhancement of the tumor deep to the sternocleidomastoid muscle (*arrow*). Note the low signal intensity strands within the lesion on both [*arrowheads*] [*A*, *B*]), which likely represent collagen, and when extensive suggest the diagnosis of desmoid-type fibromatosis.

and separated by thick bands of collagenous stroma and interspersed large branching, or staghorn-shaped, thin-walled hemangiopericytic vessels. Benign, intermediate (rarely metastasizing), and malignant forms of SFTs are described. Genetically, SFTs consistently are associated with NAB2-STAT6 gene fusions arising from recurrent intrachromosomal rearrangements on chromosome 12q. Tumors once considered distinct entities, such as hemangiopericytomas and giant cell angiofibromas, now fall under the category of SFT.[104] These tumors usually occur in middle-aged adults (range 20–70 years)[105] and typically present as slowly growing, painless masses that may be locally infiltrative. In rare cases, they may be associated with symptoms of hypoglycemia due to the production of insulinlike growth factors.[104,106] In the head and neck, SFTs arise most frequently in the sinonasal tract, orbits, oral cavity, and salivary glands but also are reported to occur in the meninges, pharynx, larynx, parapharyngeal space, thyroid, subcutaneous tissues, and, rarely, in the skin.[100,104,107,108] Orbital lesions are more common in men, whereas extraorbital lesions occur more commonly in women.[108] These tumors may grow rapidly, simulating a more malignant tumor, or may have an indolent course with slow growth over many years.

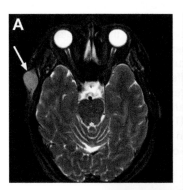
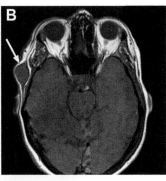
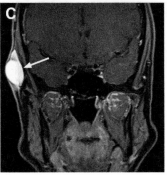

Fig. 11. DFSP in a 61-year-old woman presenting with an enlarging right temporal mass with overlying skin discoloration. (*A*) Axial T2-weighted and (*B*) axial T1-weighted MR images demonstrate a circumscribed subcutaneous mass (*arrows*), which is homogeneously hyperintense on T2-weighted imaging and isointense on T1-weighted imaging relative to muscle. (*C*) Coronal contrast-enhanced, fat-suppressed, T1-weighted image demonstrates intense homogeneous enhancement of the mass. (Images courtesy of Dr. Nandita Guha-Thakurta, MD Anderson Cancer Center, Houston, TX.)

SFTs, like other soft tissue tumors, have nonspecific imaging characteristics on MR imaging. They usually demonstrate heterogeneous, hyperintense signal intensity relative to muscle on T2-weighted sequences and isointense signal on unenhanced T1-weighted images. On both T1-weighted and T2-weighted images, linear or curvilinear low-signal-intensity lines may be observed within the tumors, potentially reflecting the hypocellular but more collagenous areas (similar to desmoid-type fibromatosis).[107] T2-weighted images also may show a low signal rim representing a pseudocapsule around the lesion[109] (Fig. 12). Stippled low signal voids likely corresponding to pseudovascular spaces also may be evident.[108] There usually is intense enhancement following contrast administration.

IMT, also commonly referred to as inflammatory pseudotumor and plasma cell granuloma, is an intermediate-grade, rarely metastasizing neoplasm composed of myofibroblastic and fibroblastic spindle cells accompanied by an inflammatory infiltrate of plasma cells, lymphocytes, and/or eosinophils.[1] Anywhere from 50% to 70% of IMTs harbor a rearrangement of the anaplastic lymphoma kinase gene on chromosome 2p23.[1,110] There appears be substantial confusion surrounding the use of the term, inflammatory pseudotumor, which historically has been used to designate various possibly distinct entities, including notably IMT as well as immunoglobulin G4 (IgG4)-related sclerosing disease.[110,111] IMTs are much more likely to show ALK expression and a relatively low level of IgG4-positive cell infiltration compared with the lesions of IgG4-related sclerosing disease, and patients with IMTs tend to be younger. There also appears to be some question as to whether there actually exist inflammatory pseudotumors that are distinct entities from both IMT and IgG4-related sclerosing disease (ie, lesions that are non–ALK-overexpressing show a paucity of IgG4 plasma cells), but it appears that for the time being, the WHO considers these lesions within the category of IMT.[112]

Most cases of IMT are diagnosed in children and young adults, but these tumors can occur across a wide age range. Treatment of IMTs includes corticosteroids and/or surgical resection. Approximately 80% of inflammatory pseudotumors respond corticosteroid treatment, but there is a 50% to 60% chance of disease recurrence. Maintenance-dose corticosteroids are recommended for at least 6 months to prevent recurrence of disease.[113]

IMTs arise most commonly in the abdominal soft tissues followed by the lung, mediastinum, and head and neck. Up to 15% of IMTs occur in the head and neck, where they are more common in adults.[100] Orbital involvement with IMT (orbital pseudotumor) is well known among radiologists as a common cause of unilateral proptosis and painful ophthalmoplegia in adults. It constitutes approximately 9% of all orbital lesions and usually is unilateral.[114,115] Patients classically present with acute or subacute eye pain associated with ophthalmoplegia, decreased vision, or proptosis, which respond rapidly to steroids. Uveal and scleral thickening is seen in 33% of patients with orbital pseudotumor and is thought to be a specific sign.[114] There are several different distributions of inflammation described in orbital pseudotumor, which are defined by the anatomic structures that are involved and that frequently overlap. The myositic form, which is the most common, affects the extraocular muscles; the dacryoadenitis form affects the lacrimal glands; the neuritis form affects the optic nerve sheath; the apical form affects the structures of the orbital apex; the episcleral form affects the anterior orbit, including the sclera and preseptal soft tissues; and, finally, the diffuse form affects the entire orbit.[116]

Extraorbital IMTs of the head and neck arise most frequently in the nasal cavity and paranasal sinuses but also occur in the nasopharynx, skull

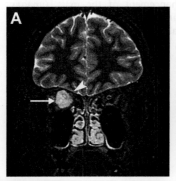
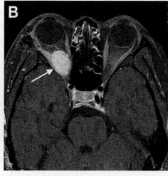

Fig. 12. SFT of the orbit in a 35-year-old woman who initially presented with declining visual acuity in the right eye. (A) Coronal STIR image demonstrates a lobulated hyperintense intraconal mass in the right orbit (arrow), which displaces the optic nerve (arrowhead) superomedially. (B) Axial contrast-enhanced, fat-suppressed, T1-weighted image demonstrates the mass (arrow) to be avidly and homogeneously enhancing.

base, temporal bone, larynx, trachea, thyroid gland, and salivary glands.[112,117] Perineural spread along maxillary, mandibular, and hypoglossal nerves and internal carotid occlusion can occur. Sinonasal pseudotumor usually is more aggressive appearing than orbital pseudotumor and commonly causes bony erosion, remodeling, and sclerosis. Extraorbital IMTs are less responsive to steroids than the orbital form; however, prognosis still is good if the lesion is resected completely.

On imaging, IMTs have nonspecific imaging features and mimic other tumors. They may be circumscribed or poorly defined and infiltrative with extensive surrounding inflammatory-appearing changes or erosion of adjacent bone. IMTs usually are isointense to hypointense relative to muscle on T1-weighted images and hypointense to only mildly hyperintense on T2-weighted images[115] (Fig. 13). Hypointensity on T2-weighted imaging may be related to the fibrous nature of the lesion. Variable but usually marked contrast enhancement can be seen.

Fibrosarcomas can be divided into adult and infantile varieties. The adult form of fibrosarcoma once was believed the most common soft tissue tumor in adults, but changes in diagnostic criteria have made this a diagnosis of exclusion, with most tumors previously classified as fibrosarcomas in adults now considered other spindle

cell sarcomas. It now is thought that adult fibrosarcomas account for fewer than 1% of adult soft tissue sarcomas.[1]

Infantile fibrosarcomas are malignant tumors diagnosed most frequently during infancy. These tumors are histologically identical to adult fibrosarcomas but generally have a much more favorable prognosis. Approximately one-third of infantile fibrosarcomas are diagnosed antenatally or in the first month of life, with 14% initially detected on prenatal US.[118] Only 12% occur after 1 year of life. The infantile form of fibrosarcoma is associated most frequently with ETV6–neurotrophic tyrosine receptor kinase (NTRK) 3 gene fusions, but other gene fusions or rearrangements involving NTRK1, BRAF, and MET also are described.[1]

Up to 15% of infantile fibrosarcomas occur in the head and neck, with reported sites including the scalp, tongue, parotid, and orbit.[100] The tumor typically presents as a rapidly enlarging painless mass with erythematous and often ulcerated overlying skin. Local recurrence following resection occurs in up to 40% of cases with metastases occurring in up to 13%.[119] These tumors usually are large at presentation with a mean size of 5 cm to 6 cm.[100] On MR imaging, infantile fibrosarcomas are heterogeneous masses that may have well-defined or infiltrative margins. They are predominantly isointense to muscle on T1-weighted imaging and hyperintense on T2-weighted

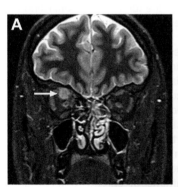
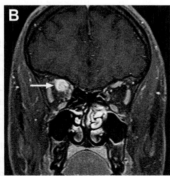
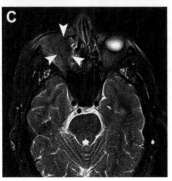

Fig. 13. IMT in a 21-year-old man presenting with right eye pain and ptosis as well as diplopia with downward gaze. (A) Coronal STIR MR image demonstrates a mildly hyperintense mass centered in the superior rectus muscle (arrow). On the corresponding coronal contrast-enhanced, fat-suppressed, T1-weighted image (B), the mass enhances avidly (arrow). The patient's symptoms improved after a course of steroids. (C) Axial T2-weighted image in a different patient with an IMT demonstrates a low signal mass (arrowheads) in the inferomedial aspect of the right orbit protruding into the adjacent ethmoid sinus region.

imaging, although they may demonstrate hypointense regions related to fibrous components. The tumors enhance heterogeneously with contrast. Internal hemorrhage and focal regions of necrosis may be evident in larger tumors.[78]

LGFMS is a malignant fibroblastic/myofibroblastic tumor that typically behaves in an indolent fashion early but has a propensity for late local recurrences and metastases occurring up to 15 years after completion of therapy.[78,100] It predominantly affects young adults in the third and fourth decades of life, but up to 20% of cases occur in the pediatric population.[120] LGFMSs are characterized histologically by alternating collagenous and myxoid areas, deceptively bland spindle cells with a whorling growth pattern, and arcades of small blood vessels, and they consistently have either FUS-CREB3L2 or FUS-CREB3L1 gene fusions.[1]

These tumors occur most commonly in the trunk and extremities, although head and neck involvement has been described, with reported sites including the face, mandible, larynx, neck, sternocleidomastoid muscle, and maxillary sinus.[121] They tend to be heterogeneous on MR imaging and may demonstrate hypointense regions on T1-weighted and T2-weighted images due to fibrous components as well areas which are hypointense on T1-weighted images and hyperintense on T2-weighted images owing to myxoid components. The resultant alternating appearance of alternating high and low signal areas on T2-weighted imaging has been described as having an appearance similar to cerebriform gyri.[122] Enhancement is heterogeneous with evidence of mixed solid and cystic areas or areas of gyriform enhancement.[78]

Finally, MFS is a malignant fibroblastic/myofibroblastic tumor that comprises a spectrum of tumors with variably myxoid stroma, pleomorphism, and the presence of characteristic prominent elongated, curvilinear, thin-walled blood vessels with a perivascular condensation of tumor cells or inflammatory cells.[1] Most MFSs arise in the limbs, but there have been occasional reports of these tumors in the head and neck, including in the maxillary sinus, sphenoid sinus, orbit, maxilla, esophagus, hypopharynx, neck, larynx, parotid, mandible, and infratemporal fossa.[123] Local, often repeated recurrences, apparently unrelated to histologic grade, can be seen in 30% to 40% of cases. Incidence of metastases is related to the tumor grade, with individuals with high-grade MFSs developing metastases in 20% to 35% of cases.[1] On MR imaging, MFSs are characterized by T2-weighted signal intensity, which is higher than that of muscle and fat, often markedly so, with

signal intensities similar to fluid due to the tumors' myxoid components (see **Fig. 2**). Signal intensity on T1-weighted images is lower than muscle with enhancement greater than muscle.[124]

So-called Fibrohistiocytic Tumors

So-called fibrohistiocytic tumors became a category when electron microscopy, immunohistochemistry, and genetics revealed that tumors initially considered fibrohistiocytic based on histology actually were not histiocytic in origin. This category, therefore, collects a group of heterogeneous lesions, many of which likely are unrelated.[125] There were no significant changes to this group of tumors in the most recent WHO update, which again contains 4 tumors: TGCT, deep benign fibrous histiocytoma, plexiform fibrohistiocytic tumor, and giant cell tumor of soft tissue (GCT-ST).[1]

TGCTs encompass a range of benign and malignant lesions arising from the synovial membrane of joints, tendon sheaths, and bursae.[1] This entity includes what had referred to in the past as pigmented villonodular synovitis, but usage of that term no longer is recommended. Cytogenetic studies most often have demonstrated a translocation of the CSF1 gene, which encodes colony-stimulating factor 1 (CSF1). Within tumors with CSF1 translocations, only a small subset of cells actually harbors this mutation, with a majority of the cells making up the tumor mass consisting of macrophages present in response to high CSF1 levels.[126]

TGCTs are classified based on anatomic location (intra-articular vs extra-articular) and pattern of growth (localized vs diffuse). The localized form usually occurs in patients aged 30 to 50 with a female predominance, whereas the diffuse type usually affects adults under the age of 40. A majority of these tumors occur in the fingers, but cases have been reported to arise in the TMJ and cervical spine facet joints.[127] TGCTs of the TMJ show 2 patterns of spread: anterior and medial to the TMJ, involving the lateral temporal bone, infratemporal fossa, and greater wing of the sphenoid; or circumferential growth from the TMJ, involving the sites, discussed previously, as well as the external auditory canal, middle ear, and mastoid. Surgery, consisting of wide local resection, is treatment of choice for these lesions.

On MR imaging, these tumors demonstrate marked T1 and T2 hypointense signal with variable T1 contrast uptake[127] (see **Fig. 1**). Heavy hemosiderin deposition in these lesions leads to a blooming artifact on gradient recalled echo and susceptibility weighted imaging sequences. Imaging should be reviewed carefully for involvement of the facial or trigeminal nerves, labyrinth, petrous carotid artery, or intradural extension.

Deep fibrous histiocytomas are benign, well-circumscribed lesions located in the subcutaneous or deep tissues.[1] They account for 1% to 2% of all benign fibrous histiocytomas. Most arise in the extremities, but the second most common region of involvement is the head and neck, where they have been reported in various locations, including the scalp, ear, face, neck, oral cavity, salivary glands, pharynx, paranasal sinuses, and larynx.[128–130] These tumors occur predominantly in men in second to fourth decades of life.[129] Treatment of choice is complete resection with negative margins because the recurrence rate is higher than that for cutaneous fibrous histiocytomas. The imaging features of deep fibrous histiocytomas are nonspecific and scarcely described. On MR imaging, these tumors are hypointense on T1-weighted sequences and hyperintense on T2-weighted sequences and have been reported to show peripheral contrast enhancement.[131]

Plexiform fibrohistiocytic tumor is a rare, slow-growing lesion arising at the dermal-subcutaneous junction. The tumor occurs most frequently in upper limbs followed by the lower limbs, with the head and neck area affected less frequently.[1] Children and young adults are affected most often with a median age of between 15 years and 20 years. These lesions have an intermediate malignant potential, with up to a 37.5% likelihood of local recurrence and nodal or distant metastases rarely reported.[132–134] Imaging demonstrates cutaneous or subcutaneous lesions with a plaque-like or infiltrative morphology, but the MR imaging characteristics of these tumors are not specific, with lesions predominantly demonstrating signal isointense to muscle on T1-weighted sequences with contrast enhancement and hyperintense signal on T2-weighted and short tau inversion recovery (STIR) sequences.[132]

GCT-STs are benign tumors located in the superficial soft tissue and occur in the head and neck in 7% of cases, with the extremities affected much more commonly.[1] These lesions generally occur in the fifth decade of life but can occur at virtually any age with an equal occurrence in men and women.[135] Although these tumors appear morphologically similar to giant cell tumors of bone, they lack the mutations of the H3F3A gene that usually are present in the latter, suggesting a different pathogenesis.[136] In the head, multiple sites have been reported to be involved, including the neck, forehead, temporal area, parotid, lips, nasal cavity, and ear.[137] MR imaging demonstrates a solid, heterogenous and frequently

hemorrhagic mass. Peripheral calcification is common, and fluid-fluid levels may be evident, presumably related to hemorrhage or necrosis.[135]

Vascular Tumors

Vascular soft tissue tumors described in the WHO classification arising in the head and neck include various types of hemangiomas, lymphangiomas, kaposiform hemangioendothelioma, Kaposi sarcoma, and angiosarcoma.[1] New to the fifth edition is the introduction of an uncommon but novel epithelioid hemangioendothelioma (EHE) subtype, which is associated with YAP1-TFE3 gene fusions rather than the more common WWTR1-CAMTA1 gene fusion found in more than 90% of EHEs.[83] EHEs arise most often in the lungs liver and bones and occur rarely in the head and neck.[1,138] Because vascular tumors are covered in another article in this issue, they are not discussed further.

Pericytic/Perivascular Tumors

Pericytic tumors are a group of lesions composed of modified vascular smooth cells that grow circumferentially around blood vessels. This group includes 3 types of tumors, which remain unchanged in the current WHO classification: myopericytoma (including myofibroma), angioleiomyoma, and glomus tumor.[1]

Despite its name, myofibroma is considered a pericytic tumor rather than a myofibroblastic tumor in the current WHO classification. Myofibromas fall under the umbrella of myopericytomas, which are distinctive perivascular myoid neoplasms composed of cytologically bland, oval to spindle-shaped, myoid tumor cells with characteristic multilayered, concentric growth around numerous small vessels. Subtypes of myopericytoma include the aforementioned myofibroma, myofibromatosis, and infantile myofibromatosis, with the former referring to a solitary lesion and the term, myofibromatosis, used to indicate multicentric lesion involvement.[1] Myofibromas are the most common fibrous tumors in infants, in whom they usually develop in the first 2 years of life, although they can occur at any age. The tumors often present as a slowly growing, asymptomatic single mass or multiple nodules in the dermis and subcutaneous tissues of the head and neck region but also can affect the trunk, extremities, skeletal muscles, bones or internal organs.[78,139] Approximately one-third of myofibromas arise in the head and neck, with involvement in the subcutaneous soft tissues, nasopharynx, oral cavity, mandible, tongue base, paranasal sinuses, infratemporal fossa and mastoid having been reported.[140–142] Boys tend to have solitary lesions, whereas multicentric lesions are more common in girls.[78] Both autosomal dominant and autosomal recessive inheritance have been reported, with mutations in PDGFRB, NOTCH3, and PTPRG associated with autosomal dominant multicentric myofibromatosis.[139] SRF and RELA gene rearrangements also have been reported in cellular/atypical myofibromas.[143]

On imaging, the lesions are round or lobulated and may be well defined or ill defined. Invasion of subcutaneous muscle or bone may be evident. They are isointense to slightly heterogeneously hyperintense compared with muscle on T1-weighted images and hyperintense on T2-weighted sequences. Most tumors also show irregular or patchy regions of hypointensity on both T1-weighted and T2-weighted pulse sequences. Enhancement often is intense and lesions occasionally demonstrate target-like enhancement[139] (Fig. 14).

Angioleiomyoma, also referred to as vascular leiomyoma, is a benign tumor composed of mature smooth muscle bundles surrounding vascular channels. They can be subclassified into the 3 histologic subtypes (solid, venous, and cavernous) on the basis of their vascular morphologies. Solid-type angioleiomyomas have closely compacted bundles of smooth muscle cells with intervening thin-walled, slitlike vascular channels; venous-type angioleiomyomas are characterized by thick muscle-coated blood vessels with smooth muscle cells of the vascular walls swirling and blending with intervascular smooth muscle bundles; cavernous-type angioleiomyoma is composed of dilated vascular channels with a proliferation of smooth muscle bundles in the intervascular spaces. Tumors showing a mixture of these morphologies can also be seen.[1] Immunohistochemically, the tumor cells are diffusely positive for smooth muscle actins and calponin and usually are strongly positive for h-caldesmon.[144] These tumors occur most commonly between the third and sixth decades, with a mean age at presentation in the mid-50s. Clinically, angioleiomyomas present as slow-growing, firm, sometimes painful masses, most commonly in the subcutis or dermis of the extremities.[145–147] Approximately 10% of angioleiomyomas are found in the head and neck region, with sites of occurrence, including the oral cavity, sinonasal cavities, lip, auricle, submandibular region, buccal space, larynx, parotid gland, and masticator space.[145,148–151]

On MR imaging, angioleiomyomas typically are well-defined oval masses that are isointense to muscle on T1-weighted images and usually show avid enhancement following contrast administration. On T2-weighted images, they show heterogeneous signal intensities including areas that are hyperintense and isointense to muscle[147]

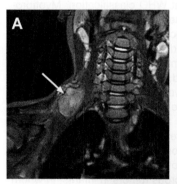
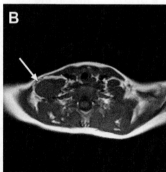
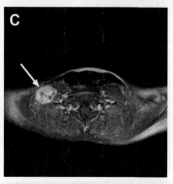

Fig. 14. Myofibroma in a 2-year-old boy presenting with a right supraclavicular mass. (A) Coronal STIR and (B) unenhanced axial T1-weighted, and axial contrast-enhanced, fat-suppressed, T1-weighted images demonstrate an ovoid mass (arrows) in the right neck situated between the lateral margins of the anterior and middle scalene muscles. The mass is heterogeneously hyperintense with some linear areas of lower signal (A), very slightly hyperintense compared with the adjacent anterior scalene muscle (B), and enhances heterogeneously with several low signal intensity, nonenhancing foci (C).

(Fig. 15). One potentially characteristic appearance that has been described on T2-weighted, fat-suppressed, and STIR images is that of a mass that is predominantly isointense to surrounding fat but has extensive areas of internal linear and branching hyperintensity, which may represent patent blood vessels.[152]

Glomus tumors, which are a distinct entity from the more common head and neck paragangliomas that also frequently are referred to as glomus tumors (eg, glomus tympanicum, glomus vagale, and glomus jugulare), are rare tumors composed of cells resembling the perivascular modified smooth muscle cells of a normal glomus body. Also referred to as glomangiomas, these tumors account for fewer than 2% of soft tissue tumors and most commonly occur in the distal extremities, with fewer than 1% arising in the head and neck.[153] They occur at any age, but most are diagnosed in young to middle-aged adults.[1,154] Malignant glomus tumors are rare but exist, with metastases or death reported in up to 40% of patients with the malignant form of the tumor[155]; 10% of patients with glomus tumors may have multiple lesions, and there is a syndrome of multiple familial glomus tumors caused by inactivating mutations in the globulin gene (GLMN), which is inherited in an autosomal dominant pattern.[156] Sporadic glomus tumors harbor recurrent NOTCH gene family rearrangements with MIR143-Notch1/ 2/3 fusion genes observed in more than half of cases.[157]

Glomus tumors of the head and neck are reported to arise primarily in the oral cavity, with the most common locations the lips, buccal mucosa, tongue, and hard palate. In this region, they have an average diameter of 1 cm to 1.5 cm, larger than glomus tumors found elsewhere in the body.[153] Other reported head and neck sites include the middle ear and mastoid, larynx, nasal cavity, and neck.[154,157–159] On MR imaging, glomus tumors demonstrate intermediate signal on T1-weighted images and markedly high signal intensity on T2-weighted images with uniform and marked enhancement. A high signal nidus surrounded by a rim of lower signal intensity has been suggested as specific for glomus tumors in the digits, but this finding is not universally present.[160]

Smooth Muscle Tumors

Tumors of smooth muscle origin include leiomyoma, LMS, and 2 entities newly introduced in the fifth edition WHO classification of soft tissue tumors: Epstein-Barr virus (EBV)-associated smooth muscle tumor and inflammatory LMS.[1]

Leiomyomas are benign tumors composed of cells that closely resemble normal smooth muscle cells with little or no nuclear atypia and, at most,

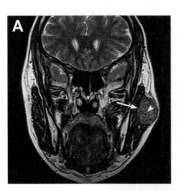
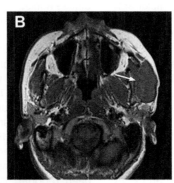
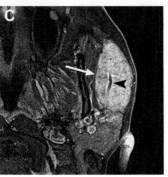

Fig. 15. Angioleiomyoma in a 44-year-old woman with a 1-year history of a slowly growing left facial mass. (A) Coronal T2-weighted, (B) axial unenhanced T1-weighted, and (C) axial contrast-enhanced, fat-suppressed, T1-weighted MR images demonstrate a lobulated mass (arrows) in the subcutaneous tissues of the left cheek superficial to the masseter muscle. The mass is heterogeneously hyperintense relative to muscle on T2-weighted imaging (A) and isointense in T1-weighted imaging (B) and enhances avidly (C). (A, C) A prominent vessel can be seen coursing through the center of the mass (arrowhead), and additional scattered hypointense punctate and curvilinear flow voids also are evident.

extremely low levels of mitotic activity. These tumors usually are found in the uterus, the retroperitoneum and abdominal cavity, and deep somatic soft tissues (usually the extremities). Unlike leiomyomas of the uterus, retroperitoneum and pelvis, somatic leiomyomas appear less likely to express estrogen and progesterone receptor proteins.[161] Fewer than 1% of leiomyomas occur in the head and neck, with the peak incidence occurring in the fifth decade.[162] The most common site of head and neck involvement is the esophagus, followed by the skin of the head and neck, the oral cavity, larynx, orbit, and nasal cavity.[163] Other reported sites include the auricle, the larynx, the orbit, trachea, salivary glands, paranasal sinuses, thyroid gland, and within the maxilla and mandible.[162,163] On MR imaging, leiomyomas appear as homogeneous masses demonstrating signal intensity hypointense or isointense to muscle on T1-weighted images and isointense to mildly hyperintense on T2-weighted images with marked postcontrast enhancement.[164,165] These tumors can demonstrate calcification or ossification.

LMS is a malignant tumor that accounts for between 4% and 15% of all soft tissue sarcomas.[166] They are believed to originate mainly from smooth muscle cells within blood vessel walls, but they also may arise from undifferentiated mesenchymal cells. Approximately 4% of LMSs occur in the head and neck, primarily in the oral cavity (most commonly involving the tongue), superficial soft tissues, paranasal sinuses, and jaws, but other reported sites of involvement include the pharynx, larynx, trachea, maxilla, thyroid, and ear.[166–169] Overall, the incidence of LMS increases with age, peaking in the seventh decade of life,[1] but, of cases reported in the head and neck, there may be a bimodal age distribution, with 1 peak in children and young adults (age 1–29) and the second in older adults (ages 51–67).[166] Predisposing conditions to the development of LMS include Li-Fraumeni syndrome, hereditary retinoblastoma, and radiation exposure.[1] Whole-exome and RNA sequencing studies have shown that LMSs are characterized by substantial mutational heterogeneity, with a high frequency of inactivation of the TP53 and RB1 tumor suppressor genes.[170] Most head and neck LMSs are of moderate grade or high histologic grade, and these tumors are clinically aggressive, showing little response to chemotherapy or radiation with frequent local recurrences and regional and distant metastases.[1,167]

The imaging features of LMS are nonspecific. On MR imaging, LMSs typically are isointense to hypointense relative to muscle on T1-weighted

images and variably hyperintense on T2-weighted images, with prominent contrast enhancement. Large lesions usually are more heterogeneous due to the presence of hemorrhage, necrosis, and cystic change[169,171,172] (Fig. 16). In the literature on uterine smooth muscle tumors, ill-defined margins, low ADC along with lack of central contrast enhancement, and presence of corresponding areas of high signal intensity on both T1-weighted and T2-weighted imaging favor a diagnosis of LMS over leiomyoma[173]; however, it has yet to be shown that these features also apply to LMS of the head and neck. Calcification in LMS is uncommon.

EBV-associated smooth muscle tumor (EBV-SMT) is a newly added tumor to the recent WHO update. These rare tumors typically manifest in immunodeficient individuals, including those with human immunodeficiency virus (HIV) infection, post-transplant patients with drug-related immunosuppression, and those with congenital immunodeficiency.[174] Histologically, these tumors can appear similar to other smooth muscle tumors, including leiomyoma and LMS, but are characterized by 2 unique and defining features: the first is the presence of variable numbers of intratumoral lymphocytes (composed predominantly of T cells) and the second the presence clusters of primitive-appearing round cells arising in a backdrop of more well-differentiated smooth muscle cells.[175] Diagnosis can be confirmed by demonstrating diffuse nuclear positivity for EBV-encoded ribonucleic acid by in situ hybridization.[125]

EBV-SMT can arise in a range of anatomic sites, and simultaneous involvement of multiple locations is not uncommon. Unlike traditional smooth muscle tumors, which follow the distribution of smooth muscle in the body, EBV-SMTs have a predilection for arising in unusual sites, including those with little smooth muscle, such as the brain and dura.[175] It is thought that they are derived from aberrant myogenous vascular smooth muscle cells.[174] In the head and neck, EBV-SMTs have been reported in the pharynx, larynx, eye and orbit, sinonasal tract, trachea, spine, dura, and cavernous sinus.[176–181] Different treatment modalities have been described for EBV-SMT, including chemotherapy, surgical resection, antiviral therapy, and reduced immunosuppression; however, there is no universally accepted approach to treat these tumors.[174] Prognosis depends on a patient's immune condition. Patients with HIV-associated EBV-SMT tend to have the poorest prognosis. The imaging features of these tumors is nonspecific and mimic those of other smooth muscle and mesenchymal tumors in the head and neck. Intracranial EBV-SMTs are described as

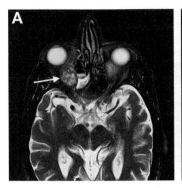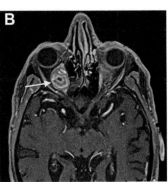

Fig. 16. Metastatic LMS to the orbit in a 77-year-old man with a history of a previously resected LMS of the left neck presenting now with diplopia. (A) Axial T2-weighted image demonstrates a mass in the right orbit (*arrow*), which is heterogeneously hyperintense centrally with a peripheral rind of more intermediate signal intensity tissue. (B) Axial contrast-enhanced, fat-suppressed, T1-weighted image demonstrates the mass (*arrow*) to enhanced heterogeneously with a central area of nonenhancement suggesting necrosis.

isointense to mildly hyperintense to white matter on T2-weighted images, isointense on T1-weighted images with variable enhancement, and occasional hemorrhage.[174]

Inflammatory LMS is the other new smooth muscle neoplasm in the updated WHO soft tissue tumor classification. It is an extremely rare malignant neoplasm sharing morphologic features with conventional LMS but also shows a prominent inflammatory infiltrate and a distinctive near-haploid genotype. These tumors occur in the deep soft tissues, most commonly of the lower limb, trunk, and retroperitoneum.[1] To date, only 2 cases of inflammatory LMS have been reported, 1 occurring in the parapharyngeal space[182] and 1 arising in the common carotid artery.[183]

Skeletal Muscle Tumors

The skeletal muscle tumors in the WHO classification of soft tissue tumors include rhabdomyoma, RMS, and ectomesenchymoma.

Rhabdomyoma is the one benign entity in the skeletal muscle tumor category. This tumor is considered a true neoplasm and is distinct from the more common hamartomatous cardiac rhabdomyoma, which frequently is associated with tuberous sclerosis. Overall, extracardiac rhabdomyomas account for fewer than 2% of striated muscle tumors.[184] Fetal, adult, and genital rhabdomyoma subtypes are recognized, with most nongenital rhabdomyomas occurring in the head and neck region.[1]

Adult rhabdomyomas are the most common rhabdomyoma subtype, occurring at a median age of 60 years and affecting men 2 times as frequently as women. These tumors present as painless, slow-growing masses, and, because of their slow rate of growth, they often are quite large at presentation; 90% of adult rhabdomyomas are found in the head and neck, and common sites

of involvement include the larynx, pharynx, and floor of the mouth. Other reported sites of origin include the parapharyngeal space, submandibular region, paratracheal region, and tongue.[184,185] In approximately 15% of cases, adult rhabdomyomas may be multicentric.[185] The fetal type of rhabdomyoma, composed of immature skeletal muscle cells, is diagnosed at a mean age of approximately 4.5 years and often is present at birth.[1,184,186] Like adult rhabdomyomas, these tumors also arise more commonly in boys. They may occur association with basal cell nevus syndrome, due to loss of function mutations of the tumor suppressor gene PTCH1, which encodes an inhibitory receptor in the sonic hedgehog signaling pathway.[187] Fetal rhabdomyomas arise most frequently in the periauricular region and face[186] but also have been reported in the nasopharynx, neck, tongue, buccal space, orbit, soft palate, larynx, and infratemporal fossa.[186,188]

On MR imaging, both fetal and adult type rhabdomyomas are homogenous lesions that do not invade surrounding soft tissue structures. They typically appear isointense or slightly hyperintense to muscle on T1-weighted and T2-weighted imaging with homogeneous enhancement[184] (**Fig. 17**).

RMS is a malignant tumor with cells showing a propensity for myogenic differentiation. RMS is predominantly a pediatric tumor, representing approximately half of soft tissue sarcomas in this population, but it also may affect adults.[189,190] The current WHO soft tissue classification recognizes 4 distinct types of RMS: embryonal (ERMS), alveolar (ARMS), pleomorphic, and spindle cell/sclerosing types.[1] Of these, the ERMS and ARMS represent the 2 most common major subtypes. Pleomorphic RMS is a rare adult variant of RMS of uncertain pathogenesis, generally arising in older adult men and most often involving the extremities. The spindle cell/sclerosing type of RMS is characterized by having a fascicular

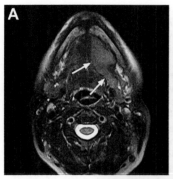
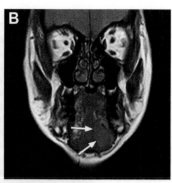
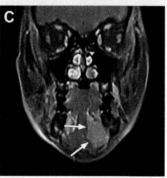

Fig. 17. Rhabdomyoma in a 53-year-old woman with a slowly enlarging submucosal mass in the left floor of mouth. (*A*) Axial T2-weighted, (*B*) coronal T1-weighted, and (*C*) coronal contrast-enhanced, fat-suppressed, T1-weighted images demonstrate a mass (*arrows*) in the left sublingual space with insinuates around but does not definitely invade the deep muscles of the tongue. The mass is hyperintense relative to muscle on both T2-weighted and T1-weighted sequences (*A, B*) and enhances homogeneously (*C*).

spindle cell and/or sclerosing morphology and occurs most commonly in the head and neck region, followed by the extremities.[1] Spindle cell RMSs can be categorized genetically into 3 groups: (1) a congenital/infantile group that shows gene fusions involving the VGLL2, SRF, TEAD1, NCOA2, and CITED2 genes; (2) an adolescent and adult group showing MYOD1 mutations; and (3) a group showing no recurrent identifiable genetic alterations. Tumors in the first group generally have a favorable prognosis, whereas MYOD1-mutant tumors follow a more aggressive course.[1,190] Given the rarity of the latter 2 subtypes of RMS, this discussion focuses on the ERMS and ARMS types.

Of the 2 major RMS subtypes, ERMS is by far the more common, occurring approximately 2.5 times more frequently than ARMS.[191] ERMS appears to have a bimodal age distribution with a first peak in early childhood and a second peak in early adolescence, whereas ARMS seems to have a constant incidence throughout childhood and adolescence.[190] ERMS, in particular, is observed with increased frequency in individuals with certain genetic disorders compared with the general population. Disorders associated most commonly with ERMS include Li-Fraumeni syndrome, NF1, Costello syndrome, Noonan syndrome, Beckwith-Wiedemann syndrome, and the DICER1 syndrome; however, only approximately 5% of patients with RMS have comorbid germline susceptibility syndromes.[190]

In addition to having different histologic features, ARMS and ERMS now are recognized as each having a distinct pathogenesis. ARMS tumor cells usually contain balanced chromosomal translocations—usually between FOXO1 and the PAX3 or PAX7 genes—producing an oncogenic fusion protein (PAX3-FOXO1 or PAX7-FOXO1), which is absent in ERMS. Approximately 20% of tumors classified as ARMS using current criteria do not harbor these fusions and behave more like ERMS clinically and molecularly, leading some authors to advocate for classifying RMS as being fusion protein positive or fusion protein negative rather than based on their histologic phenotype.[190] In ERMS, various mutations have been identified, which mostly converge on a limited number of pathways including the RAS-PI3K pathway or genes that control the cell cycle.[1]

ERMS arises most commonly in the head and neck, whereas ARMS arises more frequently occurs in the extremities, with a smaller proportion occurring in the head and neck.[190] Classically, RMS involvement in the head and neck is categorized as parameningeal (50%), nonparameningeal (25%), and orbital (25%) disease. Parameningeal lesions arise from sites with a close anatomic relationship to the meninges, including the skull base, nasopharynx and nasal cavity, middle ear and mastoid, paranasal sinuses, and the pterygopalatine and infratemporal fossae; these generally carry a worse prognosis than tumors arising from other sites.[192] Orbital RMSs tend to have a more obvious presentation with proptosis and, therefore, may be detected earlier than those at other sites, potentially leading to improved outcomes.[193] Approximately 10% to 20% of patients with RMS develop metastatic cervical adenopathy, and distant metastases are seen in approximately 15% of cases at the time of presentation.[91,189,194]

RMSs frequently are relatively well-circumscribed but often erode adjacent bone and perineural tumor spread through the skull base may be observed. On MR imaging, the signal characteristics of RMS largely are nonspecific, usually consisting of intermediate signal intensity on T1-weighted images and variable but generally intermediate to high signal intensity on T2-weighted images (**Fig. 18**). Enhancement can be variable, but often there is strong or avid enhancement following gadolinium administration. Hemorrhage, necrosis, and calcifications also may be present, resulting in a more heterogeneous enhancement pattern.[194] These tumors usually show restricted diffusion on DWI.[193]

Ectomesenchymoma is a rare, malignant multiphenotypic tumor composed of areas resembling RMS intermixed with variable neuronal or neuroblastic elements.[1] It formerly was listed as a peripheral nerve sheath tumor in the previous edition of the WHO classification but since has been reclassified as a skeletal muscle tumor. Cytogenetic studies show findings that overlap those of ERMSs, and the prognoses for both tumors are comparable. Most ectomesenchymomas develop in the first 2 decades of life, usually before 5 years of age. The head and neck are the second most common sites of involvement following the pelvis and perineum. Reported sites of head and neck involvement include the face, lips, nose, paranasal sinuses, nasal cavity ear, nasopharynx, scalp, orbit, and dura.[195–199] Ectomesenchymomas are indistinguishable from other RMSs on imaging.

Gastrointestinal Stromal Tumor

Gastrointestinal stromal tumors (GISTs) are morphologically diverse mesenchymal neoplasms originating from specialized cells in the alimentary tract known as the interstitial cells of Cajal. These tumors arise anywhere along the gastrointestinal tract, with a majority arising in the stomach followed in frequency by the small bowel.[1] A quarter of GISTs are clinically malignant and metastasize, usually to the liver and abdominal viscera; however, there are rare reports of metastasis of GIST to the head and neck region, with reported sites including bone (skull, orbit, temporal bone, and mandible), the maxillary sinus, and the oral cavity.[200,201] MR imaging appearance of GIST can be variable secondary to the necrosis,

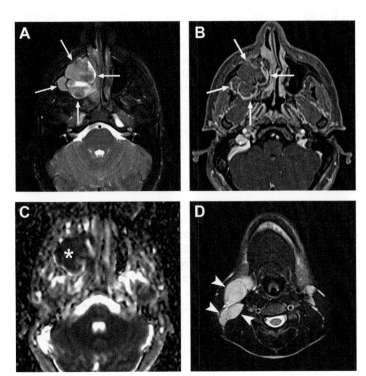

Fig. 18. ARMS in a 20-year-old man initially presenting with a right-sided neck mass and facial swelling with recurrent epistaxis. (*A*) Axial T2-weighted and (*B*) axial contrast-enhanced, fat-suppressed, T1-weighted images demonstrate a destructive, nonparameningeal mass (*arrows*) centered in the right maxillary sinus showing heterogeneous hyperintense T2-weighted signal and mild contrast enhancement. On the ADC map (*C*), the tumor demonstrates diffuse low signal (*asterisk*), indicating restricted diffusion. (*D*) Axial T2-weighted image through the upper neck also demonstrates multiple enlarged right cervical lymph nodes (*arrowheads*), representing nodal metastases.

hemorrhage, cystic changes, or calcification. As with other mensenchymal tumors, GISTs typically are hypointense on T1-weighted sequences and hyperintense on T2-weighted images with variable enhancement.[202]

Chondro-osseous Tumors

The chondro-osseous category consists of 2 uncommon tumors: soft tissue chondroma and extraskeletal osteosarcoma, and this section also discusses of mesenchymal chondrosarcoma.[1] Soft tissue chondroma is a benign cartilaginous tumor thought to arise from fetal cartilage or pluripotential mesenchyme that differentiates into cartilage secondary to an irritative stimulus.[203] These well-circumscribed, solid masses usually occur in the fingers, but rare case reports have described them arising in the external ear, lip, cheek, parotid gland, tongue, neck, and eyelid.[203–208] Soft tissue chondroma occurs predominately in the third and fourth decades of life with a slight male predominance.[209] In approximately 50% of cases, FN1 gene rearrangements can be identified.[210] The tumor typically presents as a slowly growing, painless mass, and excision is the treatment of choice. CT scan demonstrates a well-circumscribed, heterogeneously enhancing mass that often contains coarse calcifications and endochondral ossification appearing as punctate, curvilinear, or ringlike calcifications.[211] MR imaging shows a multilobulated lesion with low to intermediate T1-weighted signal intensity and T2-weighted hyperintensity relative to muscle. Low signal intensity foci on both sequences corresponding to calcifications may be evident on both T1-weighted and T2-weighted sequences.[212]

Extraskeletal osteosarcoma, also known as extraosseous osteosarcoma and soft tissue osteosarcoma, is a malignant tumor that arises independently from bone or periosteum. This tumor is extremely rare overall, accounting for fewer than 1% of all sarcomas and 4% of all osteosarcomas.[1] This tumor presents later in life, fifth to seventh decades, usually with a progressively enlarging mass that is located deep in the soft tissues.[1] These have been reported to occur in the parapharyngeal area, parotid gland, neck, optic nerve, and scalp.[213–217] Predisposing factors to the development of this tumor include trauma and, in 5% to 10% of cases, radiation.[218] Long-term prognosis is poor with a 5-year survival rate between 37% and 52%.[1] CT demonstrates a heterogenous, enhancing mass, occasionally showing central areas of low attenuation and mineralization.[219] The bone present in extraskeletal osteosarcomas often is amorphous and usually prominent

centrally.[220] MR imaging also demonstrates a heterogenous mass that usually is isointense on T1 and hyperintense on T2 studies with postcontrast enhancement.[219] MR imaging findings vary with the amount of cellular differentiation, extracellular matrix, hemorrhage, or necrosis.

Although technically listed as a tumor of bone in the WHO classification, mesenchymal chondrosarcoma is discussed, because approximately 40% of these tumors occur in the somatic soft tissues.[1] This high-grade malignant tumor accounts for 2% to 4% of all chondrosarcomas and has a characteristic biphasic pattern on histology composed of a cellular poorly differentiated small round blue cell component interspersed with islands of well-differentiated hyaline cartilage.[1,221] A recurrent gene fusion between HEY1 and NCOA2 is found in virtually all of these tumors, which is helpful in confirming a diagnosis.[222] These tumors occur across wide age range with a median age of 30 years. Approximately 15% of patients present with metastases at diagnosis.[223] Extraskeletal involvement tends to occur in the meninges, but approximately 15% occur in the head and neck, including in the craniofacial region (the most common head and neck site), the sinonasal tract, orbit, and thyroid gland.[224–226] On imaging, mesenchymal chondrosarcomas usually are large at presentation. Chondroid-type ring-and-arc calcifications are seen in up to two-thirds of cases, although they are not extensive. On MR imaging, mesenchymal chondrosarcomas usually demonstrate nonspecific features, including low to intermediate signal intensity on T1-weighted sequences and intermediate signal on T2-weighted sequences, with variable enhancement that often is more diffuse and lacks the typical cartilaginous septal and peripheral enhancement of conventional chondrosarcomas (**Fig. 19**). Some lesions may demonstrate low-signal intensity flow voids.[227] Restricted diffusion also may be seen on DWI.

Peripheral Nerve Sheath Tumors

Tumors in the peripheral nerve sheath category are of neuroectodermal origin and may occur anywhere that nerves are found. A vast majority of these tumors (90%–95%) are benign, with most representing schwannomas and neurofibromas. Malignant tumors in this category are rare with MPNST the one most frequently encountered. Other uncommon peripheral nerve sheath tumors described in the WHO soft tumor classification include granular cell tumor, solitary circumscribed neuroma, ectopic meningioma, benign Triton tumor (BTT), and a newly described entity, malignant melanotic nerve sheath tumor (MMNST).[1]

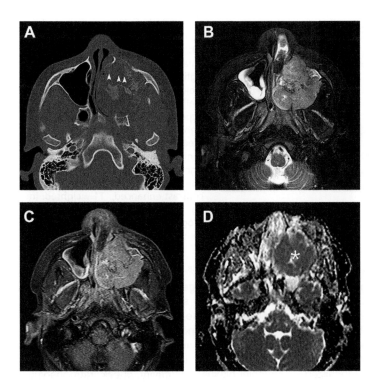

Fig. 19. Mesenchymal chondrosarcoma in a 12-year-old girl who presented initially with nasal congestion and epistaxis. (A) Axial bone window CT image demonstrates an expansile mass centered in and eroding the walls the left maxillary sinus. The mass shows internal calcifications, including some punctate and curvilinear chondroid type calcifications (arrowheads). (B) Axial T2-weighted image demonstrates the tumor to be intermediate in signal between that of muscle and the nasal mucosa, with a few areas of low signal, likely reflecting the internal calcifications. (C) Axial contrast-enhanced, fat-suppressed, T1-weighted image demonstrates diffuse, mostly homogeneous enhancement of the mass. (D) The corresponding ADC map shows low signal intensity in the tumor (asterisk) indicated restricted diffusion.

Schwannomas, which are the most common solitary nerve sheath tumors, are benign neoplasms that exhibit differentiation toward Schwann cells. Greater than 90% of these tumors are solitary sporadic, but there is an association with neurofibromatosis type 2 (NF2) and schwannomatosis, which both feature multiple schwannomas.[1] Sporadic schwannomas may affect all ages but have a peak incidence in the fourth to sixth decades of life, whereas those associated with NF2 commonly present before 30 years of age. Tumorigenesis is linked to loss of expression of merlin, the protein product of the NF2 tumor suppression gene.[228] In addition, germline mutations of either the SMARCB1 or LZTR1 tumor suppressor gene are found in 86% of familial and 40% of sporadic schwannomatosis patients.[229] Various subtypes of schwannoma are recognized. Classic schwannomas are well-encapsulated, biphasic tumors with compact (Antoni A) areas showing occasional nuclear palisading (Verocay bodies), alternating with more loosely arranged (Antoni B) tissue. Grossly, uninvolved nerve fascicles often can be found draped around the tumor capsule. Various morphologic schwannoma variants exist, which deviate from the classic schwannoma description, including ancient, cellular, plexiform, epithelioid, and microcystic/reticular subtypes.[1]

Between 25% and 45% of schwannomas arise in the head and neck region.[230] Among those located in the extracranial head and neck, approximately half occur in the superficial neck. Other relatively common sites of involvement include the parapharyngeal space, oral cavity, and nasal cavity, whereas less frequent sites include the parotid gland, larynx, skull base, and middle ear.[231,232] The most common nerves of origin in one series of schwannomas were the sympathetic trunk (33%), the vagus nerve (20%), and the facial nerve (10%), but in 17% of cases the tumor may arise from a minor nerve, or the nerve of origin cannot be identified.[231]

On MR imaging, schwannomas typically are well-defined masses, which are heterogeneously hyperintense relative to muscle on T2-weighted images and of low to intermediate signal intensity on T1-weighted images, with avid enhancement (Fig. 20). Heterogeneity on T2-weighted sequences likely reflects the biphasic composition of these tumors. A target appearance has been described with a central region of low signal intensity with peripheral high signal intensity on T2-weighted images, but this finding is seen more commonly in neurofibromas. Larger schwannomas may show contain cysts or foci of hemorrhage. These tumors do not show restricted diffusion on DWI and tend to show delayed enhancement on DCE imaging.[230]

Neurofibromas are benign peripheral nerve sheath tumors that consist of differentiated

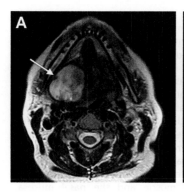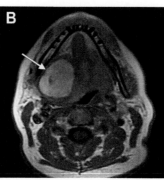

Fig. 20. Schwannoma of the sublingual space in a 48-year-old woman who presented with a gradually enlarging submucosal mass in the right floor of mouth. (*A*) Axial T2-weighted image demonstrates a well-circumscribed heterogeneously hyperintense mass (*arrow*) in the right sublingual space. Low signal areas are thought to be related to Antoni A regions, whereas the higher signal regions are thought to reflect less compact Antoni B tissue. (*B*) Axial contrast-enhanced, T1-weighted image demonstrates diffuse, mildly heterogeneous enhancement of the tumor (*arrow*).

Schwann cells, perineurial or perineurial-like cells, fibroblasts, mast cells, and residual interspersed axons embedded in a myxoid and collagenous extracellular matrix. They are the most common peripheral nerve sheath tumors, with the majority occurring as sporadic solitary lesions. Less frequently, multiple neurofibromas occur in individuals with NF1.[1] Presence of 2 or more localized cutaneous/subcutaneous neurofibromas or 1 plexiform neurofibroma is a major diagnostic criterion for the diagnosis of NF1.[233] Complete biallelic loss of function of function of the NF1 gene product, neurofibromin, is a prerequisite for development of neurofibromas.[234]

Five different macroscopic forms are recognized including localized cutaneous, diffuse cutaneous, localized intraneural, plexiform intraneural, and massive diffuse neurofibromas.[1] The localized forms are the most common type, accounting for approximately 90% of neurofibromas and occurring mostly in patients without NF1.[230,235] Localized cutaneous neurofibromas, which make up 90% of the cutaneous types, are nodular or polypoid lesions measuring up to 2 cm in size, whereas diffuse cutaneous neurofibromas can have a variety of appearances, including flat, sessile, globular, and pedunculated lesions.[236] Approximately 10% of diffuse cutaneous neurofibromas occur in the setting of NF1, and this form usually does not undergo malignant transformation.[235,237] Intraneural neurofibromas present as solitary fusiform masses or, when plexiform, as ropy or wormlike growths. Virtually all patients with NF1 develop cutaneous neurofibromas, which usually begin to appear in the second half of the first decade of life, and up to 50% ultimately show evidence of plexiform neurofibromas on imaging, which usually are evident by the age of 18.[233] Both types of intraneural neurofibromas are associated with an increased risk of malignant

transformation.[238,239] Massive soft tissue neurofibromas may range in shape from a relatively uniform regional soft tissue enlargement to pendulous baglike or capelike masses.[1]

In the head and neck, neurofibromas can be seen in virtually any space, with common areas of involvement including the carotid space, brachial plexus, oral cavity, cheek, retropharyngeal space, and posterior cervical space. In the carotid space, these tumors usually arise from the vagus nerve or sympathetic chain. Spine involvement also is common in the cervical region.[230]

On MR imaging, localized neurofibromas show low to intermediate signal on T1-weighted images, with variable enhancement after contrast administration. On T2-weighted sequences, they may be either homogeneously hyperintense or in some cases may demonstrate a characteristic target sign with a hyperintense ring of myxoid material and surrounding a hypointense region composed of fibrous tissue[230] (**Fig. 21**). On contrast-enhanced images, a reverse target sign can be seen with central enhancement surrounded by nonenhancing tissue peripherally.[235] Solitary localized neurofibromas may be difficult to differentiate from schwannomas on conventional imaging; however, as discussed previously, DTI tractography may be helpful for differentiating between the 2 tumors, because schwannomas more likely to be located eccentrically to the nerve with fascicles draped around the tumor than are neurofibromas.[48]

Plexiform neurofibromas manifest as ill-defined lesions that follow the course of a major nerve distribution. Best seen on fat-suppressed, T2-weighted MR imaging, they appear as multinodular confluent masses often with multiple target signs. They can cause significant disfigurement, crossing tissue planes to involve of multiple spaces in the neck and eroding adjacent bones.

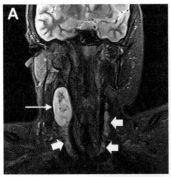
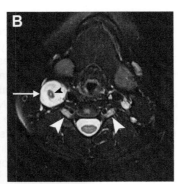
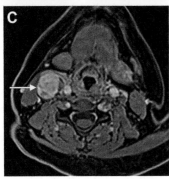

Fig. 21. Neurofibromas in a 16-year-old woman with NF1. (*A*) Coronal STIR and (*B*) axial T2-weighted images demonstrate a predominantly hyperintense mass in the right neck (*thin arrows*). On the axial image (*B*), there is a central area of low signal intensity (*black arrowhead*), likely reflecting a region of fibrous tissue surrounded by more hyperintense myxoid tissue peripherally, a finding known as the target sign. Additional wormlike plexiform neurofibromas can be seen in (*A*) along the course of the bilateral vagus nerves or sympathetic chains (*short thick arrows*), and neurofibromas also can be seen (*B*) in the bilateral neural foramina (*white arrowheads*). (*C*) Contrast-enhanced, fat-suppressed, T1-weighted image demonstrates heterogeneous enhancement of the larger neurofibroma (*arrow*).

On T1-weighted images they may be heterogeneous and show variable enhancement with contrast.[230,235]

Diffuse cutaneous neurofibromas appear as a poorly defined lesions that spread along the skin or subcutaneous connective tissue septa and surround rather than destroy adjacent structures. They are slow-growing lesions, usually measuring less than 5 cm at presentation. On MR imaging, they can have a plaque-like or infiltrative pattern of growth. Plaquelike lesions appear isointense to muscle on T1-weighted images and hyperintense on T2-weighted images. They show intense enhancement and prominent internal vascularity; however, the flow voids seen in diffuse plaque-like neurofibromas are less prominent compared with vascular lesions.[230] Infiltrative diffuse neurofibromas appear as reticulated lesions in the subcutaneous tissues, demonstrating corresponding reticulated enhancement on contrast-enhanced, fat-suppressed, T1-weighted imaging.[235]

MPNSTs in the head and neck are highly aggressive soft tissue sarcomas that show overlapping morphologic and immunophenotypic features with melanoma and other high-grade sarcomas and are associated with high rates of locoregional recurrence, distant metastases, and mortality.[240] MPNSTs may arise de novo in a peripheral nerve or from a preexisting benign nerve sheath tumor, with an increased incidence in patients with NF1 and following radiation therapy. NF1 associated tumors are estimated to account for 37% to 64% MPNSTs, whereas radiation-associated tumors account for only approximately 1%.[241] There also is a rare epithelioid subtype (making up <5%), which is the most common type to arise from schwannomas and is not associated with NF1.[242] MPNSTs typically are seen in patients aged 20 years to 50 years, and they rarely arise in children, except in the setting of NF1.[1] Frequent and concurrent mutations in 3 pathways have been demonstrated in MPNSTs: NF1, CDKN2A/CDKN2B, and PRC2. Approximately 80% of all high-grade MPNSTs exhibit complete loss of PRC2 activity and complete loss of H3K27me3 expression, the latter of which is an independent poor predictor of survival and has become a useful tool for diagnosing high-grade MPNSTs.[241,243–245]

In the head and neck, MPNSTs are reported in a wide range of locations, including the neck, tongue, cheek, parapharyngeal space, infratemporal fossa, brachial plexus, orbit, paranasal sinuses, scalp, and parotid gland.[230,240,246–248] In patients with NF1, they may arise anywhere there is a preexisting neurofibroma. In these patients, development of pain or a rapid increase in size in a preexisting neurofibroma should be viewed with a high degree of suspicion. On MR imaging, MPNSTs have nonspecific features and usually appear isointense to muscle on T1-weighted images with occasional areas of hyperintensity that may represent hemorrhage. On T2-weighted images, they are heterogeneously hyperintense and may feature areas of necrosis or cystic changes. Perilesional edema is a common finding, and these tumors show heterogeneous contrast enhancement[230] (**Fig. 22**). Features that suggest a diagnosis of MPNST over neurofibroma include size greater than 5 cm, a peripheral pattern of enhancement, the presence of perilesional edema, the presence of intratumoral cysts, ill-defined margins, intratumoral lobulations, and adjacent bone destruction.[230,249,250] MPNSTs also are unlikely to demonstrate a target sign. On DWI, MPNSTs are more likely to show low ADC values, whereas on DCE–MR imaging, they usually show early arterial enhancement with washout.[230,251,252]

A newly included entity in the peripheral nerve sheath tumor category is the MMNST, which is a rare tumor (<1% of peripheral nerve sheath tumors) composed of Schwann cells showing melanocytic differentiation, usually arising from spinal or autonomic nerves.[1] These tumors alternatively are referred to as melanotic schwannomas and can be subdivided further into psammomatous and non-psammomatous forms. MMNSTs are associated with the Carney complex in approximately 10% of cases, but in at least 1 series, the association was seen in 55% of cases.[253–255]

The tumor occurs chiefly in adults, with those occurring in the setting of Carney complex occurring at a slightly younger age (mean 22.5 years).[1] Local recurrences and metastases are common occurring at a rate of 26% to 44%. In Carney complex–associated tumors, alterations to the PRKAR1A and CNC2 genes have been identified.[1]

MMNSTs arise most frequently from the dorsal spinal nerve roots but can occur other paraspinal locations, including the sympathetic chain in the neck.[256,257] Lesions also may be multiple in up to 20% of cases.[258] The tumors characteristically demonstrate homogeneous hyperintense signal on T1-weighted images, due to the melanin content of the tumor, with more variable T2-weighted signal characteristics. T2-weighted and STIR images also may demonstrate a peripheral lobulated rim of very low signal (**Fig. 23**). Enhancement of these lesions is variable.[258]

BTT is an intraneural mass composed of both mature neural and skeletal tissue, usually involving large nerves and plexuses, including the brachial plexus. In the head and neck, 2 groups of BTTs have been proposed: (1) an aggressive central type that usually affects infants and children and involves large intracranial nerves or nerve trunks in the infratemporal fossa, and (2) a nonaggressive peripheral type characterized by subcutaneous or submucosal lesions found in older patients, including adults.[259,260] The aggressive form of

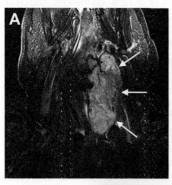
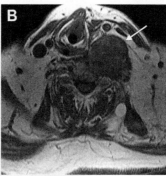
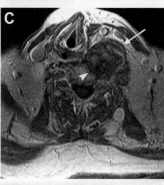

Fig. 22. MPNST in a 34-year-old man with NF1. (*A*) Coronal STIR image demonstrates a large heterogeneous hyperintense mass in the deep left neck (*arrows*). Note the lack of an obvious target sign. (*B*) Axial unenhanced, T1-weighted image demonstrates the mass (*arrow*) to be similar in intensity to muscle but mildly heterogeneous with scattered regions of higher signal intensity. The mass is inseparable from and may be invading the adjacent prevertebral musculature. On the contrast-enhanced, T1-weighted image (*C*), there is patchy heterogeneous enhancement of the mass (*arrow*). Note how the mass appears to be scalloping the adjacent vertebral body (*arrowhead*).

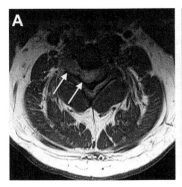 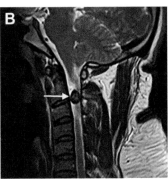

Fig. 23. Malignant melanotic peripheral nerve sheath tumor in a 41-year-old man with progressive neck pain and worsening right arm and bilateral lower extremity pain. (*A*) Axial T1-weighted MR image demonstrates bilobed mass in the cervical spinal canal extending through the right neural foramen (*arrows*), which is intrinsically hyperintense relative to muscle due to the melanocytic nature of the tumor. (*B*) Sagittal T2-weighted image demonstrates heterogeneous signal in the mass (*arrow*) with a peripheral rim of low signal intensity.

the disease commonly involves the trigeminal nerve in or near the middle cranial fossa with extension through foramen ovale into the infratemporal fossa and may result in destructive growth. Orbital involvement also is reported.[261] Most BTTs show CTNNB1 mutations similar to those of sporadic desmoids.[262] On MR imaging, these tumors have been reported as hypointense on T1-weighted images with mild to avid enhancement and to show intermediate or even profoundly hypointense signal on T2-weighted images, which may help distinguish these tumors from schwannomas, which usually are of high signal intensity on T2-weighted sequences.[263]

Other rare peripheral nerve sheath tumors that occasionally are encountered in the head and neck area include granular cell tumor, perineuroma, and solitary circumscribed neuroma.[1] Granular cell tumors are neoplasms showing neuroectodermal differentiation commonly featuring loss-of-function mutations involving the V-ATPase genes, ATP6AP1 and ATP6AP2.[264] They most commonly affect the deep dermis and subcutaneous tissues, particularly in the head and neck, where the most common sites are the tongue followed by the larynx, but they also have been reported in the trachea, esophagus, cricopharyngeus, deep neck, gingiva, scalp, orbit, and trigeminal and facial nerves.[265] Granular cell tumors have been reported to appear hypointense on both T1-weighted and T2-weighted imaging due to the presence of abundant interstitial collagen fibers and to have low to intermediate ADC values because of their higher cellularity.[230]

Solitary circumscribed neuromas are benign, usually cutaneous proliferations of nerve fibers, which involve the skin of the face in 90% of cases (usually nose, forehead, and lips).[266] Perineuromas usually are benign tumors composed entirely of perineurial cells, which present as painless masses and arise most commonly in the limbs

although the head and neck region rarely may be affected.[1] The imaging features of these latter 2 tumor types is not specific, and more superficial tumors rarely undergo imaging.

Tumors of Uncertain Differentiation

Tumors in the tumors of uncertain differentiation include benign as well as malignant soft tissue tumors that have an undetermined cellular differentiation. This results in an eclectic grouping of entities. The most common benign tumor in this category is a myxoma, whereas synovial sarcoma is the most common malignant tumor.[18] The fifth edition tumor classification added 2 new tumors to the subtype of tumors of uncertain differentiation: NTRK-rearranged spindle cell neoplasm and undifferentiated sarcoma. In addition, 2 tumors that were present in the previous edition—ectopic hamartomatous thymoma and malignant mesenchymoma—have been removed.

Intramuscular myxomas are benign, slow-growing relatively hypocellular tumors, which classically are composed of bland spindle-shaped cells in an abundant hypovascular myxoid stroma.[1] They typically arise in the large muscles of the thigh, shoulder, buttock, and upper arm and rarely involve the head and neck region.[1,267] These tumors usually affect middle-aged adults and are approximately 2 times more common in women than men. Approximately a third recur locally after excision.[267] Multiple intramuscular myxomas can develop in individuals with Mazabraud syndrome (intramuscular myxomas associated with fibrous dysplasia) as well as in McCune-Albright syndrome.[268] In greater than 90% of sporadic cases of intramuscular myxoma and in all cases associated with Mazabraud syndrome, an activating point mutation in GNAS leading to downstream activation of c-FOS can be identified.[269–271] In addition to the large muscles in the neck, they are reported to involve the geniohyoid, masseter, digastric, tongue, temporalis, hyoglossus, and mimetic muscles of the nasal vestibule.[268,272]

Juxta-articular myxoma is a rare, benign tumor arising from the connective tissue of large joints, which is morphologically similar to intramuscular myxomas but lacks the GNAS mutation.[1,267] Clinically, this tumor presents as a swollen joint with occasional functional limitation. It typically presents in the third to fifth decades of life and, unlike intramuscular myxomas, has a male predominance.[273,274] Although occurring most frequently in the knee, case reports exist of juxta-articular myxoma occurring in the TMJ.[275]

Myxomas on imaging usually are well-circumscribed, oval-shaped masses. Imaging features are similar between intramuscular and juxta-articular with the differentiation based on location.[276] CT imaging demonstrates fluid attenuation, whereas on MR imaging signal intensity similar to fluid is seen on unenhanced sequences. These tumors are hypointense compared with muscle on T1-weighted images and hyperintense on T2-weighted images (**Fig. 24**). A peritumoral fat rind may be evident on T1-weighted imaging, and T2-weighted images may show perilesional hyperintensity. These 2 findings may be helpful for distinguishing intramuscular myxomas from other soft tissue myxoid lesions. Most intramuscular myxomas show some enhancement with contrast.[268,277]

Synovial sarcomas account for approximately 10% of all sarcomas, with approximately 3% occurring in the head and neck. These tumors are characterized by a specific mutation in which SS18 is fused to 1 of the SSX genes (SSX1, SSX2, or SSX4). Histologically they appear as monomorphic blue spindle cell tumors with variable epithelial differentiation and diffuse, strong staining for TLE1. Despite their name, these tumors do not derive from synovial tissue but instead may arise from pluripotent mesenchymal cells. Synovial sarcomas most often affect adolescents and young adults, and approximately three-quarters of cases occur before the age of 50 years.[1] Most arise in the upper and lower extremities, often in a juxta-articular location. Approximately 7% arise in the head and neck, where the most frequently involved sites include the pharynx (specifically the hypopharynx) and the parapharyngeal and retropharyngeal spaces.[278–280] Other less common locations in the head and neck include the sinonasal region and masticator space. Following resection, these tumors often recur, at a rate of 50% in the first 2 years. Moreover, they metastasize in up 40% of cases, most commonly to the regional lymph nodes, lungs, and bone.[279]

Synovial sarcomas predominately are solid masses on imaging. On both CT and MR imaging, they demonstrate well-defined smooth margins and rarely infiltrate adjacent structures. Depending on the degree of internal hemorrhage and/or hemorrhage, they can appear either homogeneous or heterogeneous in nature and thus this should not be used as a distinguishing feature. Most synovial sarcomas are isointense to slightly hypertense to muscle on T1-weighted sequences. Features on T2-weighted sequences are more variable. These tumors often demonstrate heterogeneous, predominantly increased signal on T2-weighted sequences intermixed with areas of low and intermediate signal (described as the triple sign).[281] Although frequently seen in synovial sarcomas, the triple sign is not specific, however, and can be seen in other sarcomas.[282] Prominent and usually heterogeneous enhancement is seen in these tumors following contrast administration, and the tumors may demonstrate nonenhancing regions of necrosis, cystic change, or hemorrhage

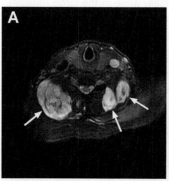 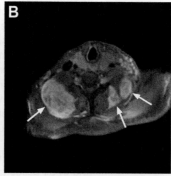

Fig. 24. Multiple intramuscular myxomas in a 59-year-old woman with a several-year history of multiple firm, rubbery subcutaneous nodules on neck, left arm, chest, and lower extremities. Axial (A) T2-weighted and (B) contrast-enhanced, fat-suppressed, T1-weighted MR images demonstrate 3 circumscribed masses in the bilateral paraspinous muscles (*arrows*). The masses demonstrate very high, but heterogeneous, signal (A) and avid postcontrast enhancement (B). The presence of multiple intramuscular myxomas should raise the possibility of an underlying genetic disorder, such as Mazabraud syndrome.

(Fig. 25). Calcifications are seen in up to 30% of cases.[282,283]

Alveolar soft part sarcomas (ASPSs) make up fewer than 1% of soft tissue sarcomas. They are characterized by a specific mutation, resulting in fusion of the ASPSCR1 and TFE3 genes. Although they occur across a broad age range, more than 70% occur in patients under the age of 30 years.[1] These tumors usually arise in the deep soft tissues of the extremities, but approximately 9% occur in the head and neck, where the most common sites of involvement are the orbit and tongue.[284,285] Other reported sites include the larynx, buccal space, and paravertebral space. On MR imaging, ASPSs have been described as showing high signal intensity on both T1-weighted and T2-weighted sequences and demonstrating strong enhancement. They frequently show flow voids and central necrosis.[284]

Molecular analysis of tumors has led to the emerging category of NTRK-rearranged spindle cell neoplasms, which encompasses tumors with a wide spectrum of morphologies and histologic grades. These tumors all harbor NTRK fusions with a variety of partner genes. Most occur in the first 2 decades of life.[1] Prognosis of NTRK-rearranged tumors appears to be related to histologic grade, and molecular biology ideally allows for predicting sensitivity to treatment, thus potentially predicting efficacy of the recently available NTRK inhibitors in this tumor class.[286,287] As a recently identified tumor type, there are no reports to the authors' knowledge of this type of tumor occurring in the head and neck, with most instead involving the extremities, trunk, and bone.[287]

The other new category is undifferentiated soft tissue sarcoma, which essentially is a diagnosis of exclusion leading to a diverse grouping of tumors. Subtypes included in this category include undifferentiated spindle cell sarcoma, undifferentiated pleomorphic sarcoma, and undifferentiated round cell sarcoma. The round cell subtype occurs most frequently in younger patients, whereas the pleomorphic subtype occurs mostly in older adults. Although there are few defining characteristics for this group, these tumors frequently have a morphologically high grade and rapid growth rate.[1]

Undifferentiated pleomorphic sarcoma, in the past referred to as malignant fibrous histiocytoma, is the most common histologic subtype of sarcomas to occur in the head and neck in adults and is a second most common diagnosis for children after RMS.[288] It also is the most common subtype of sarcoma to be radiation-induced.[289] In the head and neck, these tumors have been described in the sinonasal cavity, craniofacial bones, larynx, soft tissues of the face and neck, major salivary glands, oral cavity, pharynx, ear, eyelid, and orbit.[290] Treatment consists of wide local excision with consideration for postoperative radiation in aggressive cases or with positive margins.[288] Imaging typically demonstrates an ill-defined mass of larger size with adjacent soft tissue and bony destruction. Precise MR imaging characteristics, including enhancement and attenuation patterns, are nonspecific. These tumors frequently demonstrate invasion of adjacent soft tissue structures and bone destruction. They usually are isointense to muscle on T1-weighted imaging and heterogeneously hyperintense on T2-weighted images and show variable enhancement, which may be nodular and peripheral (see **Fig. 3**; **Fig. 26**). Restricted diffusion may be evident on DWI. Up to 20% may contain calcifications, and areas of necrosis, hemorrhage, or myxoid material also may be evident.[290]

Undifferentiated Small Round Cell Sarcomas of Bone and Soft Tissue

Undifferentiated small round cell sarcomas are a new category in the soft tissue grouping of the

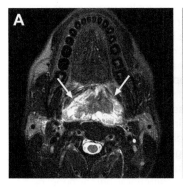
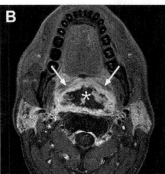

Fig. 25. Synovial sarcoma in a 38-year-old man presenting with difficulty swallowing. Axial (*A*) T2-weighted and (*B*) contrast-enhanced, fat-suppressed, T1-weighted MR images demonstrate a large mass (*arrows*) filling the oropharynx. (*A*) The mass is markedly heterogeneous with areas of low, intermediate, and high signal intensity. (*B*) Following contrast administration, the mass demonstrates irregular, predominantly peripheral enhancement with nonenhancement centrally (*asterisk*), possibly reflecting necrosis.

WHO fifth edition. Ewing sarcomas are the classic round cell tumor and previously were classified as tumors of uncertain differentiation. In recent years, it also has become increasingly apparent that there actually are several Ewing-like round cell tumors that are distinct from classic Ewing sarcoma and have unique genetic and immunohistochemical features. In addition to Ewing sarcoma, this category includes round cell sarcoma with EWSR1–non-ETS fusions, CIC-rearranged sarcoma, and sarcoma with BCOR genetic alterations.[1]

Ewing sarcomas are highly aggressive neoplasms that are seen most often in children and young adults, with a male predominace.[291] All Ewing sarcomas are associated with structural rearrangements that generate FET-ETS fusion genes.[1] Classically, they affect the diaphysis and diaphyseal-metaphysis of long bones; however, they can affect any bone and, less commonly, also can arise from soft tissues. The most common head and neck locations include the maxillofacial bones (including the paranasal sinuses), mandible, and skull base.[292] Extraskeletal involvement occurs in 12% of Ewing sarcoma patients, likely originating from neuroectodermal tissues and, in the head and neck, has been reported to occur in the nose, orbit, eyelid, submandibular region, nasopharynx, parotid, middle ear, scalp, infratemporal fossa/masticator space, carotid space,

parapharyngeal space, and cervical region.[292–295] Localized tumors have a reasonably good prognosis, with a 5-year survival of approximately 75%, but survival drops to only 30% in the setting of metastatic disease.[291]

CIC-rearranged round cell sarcoma is the most common and best characterized of the Ewing-like tumors. Characterized by the presence of recurrent CIC gene arrangements, these tumors have a predilection of young adults with a median age in the range of 25 years to 35 years, with fewer than a quarter occurring in the pediatric age group.[1] They arise most often in the deep soft tissue of the trunk, limbs, or head and neck region.[291] Skeletal involvement is uncommon in these variants. In the head and neck, these tumors have been reported in the scalp, submandibular region, tonsil, parapharyngeal space, and neck.[292] These tumors tend to have a poorer prognosis compared with classic Ewing sarcomas.[291]

Non–ETS-fused round cell sarcomas are extremely rare tumors that demonstrate rearrangements of the EWSR1 or FUS genes (both members of the FUS family of proteins) with fusion partners other than ETS. Fusion partners with EWSR1/FUS observed in these tumors include NFATc2 and PATZ1. These non–ETS-fused tumors occur tend to occur in older patients compared with traditional Ewing sarcoma. Finally, BCOR-rearranged sarcomas are variants occurring primarily in patients under the age of 20 years with a strong male predominance (approximately 4.5:1 male:female ratio).[1] The most frequently identified fusions in these tumors are BCOR-CCNB3 fusions and internal tandem (BCOR-ITD) duplications, with the BCOR-ITD variant occurring primarily in infancy. Compared with Ewing sarcoma, BCOR-rearranged sarcomas tend to demonstrate more indolent clinical behaviors.[291] Non–ETS-fused sarcomas tend to occur in long bones or in the deep soft tissues of the chest wall and abdomen, whereas BCOR-rearranged sarcomas occur more often in bone than soft tissue with a predilection for the pelvis, lower extremities, and paraspinal region. Both tumors also may rarely arise in the head and neck.[1,291]

Although each of these subtypes is genetically distinct and can have variations in morphology, their imaging appearances are indistinguishable and nonspecific. On MR imaging, they typically appear as soft tissue masses with heterogeneous signal intensity similar to muscle on T1-weighted images, intermediate to high signal intensity on T2-weighted images, and heterogeneous contrast enhancement (Fig. 27). DWI may show restricted tumor diffusion. Intratumoral hemorrhage or necrosis, or even fluid levels may be present, and

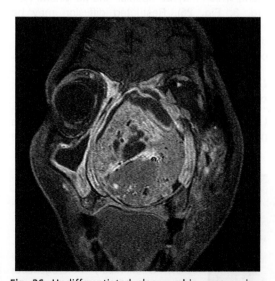

Fig. 26. Undifferentiated pleomorphic sarcoma in a 45-year-old man with an enlarging nasal mass (same patient as Fig. 3C, D). Coronal contrast-enhanced, fat-suppressed, T1-weighted image demonstrates a large heterogeneously enhancing mass with multiple nonenhancing cystic or necrotic regions filling the bilateral nasal cavities.

adjacent bone destruction or regional metastatic adenopathy may be evident in some cases. Some Ewing sarcomas also may demonstrate serpentine internal vascular flow voids.[294,296]

Other Head and Neck Soft Tissue Tumors

In addition to the previously described entities, there are several distinct soft tissue tumors of the head and neck that are not included in the *WHO Classification of Soft Tissue and Bone Tumours* but rather are described in the *WHO Classification of Head and Neck Tumours*. These include nasopharyngeal angiofibroma, sinonasal glomangiopericytoma, and BSNS.[7]

Nasopharyngeal angiofibroma, also commonly referred to as juvenile nasopharyngeal angiofibroma (JNA), is a tumor of the head and neck that is distinct from other entities that carry the angiofibroma moniker, including cellular angiofibroma (a tumor occurring in the vulva or inguinoscrotal regions), giant cell angiofibroma (now considered a type of SFT), and the aforementioned angiofibroma of soft tissue. JNA is a locally aggressive, fibrovascular neoplasm that arises in the posterolateral nasal wall, almost exclusively in adolescent boys, with a mean age of 17 years. The tumor is 20-times to 25-times more common in patients with familial adenomatous polyposis

than in the general population and appears to be associated with mutations in the beta-catenin gene (CTNNB1).[95,297,298] Evidence suggests hormonal dependency of these tumors, because growth is associated with puberty in boys, and tumor cells frequently express androgen receptors.[299]

Patients with JNA classically present in adolescence with the triad of nasal obstruction, recurrent epistaxis, and a nasopharyngeal mass, which may invade and destroy adjacent osseous structures, including the paranasal sinuses, orbit, and skull base. These tumors are believed to originate in the region of the sphenopalatine foramen and from there may extend into the nasal cavity, nasopharynx, pterygopalatine fossa, masticator space, paranasal sinuses, orbit, or middle cranial fossa. These tumors are highly vascular with a propensity for hemorrhage and, therefore, frequently are embolized prior to surgical resection.[78] On cross-sectional imaging, JNAs appear as avidly enhancing masses in the posterior nasal cavity and nasopharynx that classically widen the pterygopalatine fossa and produce anterior bowing of the posterior wall of the maxillary sinus. These tumors demonstrate signal intensity similar to muscle on T1-weighted images with intermediate to high signal intensity on T2-weighted images, although regions of the tumor may be relatively

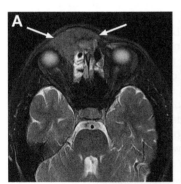
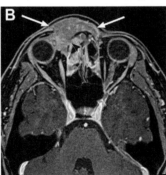
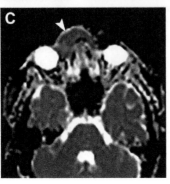

Fig. 27. Ewing sarcoma in an 18-year-old woman with a mass on the right side of the bridge of the nose, which gradually has increased size over the past 6 months. Axial (*A*) T2-weighted and (*B*) contrast-enhanced, fat-suppressed, T1-weighted images demonstrate a mass (*arrows*) in the right nasal bridge region showing intermediate T2-weighted signal intensity (isointense to gray matter and mildly hyperintense compared with muscle) and heterogeneous contrast enhancement. The mass erodes adjacent osseous structures (*black arrowhead* [*B*]) and involves the right orbit. (*C*) Axial ADC map demonstrates low signal in the mass (*white arrowhead*), indicating reduced water diffusion.

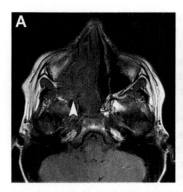 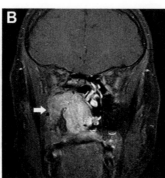

Fig. 28. Nasopharyngeal angiofibroma 13-year-old man with several year history of right nasal congestion and, more recently, several months of increasingly severe episodes of epistaxis (same patient as Fig. 3A, B). (A) Axial T1-weighted image demonstrates the right nasal cavity mass to be predominantly isointense relative to muscle. The tumor extends into and expands the right pterygopalatine fossa (PPF) (arrowhead). (B) Coronal contrast-enhanced, fat-suppressed, T1-weighted image demonstrated diffuse enhancement of the mass which extends laterally toward the masticator space (arrow) from the PPF through the pterygomaxillary fissure.

hypointense secondary to fibrous components[300] (see Fig. 3; Fig. 28). Large intratumoral flow voids also commonly are present.

Sinonasal glomangiopericytoma is a borderline/low-grade malignant soft tissue tumor of the nasal cavity characterized by perivascular myoid type differentiation, which reasonably could be considered a type of pericytic tumor.[7] This tumor in the past also has been referred to as sinonasal hemangiopericytoma and sinonasal hemangiopericytoma-like tumor. Accounting for fewer than 0.5% of sinonasal neoplasms, they have a peak incidence in the seventh decade of life but may arise at age and have a slight female predilection. These tumors are slow growing and nearly always arise unilaterally in the nasal cavity. Extension into the paranasal sinuses is common, however, and isolated paranasal sinus involvement also is reported.[301] Patients usually present with nasal obstruction or epistaxis, with an average symptom duration of up to a year. Rare instances of oncogenic osteomalacia associated with these tumors also have been reported and are thought to be caused by production of fibroblastic growth factor-23, a substance that

regulates phosphate reabsorption in the kidney.[302] Local recurrence after resection of these tumors is approximately 17%.[301] Somatic, single-nucleotide substitution, heterozygous mutations in the beta-catenin gene (CTNNB1) have been identified in sinonasal glomangiopericytomas,[303,304] and they can be distinguished from other histologically similar tumors by lack of corresponding gene fusion anomalies seen in those tumors—for example, STAT6 fusion in SFTs and MIR143-NOTCH fusion in glomus tumors.[7]

On imaging, sinonasal glomangiopericytomas present as sinonasal soft tissue masses that show indolent expansile growth with smooth bony remodeling; however, when large, these tumors can cause bone destruction with extension into the orbits and intracranial compartment.[305] On MR imaging, these lesions usually are isointense to muscle on T1-weighted images and of low to isointense signal intensity on T2-weighted sequences. Following contrast administration, they typically demonstrate avid and diffuse enhancement (Fig. 29). Larger tumors frequently demonstrate flow voids on T2-weighted images.[305,306] DWI shows increased ADC values,

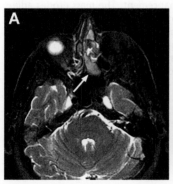 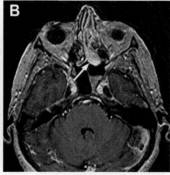

Fig. 29. Sinonasal glomangiopericytoma in an 81-year-old woman with complaints of nasal obstruction. (A) Axial T2-weighted image demonstrates a mildly hyperintense, polypoid soft tissue mass in the left posterior nasal cavity (arrow). (B) Contrast-enhanced, T2-weighted image demonstrates avid, homogeneous enhancement of the lesion (arrow).

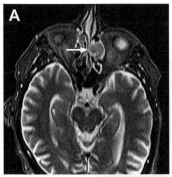
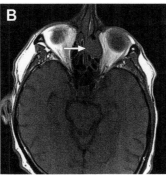
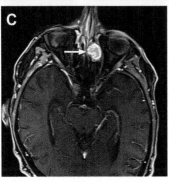

Fig. 30. BSNS isolated left ethmoid sinus mass on CT (not shown). Axial (*A*) T2-weighted, (*B*) unenhanced T1-weighted, and (*C*) contrast-enhanced, fat-suppressed, T1-weighted images demonstrate a circumscribed soft tissue mass in the left ethmoid sinuses (*arrows*), which is mildly hyperintense relative to muscle but hypointense relative to mucosa on T2-weighted imaging, shows T1-weighted signal isointense signal compared with muscle, and shows avid enhancement.

whereas DCE–MR imaging may show rapid wash-in and washout of contrast.[306]

BSNS is a relatively new entity, which was introduced in the 2017 fourth edition of the *WHO Classification of Head and Neck Tumours*.[7] BSNS is a low-grade spindle cell tumor with neural and myogenic features that exclusively involves the sinonasal region in middle-aged patients (peak incidence in the fifth decade), with a 2:1 female-to-male predilection. Diagnosis of these tumors is based on the presence of rearrangements of the PAX3 gene, with the most common rearrangement a PAX3-MAML3 fusion.[307] Clinically, these present as infiltrative tumors arising most commonly in the superior nasal cavity and ethmoid sinuses, and they often recur locally.[307,308] BSNSs tend to be well margined and slow growing but can be locally aggressive and may erode through the skull base or into the orbit. These tumors have nonspecific imaging characteristics, which are similar to those of other primary sinonasal tumors. On MR imaging, they are isointense to hypointense relative to cortex on T2-weighted imaging and enhance avidly[309] (**Fig. 30**).

SUMMARY

The head and neck region can give rise to virtually any type of soft tissue tumor. Cross-sectional imaging often plays an important role in characterizing these tumors and guiding management, with MR imaging the ideal imaging modality for these tumors given its superior contrast resolution and ability to better characterize the lesion location, extension, and involvement of nearby structures in the head and neck. In many cases, the imaging characteristics of a given soft tissue tumor is nonspecific, with definitive diagnosis requiring tissue sampling for histology, but, in certain instances, a combination of demographic, clinical, and imaging features of the tumor (some of which have been attempted to be summarized in this article) may point to a tissue specific diagnosis or significantly narrow the list of likely differential considerations. In addition, advanced MR imaging techniques, including DWI and DCE–MR imaging, may be helpful in soft tissue tumor characterization in certain instances, particularly for differentiating benign from malignant soft tissue lesions.

CLINICS CARE POINTS

- Most soft tissue tumors of the head and neck demonstrate nonspecific features on MR imaging and ultimately require biopsy for diagnosis.

DISCLOSURE

None.

REFERENCES

1. The WHO Classification of Tumours of Soft Tissue and Bone Board. The WHO classification of Tumours of soft tissue and bone. 5th edition. Lyon (France): IARC Press; 2020.
2. Laffers W, Stohr G, Goke F, et al. [Soft tissue tumors of the head and neck region]. [Weichteiltumoren des Kopf-Hals-Bereichs]. HNO 2013;61(11):928–36.
3. Fletcher CD. Distinctive soft tissue tumors of the head and neck. Mod Pathol 2002;15(3):324–30.
4. Galy-Bernadoy C, Garrel R. Head and neck soft-tissue sarcoma in adults. Eur Ann Otorhinolaryngol Head Neck Dis 2016;133(1):37–42.
5. Shellenberger TD, Sturgis EM. Sarcomas of the head and neck region. Curr Oncol Rep 2009; 11(2):135–42.
6. Tran NA, Guenette JP, Jagannathan J. Soft tissue special issue: imaging of bone and soft tissue sarcomas in the head and neck. Head Neck Pathol 2020;14(1):132–43.
7. El-Naggar AK, Chan JKC, Grandis JR, et al. The WHO classification of head and neck tumours. 4th edition. Lyon (France): IARC Press; 2017.
8. Berquist TH, Ehman RL, King BF, et al. Value of MR imaging in differentiating benign from malignant soft-tissue masses: study of 95 lesions. AJR Am J Roentgenol 1990;155(6):1251–5.
9. Gielen JL, De Schepper AM, Vanhoenacker F, et al. Accuracy of MRI in characterization of soft tissue tumors and tumor-like lesions. A prospective study in 548 patients. Eur Radiol 2004;14(12):2320–30.
10. Crim JR, Seeger LL, Yao L, et al. Diagnosis of soft-tissue masses with MR imaging: can benign masses be differentiated from malignant ones? Radiology 1992;185(2):581–6.
11. Kransdorf MJ, Jelinek JS, Moser RP Jr, et al. Soft-tissue masses: diagnosis using MR imaging. AJR Am J Roentgenol 1989;153(3):541–7.
12. Sundaram M, McLeod RA. MR imaging of tumor and tumorlike lesions of bone and soft tissue. AJR Am J Roentgenol 1990;155(4):817–24.
13. Brisse H, Orbach D, Klijanienko J, et al. Imaging and diagnostic strategy of soft tissue tumors in children. Eur Radiol 2006;16(5):1147–64.
14. Neuhaus SJ, Pinnock N, Giblin V, et al. Treatment and outcome of radiation-induced soft-tissue sarcomas at a specialist institution. Eur J Surg Oncol 2009;35(6):654–9.
15. Xi M, Liu MZ, Wang HX, et al. Radiation-induced sarcoma in patients with nasopharyngeal carcinoma: a single-institution study. Cancer 2010; 116(23):5479–86.
16. Correa R, Salpea P, Stratakis CA. Carney complex: an update. Eur J Endocrinol 2015;173(4):M85–97.
17. Munksgaard PS, Salkus G, Iyer VV, et al. Mazabraud's syndrome: case report and literature review. Acta Radiol Short Rep 2013;2(4). 2047981613492532.
18. De Schepper AM, Bloem JL. Soft tissue tumors: grading, staging, and tissue-specific diagnosis. Top Magn Reson Imaging 2007;18(6):431–44.
19. Wu JS, Hochman MG. Soft-tissue tumors and tumorlike lesions: a systematic imaging approach. Radiology 2009;253(2):297–316.
20. Baheti AD, Tirumani SH, Rosenthal MH, et al. Myxoid soft-tissue neoplasms: comprehensive update of the taxonomy and MRI features. AJR Am J Roentgenol 2015;204(2):374–85.
21. Miller TT, Sofka CM, Zhang P, et al. Systematic approach to tumors and tumor-like conditions of soft tissue. In: Bonakdarpour A, Reinus WR, Khurana JS, editors. Diagnostic imaging of musculoskeletal diseases: a systematic approach. New York: Springer; 2010. p. 313–49.
22. Bian Y, Jin P, Wang Y, et al. Clinical applications of DSC-MRI parameters assess angiogenesis and differentiate malignant from benign soft tissue tumors in limbs. Acad Radiol 2020;27(3):354–60.
23. Costa FM, Canella C, Gasparetto E. Advanced magnetic resonance imaging techniques in the evaluation of musculoskeletal tumors. Radiol Clin North Am 2011;49(6):1325–58. vii-viii.
24. Dodin G, Salleron J, Jendoubi S, et al. Added-value of advanced magnetic resonance imaging to conventional morphologic analysis for the differentiation between benign and malignant non-fatty soft-tissue tumors. Eur Radiol 2021;31(3):1536–47.
25. Jansen JFA, Parra C, Lu Y, et al. Evaluation of head and neck tumors with functional MR imaging. Magn Reson Imaging Clin N Am 2016;24(1):123–33.
26. Nagata S, Nishimura H, Uchida M, et al. Diffusion-weighted imaging of soft tissue tumors: usefulness of the apparent diffusion coefficient for differential diagnosis. Radiat Med 2008;26(5):287–95.
27. Teixeira PA, Gay F, Chen B, et al. Diffusion-weighted magnetic resonance imaging for the initial characterization of non-fatty soft tissue tumors: correlation between T2 signal intensity and ADC values. Skeletal Radiol 2016;45(2):263–71.
28. van Rijswijk CS, Kunz P, Hogendoorn PC, et al. Diffusion-weighted MRI in the characterization of soft-tissue tumors. J Magn Reson Imaging 2002; 15(3):302–7.
29. Hong JH, Jee WH, Jung CK, et al. Soft tissue sarcoma: adding diffusion-weighted imaging improves MR imaging evaluation of tumor margin infiltration. Eur Radiol 2019;29(5):2589–97.
30. Choi YJ, Lee IS, Song YS, et al. Diagnostic performance of diffusion-weighted (DWI) and dynamic

contrast-enhanced (DCE) MRI for the differentiation of benign from malignant soft-tissue tumors.
J Magn Reson Imaging 2019;50(3):798–809.

31. Einarsdottir H, Karlsson M, Wejde J, et al. Diffusion-
weighted MRI of soft tissue tumours. Eur Radiol
2004;14(6):959–63.

32. Lee SK, Jee WH, Jung CK, et al. Multiparametric
quantitative analysis of tumor perfusion and diffusion with 3T MRI: differentiation between benign
and malignant soft tissue tumors. Br J Radiol
2020;93(1115):20191035.

33. Lee SY, Jee WH, Jung JY, et al. Differentiation of
malignant from benign soft tissue tumours: use of
additive qualitative and quantitative diffusion-
weighted MR imaging to standard MR imaging at
3.0 T. Eur Radiol 2016;26(3):743–54.

34. Oka K, Yakushiji T, Sato H, et al. Ability of diffusion-
weighted imaging for the differential diagnosis between chronic expanding hematomas and malignant soft tissue tumors. J Magn Reson Imaging
2008;28(5):1195–200.

35. Razek A, Nada N, Ghaniem M, et al. Assessment of
soft tissue tumours of the extremities with diffusion
echoplanar MR imaging. Radiol Med 2012;117(1):
96–101.

36. Song Y, Yoon YC, Chong Y, et al. Diagnostic performance of conventional MRI parameters and
apparent diffusion coefficient values in differentiating between benign and malignant soft-tissue tumours. Clin Radiol 2017;72(8):691 e1–691 e10.

37. Schnapauff D, Zeile M, Niederhagen MB, et al.
Diffusion-weighted echo-planar magnetic resonance imaging for the assessment of tumor cellularity in patients with soft-tissue sarcomas.
J Magn Reson Imaging 2009;29(6):1355–9.

38. Winfield JM, Miah AB, Strauss D, et al. Utility of
multi-parametric quantitative magnetic resonance
imaging for characterization and radiotherapy
response assessment in soft-tissue sarcomas and
correlation with histopathology. Front Oncol 2019;
9:280.

39. Dudeck O, Zeile M, Pink D, et al. Diffusion-
weighted magnetic resonance imaging allows
monitoring of anticancer treatment effects in patients with soft-tissue sarcomas. J Magn Reson Imaging 2008;27(5):1109–13.

40. Hayashida Y, Yakushiji T, Awai K, et al. Monitoring
therapeutic responses of primary bone tumors by
diffusion-weighted image: Initial results. Eur Radiol
2006;16(12):2637–43.

41. Soldatos T, Ahlawat S, Montgomery E, et al. Multi-
parametric assessment of treatment response in
high-grade soft-tissue sarcomas with anatomic
and functional MR imaging sequences. Radiology
2016;278(3):831–40.

42. Uhl M, Saueressig U, van Buiren M, et al. Osteosarcoma: preliminary results of in vivo assessment of

tumor necrosis after chemotherapy with diffusion-
and perfusion-weighted magnetic resonance imaging. Invest Radiol 2006;41(8):618–23.

43. Padhani AR, Miles KA. Multiparametric imaging of
tumor response to therapy. Radiology 2010;
256(2):348–64.

44. Baur A, Huber A, Arbogast S, et al. Diffusion-
weighted imaging of tumor recurrencies and post-
therapeutical soft-tissue changes in humans. Eur
Radiol 2001;11(5):828–33.

45. Kasprian G, Amann G, Panotopoulos J, et al. Peripheral nerve tractography in soft tissue tumors:
a preliminary 3-tesla diffusion tensor magnetic
resonance imaging study. Muscle Nerve 2015;
51(3):338–45.

46. Akter M, Hirai T, Minoda R, et al. Diffusion tensor
tractography in the head-and-neck region using a
clinical 3-T MR scanner. Acad Radiol 2009;16(7):
858–65.

47. Abdel Razek AAK. Diffusion tensor imaging in differentiation of residual head and neck squamous
cell carcinoma from post-radiation changes.
Magn Reson Imaging 2018;54:84–9.

48. Gersing AS, Cervantes B, Knebel C, et al. Diffusion
tensor imaging and tractography for preoperative
assessment of benign peripheral nerve sheath tumors. Eur J Radiol 2020;129:109110.

49. Sujlana P, Skrok J, Fayad LM. Review of dynamic
contrast-enhanced MRI: technical aspects and applications in the musculoskeletal system. J Magn
Reson Imaging 2018;47(4):875–90.

50. Tuncbilek N, Karakas HM, Okten OO. Dynamic
contrast enhanced MRI in the differential diagnosis
of soft tissue tumors. Eur J Radiol 2005;53(3):
500–5.

51. van Rijswijk CS, Geirnaerdt MJ, Hogendoorn PC,
et al. Soft-tissue tumors: value of static and dynamic gadopentetate dimeglumine-enhanced MR
imaging in prediction of malignancy. Radiology
2004;233(2):493–502.

52. Li X, Wang Q, Dou Y, et al. Soft tissue sarcoma: can
dynamic contrast-enhanced (DCE) MRI be used to
predict the histological grade? Skeletal Radiol
2020;49(11):1829–38.

53. Del Grande F, Subhawong T, Weber K, et al. Detection of soft-tissue sarcoma recurrence: added
value of functional MR imaging techniques at 3.0
T. Radiology 2014;271(2):499–511.

54. Sumi M, Nakamura T. Head and neck tumours:
combined MRI assessment based on IVIM and
TIC analyses for the differentiation of tumors of
different histological types. Eur Radiol 2014;24(1):
223–31.

55. Myhre-Jensen O. A consecutive 7-year series of
1331 benign soft tissue tumours. Clinicopathologic
data. Comparison with sarcomas. Acta Orthop
Scand 1981;52(3):287–93.

56. Razek AA, Huang BY. Soft tissue tumors of the head and neck: imaging-based review of the WHO classification. Radiographics 2011;31(7): 1923–54.

57. Rydholm A, Berg NO. Size, site and clinical incidence of lipoma. Factors in the differential diagnosis of lipoma and sarcoma. Acta Orthop Scand 1983;54(6):929–34.

58. El-Monem MH, Gaafar AH, Magdy EA. Lipomas of the head and neck: presentation variability and diagnostic work-up. J Laryngol Otol 2006;120(1): 47–55.

59. Kim KS, Yang HS. Unusual locations of lipoma: differential diagnosis of head and neck mass. Aust Fam Physician 2014;43(12):867–70.

60. Bancroft LW, Kransdorf MJ, Peterson JJ, et al. Benign fatty tumors: classification, clinical course, imaging appearance, and treatment. Skeletal Radiol 2006;35(10):719–33.

61. Cappabianca S, Colella G, Pezzullo MG, et al. Lipomatous lesions of the head and neck region: imaging findings in comparison with histological type. Radiol Med 2008;113(5):758–70.

62. Murphey MD, Carroll JF, Flemming DJ, et al. From the archives of the AFIP: benign musculoskeletal lipomatous lesions. Radiographics 2004;24(5): 1433–66.

63. Lomoro P, Simonetti I, Nanni AL, et al. Imaging of head and neck lipoblastoma: case report and systematic review. J Ultrasound 2020. https://doi.org/10.1007/s40477-020-00439-w.

64. Bartuma H, Domanski HA, Von Steyern FV, et al. Cytogenetic and molecular cytogenetic findings in lipoblastoma. Cancer Genet Cytogenet 2008; 183(1):60–3.

65. Alaggio R, Coffin CM, Weiss SW, et al. Liposarcomas in young patients: a study of 82 cases occurring in patients younger than 22 years of age. Am J Surg Pathol 2009;33(5):645–58.

66. Stanelle EJ, Christison-Lagay ER, Sidebotham EL, et al. Prognostic factors and survival in pediatric and adolescent liposarcoma. Sarcoma 2012; 2012:870910.

67. Huh WW, Yuen C, Munsell M, et al. Liposarcoma in children and young adults: a multi-institutional experience. Pediatr Blood Cancer 2011;57(7): 1142–6.

68. Dao D, Najor AJ, Sun PY, et al. Follow-up outcomes of pediatric patients who underwent surgical resection for lipoblastomas or lipoblastomatosis: a single-institution experience with a systematic review and meta-analysis. Pediatr Surg Int 2020; 36(3):341–55.

69. Tadisina KK, Mlynek KS, Hwang LK, et al. Syndromic lipomatosis of the head and neck: a review of the literature. Aesthetic Plast Surg 2015;39(3): 440–8.

70. Creytens D, Mentzel T, Ferdinande L, et al. "Atypical" pleomorphic lipomatous tumor: a clinicopathologic, immunohistochemical and molecular study of 21 cases, emphasizing its relationship to atypical spindle cell lipomatous tumor and suggesting a morphologic spectrum (Atypical Spindle Cell/Pleomorphic Lipomatous Tumor). Am J Surg Pathol 2017;41(11):1443–55.

71. Bahadir B, Behzatoglu K, Hacihasanoglu E, et al. Atypical spindle cell/pleomorphic lipomatous tumor: a clinicopathologic, immunohistochemical, and molecular study of 20 cases. Pathol Int 2018; 68(10):550–6.

72. Marino-Enriquez A, Nascimento AF, Ligon AH, et al. Atypical spindle cell lipomatous tumor: clinicopathologic characterization of 232 cases demonstrating a morphologic spectrum. Am J Surg Pathol 2017; 41(2):234–44.

73. Gritli S, Khamassi K, Lachkhem A, et al. Head and neck liposarcomas: a 32 years experience. Auris Nasus Larynx 2010;37(3):347–51.

74. Coffin CM, Alaggio R. Adipose and myxoid tumors of childhood and adolescence. Pediatr Dev Pathol 2012;15(1 Suppl):239–54.

75. Francom CR, Leoniak SM, Lovell MA, et al. Head and neck pleomorphic myxoid liposarcoma in a child with Li-Fraumeni syndrome. Int J Pediatr Otorhinolaryngol 2019;123:191–4.

76. Sinclair TJ, Thorson CM, Alvarez E, et al. Pleomorphic myxoid liposarcoma in an adolescent with Li-Fraumeni syndrome. Pediatr Surg Int 2017;33(5): 631–5.

77. Coffin CM, Dehner LP. Fibroblastic-myofibroblastic tumors in children and adolescents: a clinicopathologic study of 108 examples in 103 patients. Pediatr Pathol 1991;11(4):569–88.

78. Sargar KM, Sheybani EF, Shenoy A, et al. Pediatric fibroblastic and myofibroblastic tumors: a pictorial review. Radiographics 2016;36(4):1195–214.

79. Vilanova JC, Woertler K, Narvaez JA, et al. Soft-tissue tumors update: MR imaging features according to the WHO classification. Eur Radiol 2007; 17(1):125–38.

80. Marino-Enriquez A, Fletcher CD. Angiofibroma of soft tissue: clinicopathologic characterization of a distinctive benign fibrovascular neoplasm in a series of 37 cases. Am J Surg Pathol 2012;36(4): 500–8.

81. Carter JM, Weiss SW, Linos K, et al. Superficial CD34-positive fibroblastic tumor: report of 18 cases of a distinctive low-grade mesenchymal neoplasm of intermediate (borderline) malignancy. Mod Pathol 2014;27(2):294–302.

82. Kao YC, Flucke U, Eijkelenboom A, et al. Novel EWSR1-SMAD3 gene fusions in a group of acral fibroblastic spindle cell neoplasms. Am J Surg Pathol 2018;42(4):522–8.

83. Kallen ME, Hornick JL. The 2020 WHO classification: what's new in soft tissue tumor pathology? Am J Surg Pathol 2021;45(1):e1–23.

84. Zhao M, Sun K, Li C, et al. Angiofibroma of soft tissue: clinicopathologic study of 2 cases of a recently characterized benign soft tissue tumor. Int J Clin Exp Pathol 2013;6(10):2208–15.

85. Yamaga K, Fujita A, Osaki M, et al. Detailed analysis of a superficial CD34-positive fibroblastic tumor: a case report and review of the literature. Oncol Lett 2017;14(3):3395–400.

86. Mindiola-Romero AE, Maloney N, Bridge JA, et al. A concise review of angiofibroma of soft tissue: a rare newly described entity that can be encountered by dermatopathologists. J Cutan Pathol 2020;47(2):179–85.

87. Davids JR, Wenger DR, Mubarak SJ. Congenital muscular torticollis: sequela of intrauterine or perinatal compartment syndrome. J Pediatr Orthop 1993;13(2):141–7.

88. Coyle J, White LM, Dickson B, et al. MRI characteristics of nodular fasciitis of the musculoskeletal system. Skeletal Radiol 2013;42(7):975–82.

89. Kumar B, Pradhan A. Diagnosis of sternomastoid tumor of infancy by fine-needle aspiration cytology. Diagn Cytopathol 2011;39(1):13–7.

90. Ablin DS, Jain K, Howell L, et al. Ultrasound and MR imaging of fibromatosis colli (sternomastoid tumor of infancy). Pediatr Radiol 1998;28(4):230–3.

91. Lloyd C, McHugh K. The role of radiology in head and neck tumours in children. Cancer Imaging 2010;10:49–61.

92. Kim ST, Kim HJ, Park SW, et al. Nodular fasciitis in the head and neck: CT and MR imaging findings. AJNR Am J Neuroradiol 2005;26(10):2617–23.

93. Wagner RD, Wang EK, Lloyd MS, et al. Cranial fasciitis: a systematic review and diagnostic approach to a pediatric scalp mass. J Craniofac Surg 2016;27(1):e65–71.

94. Dinauer PA, Brixey CJ, Moncur JT, et al. Pathologic and MR imaging features of benign fibrous soft-tissue tumors in adults. Radiographics 2007;27(1):173–87.

95. Coffin CM, Alaggio R. Fibroblastic and myofibroblastic tumors in children and adolescents. Pediatr Dev Pathol 2012;15(1 Suppl):127–80.

96. Lee DG, Lee SH, Hwang SW, et al. Myositis ossificans in the paraspinal muscles of the neck after acupuncture: a case report. Spine J 2013;13(7):e9–12.

97. Kruse AL, Dannemann C, Gratz KW. Bilateral myositis ossificans of the masseter muscle after chemoradiotherapy and critical illness neuropathy–report of a rare entity and review of literature. Head Neck Oncol 2009;1:30.

98. Sarac S, Sennaroglu L, Hosal AS, et al. Myositis ossificans in the neck. Eur Arch Otorhinolaryngol 1999;256(4):199–201.

99. Kokkosis AA, Balsam D, Lee TK, et al. Pediatric nontraumatic myositis ossificans of the neck. Pediatr Radiol 2009;39(4):409–12.

100. Baranov E, Hornick JL. Soft tissue special issue: fibroblastic and myofibroblastic neoplasms of the head and neck. Head Neck Pathol 2020;14(1):43–58.

101. Lee JC, Thomas JM, Phillips S, et al. Aggressive fibromatosis: MRI features with pathologic correlation. AJR Am J Roentgenol 2006;186(1):247–54.

102. Murphey MD, Ruble CM, Tyszko SM, et al. From the archives of the AFIP: musculoskeletal fibromatoses: radiologic-pathologic correlation. Radiographics 2009;29(7):2143–73.

103. Millare GG, Guha-Thakurta N, Sturgis EM, et al. Imaging findings of head and neck dermatofibrosarcoma protuberans. AJNR Am J Neuroradiol 2014;35(2):373–8.

104. Thway K, Ng W, Noujaim J, et al. The current status of solitary fibrous tumor: diagnostic features, variants, and genetics. Int J Surg Pathol 2016;24(4):281–92.

105. Fukunaga M, Naganuma H, Nikaido T, et al. Extrapleural solitary fibrous tumor: a report of seven cases. Mod Pathol 1997;10(5):443–50.

106. Steigen SE, Schaeffer DF, West RB, et al. Expression of insulin-like growth factor 2 in mesenchymal neoplasms. Mod Pathol 2009;22(7):914–21.

107. Kim HJ, Lee HK, Seo JJ, et al. MR imaging of solitary fibrous tumors in the head and neck. Korean J Radiol 2005;6(3):136–42.

108. Keyserling H, Peterson K, Camacho D, et al. Giant cell angiofibroma of the orbit. AJNR Am J Neuroradiol 2004;25(7):1266–8.

109. Yin B, Liu L, Li YD, et al. Retroperitoneal hemangiopericytoma: case report and literature review. Chin Med J (Engl) 2011;124(1):155–6.

110. Hohne S, Milzsch M, Adams J, et al. Inflammatory pseudotumor (IPT) and inflammatory myofibroblastic tumor (IMT): a representative literature review occasioned by a rare IMT of the transverse colon in a 9-year-old child. Tumori 2015;101(3):249–56.

111. Yamamoto H, Yamaguchi H, Aishima S, et al. Inflammatory myofibroblastic tumor versus IgG4-related sclerosing disease and inflammatory pseudotumor: a comparative clinicopathologic study. Am J Surg Pathol 2009;33(9):1330–40.

112. Devaney KO, Lafeir DJ, Triantafyllou A, et al. Inflammatory myofibroblastic tumors of the head and neck: evaluation of clinicopathologic and prognostic features. Eur Arch Otorhinolaryngol 2012;269(12):2461–5.

113. Kansara S, Bell D, Johnson J, et al. Head and neck inflammatory pseudotumor: case series and review of the literature. Neuroradiol J 2016;29(6):440–6.

114. Narla LD, Newman B, Spottswood SS, et al. Inflammatory pseudotumor. Radiographics 2003;23(3): 719–29.

115. Park SB, Lee JH, Weon YC. Imaging findings of head and neck inflammatory pseudotumor. AJR Am J Roentgenol 2009;193(4):1180–6.

116. Vohra ST, Escott EJ, Stevens D, et al. Categorization and characterization of lesions of the orbital apex. Neuroradiology 2011;53(2):89–107.

117. Strianese D, Tranfa F, Finelli M, et al. Inflammatory myofibroblastic tumor of the orbit: a clinicopathological study of 25 cases. Saudi J Ophthalmol 2018;32(1):33–9.

118. Orbach D, Rey A, Cecchetto G, et al. Infantile fibrosarcoma: management based on the European experience. J Clin Oncol 2010;28(2):318–23.

119. Orbach D, Brennan B, De Paoli A, et al. Conservative strategy in infantile fibrosarcoma is possible: the European paediatric Soft tissue sarcoma Study Group experience. Eur J Cancer 2016;57:1–9.

120. Folpe AL, Lane KL, Paull G, et al. Low-grade fibromyxoid sarcoma and hyalinizing spindle cell tumor with giant rosettes: a clinicopathologic study of 73 cases supporting their identity and assessing the impact of high-grade areas. Am J Surg Pathol 2000;24(10):1353–60.

121. Cowan ML, Thompson LD, Leon ME, et al. Low-grade fibromyxoid sarcoma of the head and neck: a clinicopathologic series and review of the literature. Head Neck Pathol 2016;10(2):161–6.

122. Hwang S, Kelliher E, Hameed M. Imaging features of low-grade fibromyxoid sarcoma (Evans tumor). Skeletal Radiol 2012;41(10):1263–72.

123. Dell'Aversana Orabona G, Iaconetta G, Abbate V, et al. Head and neck myofibrosarcoma: a case report and review of the literature. J Med Case Rep 2014;8:468.

124. Waters B, Panicek DM, Lefkowitz RA, et al. Low-grade myxofibrosarcoma: CT and MRI patterns in recurrent disease. AJR Am J Roentgenol 2007; 188(2):W193–8.

125. Choi JH, Ro JY. The 2020 WHO classification of tumors of soft tissue: selected changes and new entities. Adv Anat Pathol 2021;28(1):44–58.

126. West RB, Rubin BP, Miller MA, et al. A landscape effect in tenosynovial giant-cell tumor from activation of CSF1 expression by a translocation in a minority of tumor cells. Proc Natl Acad Sci U S A 2006;103(3):690–5.

127. Carlson ML, Osetinsky LM, Alon EE, et al. Tenosynovial giant cell tumors of the temporomandibular joint and lateral skull base: review of 11 cases. Laryngoscope 2017;127(10):2340–6.

128. Bielamowicz S, Dauer MS, Chang B, et al. Noncutaneous benign fibrous histiocytoma of the head and neck. Otolaryngol Head Neck Surg 1995; 113(1):140–6.

129. Jo E, Cho ES, Kim HS, et al. Deep benign fibrous histiocytoma in the oral cavity: a case report. J Korean Assoc Oral Maxillofac Surg 2015;41(5): 270–2.

130. Gleason BC, Fletcher CD. Deep "benign" fibrous histiocytoma: clinicopathologic analysis of 69 cases of a rare tumor indicating occasional metastatic potential. Am J Surg Pathol 2008;32(3): 354–62.

131. Machiels F, De Maeseneer M, Chaskis C, et al. Deep benign fibrous histiocytoma of the knee: CT and MR features with pathologic correlation. Eur Radiol 1998;8(6):989–91.

132. Ghuman M, Hwang S, Antonescu CR, et al. Plexiform fibrohistiocytic tumor: imaging features and clinical findings. Skeletal Radiol 2019;48(3): 437–43.

133. Remstein ED, Arndt CA, Nascimento AG. Plexiform fibrohistiocytic tumor: clinicopathologic analysis of 22 cases. Am J Surg Pathol 1999;23(6): 662–70.

134. Enzinger FM, Zhang RY. Plexiform fibrohistiocytic tumor presenting in children and young adults. An analysis of 65 cases. Am J Surg Pathol 1988; 12(11):818–26.

135. Mavrogenis AF, Tsukamoto S, Antoniadou T, et al. Giant cell tumor of soft tissue: a rare entity. Orthopedics 2019;42(4):e364–9.

136. Lee JC, Liang CW, Fletcher CD. Giant cell tumor of soft tissue is genetically distinct from its bone counterpart. Mod Pathol 2017;30(5):728–33.

137. Hafiz SM, Bablghaith ES, Alsaedi AJ, et al. Giant-cell tumors of soft tissue in the head and neck: a review article. Int J Health Sci (Qassim) 2018;12(4): 88–91.

138. Naqvi J, Ordonez NG, Luna MA, et al. Epithelioid hemangioendothelioma of the head and neck: role of podoplanin in the differential diagnosis. Head Neck Pathol 2008;2(1):25–30.

139. Yi KM, Chen K, Ma Q, et al. Myofibroma/myofibromatosis: MDCT and MR imaging findings in 24 patients with radiological-pathological correlation. BMC Med Imaging 2020;20(1):100.

140. Loundon N, Dedieuleveult T, Ayache D, et al. Head and neck infantile myofibromatosis–a report of three cases. Int J Pediatr Otorhinolaryngol 1999; 51(3):181–6.

141. Lopes RN, Alves Fde A, Rocha AC, et al. Head and neck solitary infantile myofibroma: clinicopathological and immunohistochemical features of a case series. Acta Histochem 2015;117(4–5):431–6. https://doi.org/10.1016/j.acthis.2015.02.001.

142. Beck JC, Devaney KO, Weatherly RA, et al. Pediatric myofibromatosis of the head and neck. Arch Otolaryngol Head Neck Surg 1999;125(1):39–44.

143. Antonescu CR, Sung YS, Zhang L, et al. Recurrent SRF-RELA Fusions define a novel subset of cellular

myofibroma/myopericytoma: a potential diagnostic pitfall with sarcomas with myogenic differentiation. Am J Surg Pathol 2017;41(5):677–84.

144. Matsuyama A, Hisaoka M, Hashimoto H. Angioleiomyoma: a clinicopathologic and immunohistochemical reappraisal with special reference to the correlation with myopericytoma. Hum Pathol 2007;38(4):645–51.

145. Agaimy A, Michal M, Thompson LD, et al. Angioleiomyoma of the sinonasal tract: analysis of 16 cases and review of the literature. Head Neck Pathol 2015;9(4):463–73.

146. Hachisuga T, Hashimoto H, Enjoji M. Angioleiomyoma. A clinicopathologic reappraisal of 562 cases. Cancer 1984;54(1):126–30.

147. Ramesh P, Annapureddy SR, Khan F, et al. Angioleiomyoma: a clinical, pathological and radiological review. Int J Clin Pract 2004;58(6):587–91.

148. Wang CP, Chang YL, Sheen TS. Vascular leiomyoma of the head and neck. Laryngoscope 2004;114(4):661–5.

149. Aitken-Saavedra J, da Silva KD, Gomes AP, et al. Clinicopathologic and immunohistochemical characterization of 14 cases of angioleiomyomas in oral cavity. Med Oral Patol Oral Cir Bucal 2018; 23(5):e564–8.

150. Kim HY, Jung SN, Kwon H, et al. Angiomyoma in the buccal space. J Craniofac Surg 2010;21(5): 1634–5.

151. Mehta RP, Faquin WC, Franco RA. Pathology quiz case 2. Angiomyoma of the larynx. Arch Otolaryngol Head Neck Surg 2004;130(7):889, 890-1.

152. Gupte C, Butt SH, Tirabosco R, et al. Angioleiomyoma: magnetic resonance imaging features in ten cases. Skeletal Radiol 2008;37(11):1003–9.

153. Zou H, Song L, Jia M, et al. Glomus tumor in the floor of the mouth: a case report and review of the literature. World J Surg Oncol 2018;16(1):201.

154. Mravic M, LaChaud G, Nguyen A, et al. Clinical and histopathological diagnosis of glomus tumor: an institutional experience of 138 cases. Int J Surg Pathol 2015;23(3):181–8.

155. Luzar B, Martin B, Fisher C, et al. Cutaneous malignant glomus tumours: applicability of currently established malignancy criteria for tumours occurring in the skin. Pathology 2018;50(7):711–7.

156. Brouillard P, Boon LM, Mulliken JB, et al. Mutations in a novel factor, glomulin, are responsible for glomuvenous malformations ("glomangiomas"). Am J Hum Genet 2002;70(4):866–74.

157. Mosquera JM, Sboner A, Zhang L, et al. Novel MIR143-NOTCH fusions in benign and malignant glomus tumors. Genes Chromosomes Cancer 2013;52(11):1075–87.

158. Chirila M, Rogojan L. Glomangioma of the nasal septum: a case report and review. Ear Nose Throat J 2013;92(4–5):E7–9.

159. Kaufman AC, Brant JA, Luu NN, et al. Recurrent glomangioma ("true" glomus tumor) of the middle ear and mastoid. World J Otorhinolaryngol Head Neck Surg 2019;5(4):175–9.

160. Chou T, Pan SC, Shieh SJ, et al. Glomus tumor: twenty-year experience and literature review. Ann Plast Surg 2016;76(Suppl 1):S35–40.

161. Billings SD, Folpe AL, Weiss SW. Do leiomyomas of deep soft tissue exist? An analysis of highly differentiated smooth muscle tumors of deep soft tissue supporting two distinct subtypes. Am J Surg Pathol 2001;25(9):1134–42.

162. Veeresh M, Sudhakara M, Girish G, et al. Leiomyoma: a rare tumor in the head and neck and oral cavity: report of 3 cases with review. J Oral Maxillofac Pathol 2013;17(2):281–7.

163. Barnes L. Tumors and tumor like lesions of soft tissue. In: Barnes L, editor. Surgical pathology of head and neck. 2nd edition. New York: Marcel Dekker; 2001. p. 912–5.

164. Fasih N, Prasad Shanbhogue AK, Macdonald DB, et al. Leiomyomas beyond the uterus: unusual locations, rare manifestations. Radiographics 2008; 28(7):1931–48.

165. Ikeda K, Kuroda M, Sakaida N, et al. Cellular leiomyoma of the nasal cavity: findings of CT and MR imaging. AJNR Am J Neuroradiol 2005;26(6): 1336–8.

166. Yadav J, Bakshi J, Chouhan M, et al. Head and neck leiomyosarcoma. Indian J Otolaryngol Head Neck Surg 2013;65(Suppl 1):1–5.

167. Fitzpatrick SG, Woodworth BA, Monteiro C, et al. Nasal sinus leiomyosarcoma in a patient with history of non-hereditary unilateral treated retinoblastoma. Head Neck Pathol 2011;5(1):57–62.

168. Marioni G, Bertino G, Mariuzzi L, et al. Laryngeal leiomyosarcoma. J Laryngol Otol 2000;114(5): 398–401.

169. Kuo R, Huang JK, Lee KS, et al. Leiomyosarcoma in the nasopharynx: MR imaging findings. AJNR Am J Neuroradiol 2007;28(7):1373–4.

170. Chudasama P, Mughal SS, Sanders MA, et al. Integrative genomic and transcriptomic analysis of leiomyosarcoma. Nat Commun 2018;9(1):144.

171. Walker EA, Song AJ, Murphey MD. Magnetic resonance imaging of soft-tissue masses. Semin Roentgenol 2010;45(4):277–97.

172. Patel SC, Silbergleit R, Talati SJ. Sarcomas of the head and neck. Top Magn Reson Imaging 1999; 10(6):362–75.

173. Sun S, Bonaffini PA, Nougaret S, et al. How to differentiate uterine leiomyosarcoma from leiomyoma with imaging. Diagn Interv Imaging 2019;100(10): 619–34.

174. Dekate J, Chetty R. Epstein-barr virus-associated smooth muscle tumor. Arch Pathol Lab Med 2016;140(7):718–22.

175. Deyrup AT, Lee VK, Hill CE, et al. Epstein-Barr virus-associated smooth muscle tumors are distinctive mesenchymal tumors reflecting multiple infection events: a clinicopathologic and molecular analysis of 29 tumors from 19 patients. Am J Surg Pathol 2006;30(1):75–82.

176. Kim JW, Lee DK, Fishman M. Orbital smooth muscle tumor associated with epstein-barr virus in a human immunodeficiency virus-positive patient. Arch Ophthalmol 2010;128(8):1084–5.

177. Yu L, Aldave AJ, Glasgow BJ. Epstein-Barr virus-associated smooth muscle tumor of the iris in a patient with transplant: a case report and review of the literature. Arch Pathol Lab Med 2009;133(8):1238–41.

178. Hussein K, Rath B, Ludewig B, et al. Clinico-pathological characteristics of different types of immunodeficiency-associated smooth muscle tumours. Eur J Cancer 2014;50(14):2417–24.

179. Dominelli GS, Jen R, Park K, et al. Tracheal Epstein-Barr virus-associated smooth muscle tumour in an HIV-positive patient. Can Respir J 2014;21(6):334–6.

180. Raheja A, Sowder A, Palmer C, et al. Epstein-Barr virus-associated smooth muscle tumor of the cavernous sinus: a delayed complication of allogenic peripheral blood stem cell transplantation: case report. J Neurosurg 2017;126(5):1479–83.

181. Purgina B, Rao UN, Miettinen M, et al. AIDS-related EBV-associated smooth muscle tumors: a review of 64 published cases. Patholog Res Int 2011;2011: 561548.

182. Cloutier JM, Charville GW, Mertens F, et al. "Inflammatory Leiomyosarcoma" and "Histiocyte-rich Rhabdomyoblastic Tumor": a clinicopathological, immunohistochemical and genetic study of 13 cases, with a proposal for reclassification as "Inflammatory Rhabdomyoblastic Tumor". Mod Pathol 2021;34(4):758–69.

183. Morita I, Isoda R, Hirabayashi Y, et al. A long-living case of carotid aneurysm caused by inflammatory leiomyosarcoma. Asian Cardiovasc Thorac Ann 2016;24(8):801–4.

184. de Trey LA, Schmid S, Huber GF. Multifocal adult rhabdomyoma of the head and neck manifestation in 7 locations and review of the literature. Case Rep Otolaryngol 2013;2013:758416.

185. Liess BD, Zitsch RP 3rd, Lane R, et al. Multifocal adult rhabdomyoma: a case report and literature review. Am J Otolaryngol 2005;26(3):214–7.

186. Kapadia SB, Meis JM, Frisman DM, et al. Fetal rhabdomyoma of the head and neck: a clinicopathologic and immunophenotypic study of 24 cases. Hum Pathol 1993;24(7):754–65.

187. Hettmer S, Teot LA, van Hummelen P, et al. Mutations in Hedgehog pathway genes in fetal rhabdomyomas. J Pathol 2013;231(1):44–52.

188. Leboulanger N, Picard A, Roger G, et al. Fetal rhabdomyoma of the infratemporal fossa in children. Eur Ann Otorhinolaryngol Head Neck Dis 2010;127(1):30–2.

189. Stein-Wexler RMR. imaging of soft tissue masses in children. Magn Reson Imaging Clin N Am 2009; 17(3):489–507, vi.

190. Skapek SX, Ferrari A, Gupta AA, et al. Rhabdomyosarcoma. Nat Rev Dis Primers 2019;5(1):1.

191. Perez EA, Kassira N, Cheung MC, et al. Rhabdomyosarcoma in children: a SEER population based study. J Surg Res 2011;170(2):e243–51.

192. Defachelles AS, Rey A, Oberlin O, et al. Treatment of nonmetastatic cranial parameningeal rhabdomyosarcoma in children younger than 3 years old: results from international society of pediatric oncology studies MMT 89 and 95. J Clin Oncol 2009;27(8):1310–5.

193. Jawad N, McHugh K. The clinical and radiologic features of paediatric rhabdomyosarcoma. Pediatr Radiol 2019;49(11):1516–23.

194. Freling NJ, Merks JH, Saeed P, et al. Imaging findings in craniofacial childhood rhabdomyosarcoma. Pediatr Radiol 2010;40(11):1723–38 [quiz 1855].

195. Cornejo P, Egelhoff J, Kaye R, et al. Malignant Ectomesenchymoma of the Scalp. Appl Radiol 2020; 49(3):40–2.

196. Kosem M, Ibiloglu I, Bakan V, et al. Ectomesenchymoma: case report and review of the literature. Turk J Pediatr 2004;46(1):82–7.

197. Nael A, Siaghani P, Wu WW, et al. Metastatic malignant ectomesenchymoma initially presenting as a pelvic mass: report of a case and review of literature. Case Rep Pediatr 2014;2014:792925.

198. Brehmer D, Overhoff HM, Marx A. Malignant ectomesenchymoma of the nose. Case report and review of the literature. ORL J Otorhinolaryngol Relat Spec 2003;65(1):52–6.

199. Paikos P, Papathanassiou M, Stefanaki K, et al. Malignant ectomesenchymoma of the orbit in a child: case report and review of the literature. Surv Ophthalmol 2002;47(4):368–74.

200. Wu YY, Chen YY, Lee KF, et al. Maxillary sinus metastasis from gastrointestinal stromal tumor(GIST): a rare presentation and literature review. J Cancer Res Pract 2017;4(2):80–3.

201. Friedrich RE, Zustin J. Late metastasis of gastrointestinal stromal tumour to the oral cavity. Anticancer Res 2010;30(10):4283–8.

202. Yu MH, Lee JM, Baek JH, et al. MRI features of gastrointestinal stromal tumors. AJR Am J Roentgenol 2014;203(5):980–91.

203. Kamysz JW, Zawin JK, Gonzalez-Crussi F. Soft tissue chondroma of the neck: a case report and review of the literature. Pediatr Radiol 1996;26(2):145–7.

204. Lee WK, Ko HC, Kim BS, et al. Soft tissue chondroma on the lip: clinical, histopathological and

ultrasonographic findings. Australas J Dermatol 2018;59(3):e227–8.

205. Aseem F, Pace ST, Onajin O, et al. Soft tissue chondroma of the eyelid. Ophthal Plast Reconstr Surg 2018;34(5):e168–70.

206. Dimitrijevic MV, Sopta J, Ivisevic TB, et al. Chondroma of the tongue. J Craniofac Surg 2019; 30(4):e315–7.

207. Murenzi G, Kaye R, Cole A, et al. A rare case of chondroma of the parotid gland. Lab Med Spring 2014;45(2):156–60.

208. Khadim MT, Asif M, Ali Z. Extraskeletal soft tissue chondromas of head and neck region. Ann Pak Inst Med Sci 2011;7(1):42–4.

209. Chung EB, Enzinger FM. Chondroma of soft parts. Cancer 1978;41(4):1414–24.

210. Amary F, Perez-Casanova L, Ye H, et al. Synovial chondromatosis and soft tissue chondroma: extra-osseous cartilaginous tumor defined by FN1 gene rearrangement. Mod Pathol 2019;32(12):1762–71.

211. Zlatkin MB, Lander PH, Begin LR, et al. Soft-tissue chondromas. AJR Am J Roentgenol 1985;144(6): 1263–7.

212. Singh AP, Dhammi IK, Jain AK, et al. Extraskeletal juxtaarticular chondroma of the knee. Acta Orthop Traumatol Turc 2011;45(2):130–4.

213. Lyngdoh B, Mishra J, Dey B, et al. Primary extra-skeletal osteosarcoma arising from the optic nerve: a rare case report. Ocul Oncol Pathol 2018;4(5): 304–8.

214. Al-Janabi Y, Al-Janabi K, Tzafetta K, et al. Primary cutaneous osteosarcoma of the scalp. BMJ Case Rep 2018;2018. bcr2017222641.

215. Zhang JS, Wen G, Liu Y, et al. Extraskeletal osteo-sarcoma in right neck subcutaneous tissue: a case report of an extremely rare tumour. Mol Clin Oncol 2018;9(2):149–54.

216. Hamamoto T, Kono T, Furuie H, et al. Extraskeletal osteosarcoma in the parotid gland: a case report. Auris Nasus Larynx 2018;45(3):644–7.

217. Aslan M, Samdanci ET. A very rare mass mimicking paraganglioma in the parapharyngeal area: extra-skeletal osteosarcoma. Braz J Otorhinolaryngol 2020. https://doi.org/10.1016/j.bjorl.2020.11.012.

218. Hatano H, Morita T, Kobayashi H, et al. Extraskele-tal osteosarcoma of the jaw. Skeletal Radiol 2005; 34(3):171–5.

219. Roller LA, Chebib I, Bredella MA, et al. Clinical, radiological, and pathological features of extraske-letal osteosarcoma. Skeletal Radiol 2018;47(9): 1213–20.

220. Saito Y, Miyajima C, Nakao K, et al. Highly malig-nant submandibular extraskeletal osteosarcoma in a young patient. Auris Nasus Larynx 2008; 35(4):576–8.

221. Fanburg-Smith JC, Auerbach A, Marwaha JS, et al. Reappraisal of mesenchymal chondrosarcoma:

novel morphologic observations of the hyaline cartilage and endochondral ossification and beta-catenin, Sox9, and osteocalcin immunostaining of 22 cases. Hum Pathol 2010;41(5):653–62.

222. Wang L, Motoi T, Khanin R, et al. Identification of a novel, recurrent HEY1-NCOA2 fusion in mesen-chymal chondrosarcoma based on a genome-wide screen of exon-level expression data. Genes Chromosomes Cancer 2012;51(2):127–39.

223. Frezza AM, Cesari M, Baumhoer D, et al. Mesen-chymal chondrosarcoma: prognostic factors and outcome in 113 patients. A European Musculoskel-etal Oncology Society study. Eur J Cancer 2015; 51(3):374–81.

224. Pellitteri PK, Ferlito A, Fagan JJ, et al. Mesen-chymal chondrosarcoma of the head and neck. Oral Oncol 2007;43(10):970–5.

225. Saito K, Unni KK, Wollan PC, et al. Chondrosar-coma of the jaw and facial bones. Cancer 1995; 76(9):1550–8.

226. Vencio EF, Reeve CM, Unni KK, et al. Mesenchymal chondrosarcoma of the jaw bones: clinicopatho-logic study of 19 cases. Cancer 1998;82(12): 2350–5.

227. Murphey MD, Walker EA, Wilson AJ, et al. From the archives of the AFIP: imaging of primary chondro-sarcoma: radiologic-pathologic correlation. Radio-graphics 2003;23(5):1245–78.

228. Stemmer-Rachamimov AO, Xu L, Gonzalez-Agosti C, et al. Universal absence of merlin, but not other ERM family members, in schwannomas. Am J Pathol 1997;151(6):1649–54.

229. Kehrer-Sawatzki H, Farschtschi S, Mautner VF, et al. The molecular pathogenesis of schwannoma-tosis, a paradigm for the co-involvement of multiple tumour suppressor genes in tumorigenesis. Hum Genet 2017;136(2):129–48.

230. Abdel Razek AAK, Gamaleldin OA, Elsebaie NA. Peripheral nerve sheath tumors of head and neck: imaging-based review of World Health Orga-nization Classification. J Comput Assist Tomogr 2020;44(6):928–40.

231. Liu HL, Yu SY, Li GK, et al. Extracranial head and neck Schwannomas: a study of the nerve of origin. Eur Arch Otorhinolaryngol 2011;268(9):1343–7.

232. Butler RT, Patel RM, McHugh JB. Head and neck schwannomas: 20-year experience of a single insti-tution excluding cutaneous and acoustic sites. Head Neck Pathol 2016;10(3):286–91.

233. Ferner RE, Huson SM, Thomas N, et al. Guidelines for the diagnosis and management of individuals with neurofibromatosis 1. J Med Genet 2007; 44(2):81–8.

234. Pemov A, Li H, Patidar R, et al. The primacy of NF1 loss as the driver of tumorigenesis in neurofibroma-tosis type 1-associated plexiform neurofibromas. Oncogene 2017;36(22):3168–77.

235. Patel NB, Stacy GS. Musculoskeletal manifestations of neurofibromatosis type 1. AJR Am J Roentgenol 2012;199(1):W99–106.

236. Ortonne N, Wolkenstein P, Blakeley JO, et al. Cutaneous neurofibromas: current clinical and pathologic issues. Neurology 2018;91(2 Suppl 1):S5–13.

237. Ferner RE, Gutmann DH. International consensus statement on malignant peripheral nerve sheath tumors in neurofibromatosis. Cancer Res 2002;62(5):1573–7.

238. Ferner RE, Gutmann DH. Neurofibromatosis type 1 (NF1): diagnosis and management. Handb Clin Neurol 2013;115:939–55.

239. Longo JF, Weber SM, Turner-Ivey BP, et al. Recent advances in the diagnosis and pathogenesis of neurofibromatosis type 1 (NF1)-associated peripheral nervous system neoplasms. Adv Anat Pathol 2018;25(5):353–68.

240. Owosho AA, Estilo CL, Huryn JM, et al. A clinicopathologic study of head and neck malignant peripheral nerve sheath tumors. Head Neck Pathol 2018;12(2):151–9.

241. Meyer A, Billings SD. What's new in nerve sheath tumors. Virchows Arch 2020;476(1):65–80.

242. Schaefer IM, Dong F, Garcia EP, et al. Recurrent SMARCB1 inactivation in epithelioid malignant peripheral nerve sheath tumors. Am J Surg Pathol 2019;43(6):835–43.

243. Lee W, Teckie S, Wiesner T, et al. PRC2 is recurrently inactivated through EED or SUZ12 loss in malignant peripheral nerve sheath tumors. Nat Genet 2014;46(11):1227–32.

244. Prieto-Granada CN, Wiesner T, Messina JL, et al. Loss of H3K27me3 expression is a highly sensitive marker for sporadic and radiation-induced MPNST. Am J Surg Pathol 2016;40(4):479–89.

245. Schaefer IM, Fletcher CD, Hornick JL. Loss of H3K27 trimethylation distinguishes malignant peripheral nerve sheath tumors from histologic mimics. Mod Pathol 2016;29(1):4–13.

246. Vengaloor Thomas T, Abraham A, Bhanat E, et al. Malignant peripheral nerve sheath tumor of nasal cavity and paranasal sinus with 13 years of follow-up-A case report and review of literature. Clin Case Rep 2019;7(11):2194–201.

247. Hujala K, Martikainen P, Minn H, et al. Malignant nerve sheath tumors of the head and neck: four case studies and review of the literature. Eur Arch Otorhinolaryngol 1993;250(7):379–82.

248. Mullins BT, Hackman T. Malignant peripheral nerve sheath tumors of the head and neck: a case series and literature review. Case Rep Otolaryngol 2014;2014:368920.

249. Wasa J, Nishida Y, Tsukushi S, et al. MRI features in the differentiation of malignant peripheral nerve sheath tumors and neurofibromas. AJR Am J Roentgenol 2010;194(6):1568–74.

250. Yu YH, Wu JT, Ye J, et al. Radiological findings of malignant peripheral nerve sheath tumor: reports of six cases and review of literature. World J Surg Oncol 2016;14:142.

251. Ahlawat S, Blakeley JO, Rodriguez FJ, et al. Imaging biomarkers for malignant peripheral nerve sheath tumors in neurofibromatosis type 1. Neurology 2019;93(11):e1076–84.

252. Demehri S, Belzberg A, Blakeley J, et al. Conventional and functional MR imaging of peripheral nerve sheath tumors: initial experience. AJNR Am J Neuroradiol 2014;35(8):1615–20.

253. Agarwalla PK, Koch MJ, Mordes DA, et al. Pigmented lesions of the nervous system and the neural crest: lessons from embryology. Neurosurgery 2016;78(1):142–55.

254. Torres-Mora J, Dry S, Li X, et al. Malignant melanotic schwannian tumor: a clinicopathologic, immunohistochemical, and gene expression profiling study of 40 cases, with a proposal for the reclassification of "melanotic schwannoma". Am J Surg Pathol 2014;38(1):94–105.

255. Carney JA. Psammomatous melanotic schwannoma. A distinctive, heritable tumor with special associations, including cardiac myxoma and the Cushing syndrome. Am J Surg Pathol 1990;14(3):206–22.

256. Nguyen CT, Tan J, Blackwell KE, et al. Primary melanocytic schwannoma of cervical sympathetic chain. Head Neck 2000;22(2):195–9.

257. Topf MC, Pham QH, D'Souza JN, et al. Pigmented melanotic schwannoma of the neck: report of 2 cases and review of the literature. Ear Nose Throat J 2019;98(2):102–6.

258. Khoo M, Pressney I, Hargunani R, et al. Melanotic schwannoma: an 11-year case series. Skeletal Radiol 2016;45(1):29–34.

259. Amita K, Shankar SV, Nischal KC, et al. Benign triton tumor: a rare entity in head and neck region. Korean J Pathol 2013;47(1):74–6.

260. Bae DH, Kim CH, Cheong JH, et al. Adulthood benign triton tumor developed in the orbit. J Korean Neurosurg Soc 2014;56(2):146–8.

261. Coli A, Novello M, Tamburrini G, et al. Intracranial neuromuscular choristoma: report of a case with literature review. Neuropathology 2017;37(4):341–5.

262. Carter JM, Howe BM, Hawse JR, et al. CTNNB1 mutations and estrogen receptor expression in neuromuscular choristoma and its associated fibromatosis. Am J Surg Pathol 2016;40(10):1368–74.

263. Castro DE, Raghuram K, Phillips CD. Benign triton tumor of the trigeminal nerve. AJNR Am J Neuroradiol 2005;26(4):967–9.

264. Pareja F, Brandes AH, Basili T, et al. Loss-of-function mutations in ATP6AP1 and ATP6AP2 in granular cell tumors. Nat Commun 2018;9(1):3533.

265. Alessi DM, Zimmerman MC. Granular cell tumors of the head and neck. Laryngoscope 1988;98(8 Pt 1): 810–4.

266. Koutlas IG, Scheithauer BW. Palisaded encapsulated ("solitary circumscribed") neuroma of the oral cavity: a review of 55 cases. Head Neck Pathol 2010;4(1):15–26.

267. Allen PW. Myxoma is not a single entity: a review of the concept of myxoma. Ann Diagn Pathol 2000; 4(2):99–123.

268. Ishoo E. Intramuscular myxoma presenting as a rare posterior neck mass in a young child: case report and literature review. Arch Otolaryngol Head Neck Surg 2007;133(4):398–401.

269. Willems SM, Mohseny AB, Balog C, et al. Cellular/intramuscular myxoma and grade I myxofibrosarcoma are characterized by distinct genetic alterations and specific composition of their extracellular matrix. J Cell Mol Med 2009;13(7): 1291–301.

270. Okamoto S, Hisaoka M, Meis-Kindblom JM, et al. Juxta-articular myxoma and intramuscular myxoma are two distinct entities. Activating Gs alpha mutation at Arg 201 codon does not occur in juxta-articular myxoma. Virchows Arch 2002;440(1): 12–5.

271. Sunitsch S, Gilg MM, Kashofer K, et al. Detection of GNAS mutations in intramuscular/cellular myxomas as diagnostic tool in the classification of myxoid soft tissue tumors. Diagn Pathol 2018;13(1):52.

272. Li G, Jiang W, Li W, et al. Intramuscular myxoma of the hyoglossus muscle: a case report and literature review. Oncol Lett 2014;7(5):1679–82.

273. Korver RJ, Theunissen PH, van de Kreeke WT, et al. Juxta-articular myxoma of the knee in a 5-year-old boy: a case report and review of the literature (2009: 12b). Eur Radiol 2010;20(3):764–8.

274. Somford MP, de Vries JS, Dingemans W, et al. Juxta-articular myxoma of the knee. J Knee Surg 2011;24(4):299–301.

275. Ye ZX, Yang C, Chen MJ, et al. Juxta-articular myxoma of the temporomandibular joint. J Craniofac Surg 2015;26(8):e695–6.

276. King DG, Saifuddin A, Preston HV, et al. Magnetic resonance imaging of juxta-articular myxoma. Skeletal Radiol 1995;24(2):145–7.

277. Gandhi MR, Tang YM, Panizza B. Myxoma of the masticator space. Australas Radiol 2007; 51(Suppl):B202–4.

278. Fatima SS, Din NU, Ahmad Z. Primary synovial sarcoma of the pharynx: a series of five cases and literature review. Head Neck Pathol 2015;9(4):458–62.

279. Shi H, Wang S, Wang P, et al. Primary retropharyngeal synovial sarcoma. AJNR Am J Neuroradiol 2009;30(4):811–2.

280. Sultan I, Rodriguez-Galindo C, Saab R, et al. Comparing children and adults with synovial sarcoma in the Surveillance, Epidemiology, and End Results program, 1983 to 2005: an analysis of 1268 patients. Cancer 2009;115(15):3537–47.

281. Jones BC, Sundaram M, Kransdorf MJ. Synovial sarcoma: MR imaging findings in 34 patients. AJR Am J Roentgenol 1993;161(4):827–30.

282. Murphey MD, Gibson MS, Jennings BT, et al. From the archives of the AFIP: imaging of synovial sarcoma with radiologic-pathologic correlation. Radiographics 2006;26(5):1543–65.

283. Hirsch RJ, Yousem DM, Loevner LA, et al. Synovial sarcomas of the head and neck: MR findings. AJR Am J Roentgenol 1997;169(4):1185–8.

284. Kim HS, Lee HK, Weon YC, et al. Alveolar soft-part sarcoma of the head and neck: clinical and imaging features in five cases. AJNR Am J Neuroradiol 2005;26(6):1331–5.

285. Wang H, Jacobson A, Harmon DC, et al. Prognostic factors in alveolar soft part sarcoma: a SEER analysis. J Surg Oncol 2016;113(5):581–6.

286. Casali PG, Dei Tos AP, Gronchi A. When does a new sarcoma exist? Clin Sarcoma Res 2020;10:19.

287. So YK, Chow C, To KF, et al. Myxoid spindle cell sarcoma with LMNA-NTRK fusion: expanding the morphologic spectrum of NTRK-rearranged tumors. Int J Surg Pathol 2020;28(5):574–8.

288. Peng KA, Grogan T, Wang MB. Head and neck sarcomas: analysis of the SEER database. Otolaryngol Head Neck Surg 2014;151(4):627–33.

289. Patel SG, See AC, Williamson PA, et al. Radiation induced sarcoma of the head and neck. Head Neck 1999;21(4):346–54.

290. Park SW, Kim HJ, Lee JH, et al. Malignant fibrous histiocytoma of the head and neck: CT and MR imaging findings. AJNR Am J Neuroradiol 2009;30(1): 71–6.

291. Sbaraglia M, Righi A, Gambarotti M, et al. Ewing sarcoma and Ewing-like tumors. Virchows Arch 2020;476(1):109–19.

292. Owosho AA, Estilo CL, Huryn JM, et al. Head and neck round cell sarcomas: a comparative clinicopathologic analysis of 2 molecular subsets: ewing and CIC-rearranged sarcomas. Head Neck Pathol 2017;11(4):450–9.

293. Ellis MA, Gerry DR, Neskey DM, et al. Ewing sarcoma of the head and neck. Ann Otol Rhinol Laryngol 2017;126(3):179–84.

294. Ng SH, Ko SF, Cheung YC, et al. Extraskeletal Ewing's sarcoma of the parapharyngeal space. Br J Radiol 2004;77(924):1046–9.

295. Zhang WD, Chen YF, Li CX, et al. Computed tomography and magnetic resonance imaging findings of peripheral primitive neuroectodermal tumors of the head and neck. Eur J Radiol 2011; 80(2):607–11.

296. Murphey MD, Senchak LT, Mambalam PK, et al. From the radiologic pathology archives: ewing

sarcoma family of tumors: radiologic-pathologic correlation. Radiographics 2013;33(3):803–31.

297. Doody J, Adil EA, Trenor CC 3rd, et al. The genetic and molecular determinants of juvenile nasopharyngeal angiofibroma: a systematic review. Ann Otol Rhinol Laryngol 2019;128(11):1061–72.

298. Ferouz AS, Mohr RM, Paul P. Juvenile nasopharyngeal angiofibroma and familial adenomatous polyposis: an association? Otolaryngol Head Neck Surg 1995;113(4):435–9.

299. Hwang HC, Mills SE, Patterson K, et al. Expression of androgen receptors in nasopharyngeal angiofibroma: an immunohistochemical study of 24 cases. Mod Pathol 1998;11(11):1122–6.

300. Robson CD. Imaging of head and neck neoplasms in children. Pediatr Radiol 2010;40(4):499–509.

301. Thompson LD, Miettinen M, Wenig BM. Sinonasal-type hemangiopericytoma: a clinicopathologic and immunophenotypic analysis of 104 cases showing perivascular myoid differentiation. Am J Surg Pathol 2003;27(6):737–49.

302. Brandwein-Gensler M, Siegal GP. Striking pathology gold: a singular experience with daily reverberations: sinonasal hemangiopericytoma (glomangiopericytoma) and oncogenic osteomalacia. Head Neck Pathol 2012;6(1):64–74.

303. Lasota J, Felisiak-Golabek A, Aly FZ, et al. Nuclear expression and gain-of-function beta-catenin mutation in glomangiopericytoma (sinonasal-type hemangiopericytoma): insight into pathogenesis and a diagnostic marker. Mod Pathol 2015;28(5):715–20.

304. Haller F, Bieg M, Moskalev EA, et al. Recurrent mutations within the amino-terminal region of beta-catenin are probable key molecular driver events in sinonasal hemangiopericytoma. Am J Pathol 2015;185(2):563–71.

305. Palacios E, Restrepo S, Mastrogiovanni L, et al. Sinonasal hemangiopericytomas: clinicopathologic and imaging findings. Ear Nose Throat J 2005;84(2):99–102.

306. Suh CH, Lee JH, Lee MK, et al. CT and MRI findings of glomangiopericytoma in the head and neck: case series study and systematic review. AJNR Am J Neuroradiol 2020;41(1):155–9.

307. Andreasen S, Bishop JA, Hellquist H, et al. Biphenotypic sinonasal sarcoma: demographics, clinicopathological characteristics, molecular features, and prognosis of a recently described entity. Virchows Arch 2018;473(5):615–26.

308. Wang X, Bledsoe KL, Graham RP, et al. Recurrent PAX3-MAML3 fusion in biphenotypic sinonasal sarcoma. Nat Genet 2014;46(7):666–8.

309. Dean KE, Shatzkes D, Phillips CD. Imaging review of new and emerging sinonasal tumors and tumor-like entities from the fourth edition of the World Health Organization Classification of head and neck tumors. AJNR Am J Neuroradiol 2019;40(4):584–90.

MR Imaging of Vascular Malformations and Tumors of Head and Neck

Ahmed Abdel Khalek Abdel Razek, MD[a,†], Ali H. Elmokadem, MD[a],
Mosad Soliman, MD[b], Suresh K. Mukherji, MD, MBA, FACR[c,*]

KEYWORDS

• Vascular malformations • Vascular tumors • Vascular anomalies • Head and neck • Hemangioma
• Venous • Arterial • Lymphatic

KEY POINTS

- MR imaging plays a pivotal role in the diagnosis, treatment planning and follow-up of most vascular malformations and tumors of the head and neck.
- The International Society for the Study of Vascular Anomalies classified vascular lesions into malformations and tumors.
- Vascular malformations are subclassified based on type of forming vessels and flow. Vascular tumors are subclassified into benign, reactive, locally malignant, and malignant.
- Conventional MR imaging provides a differential diagnosis for an atypical lesion. Diffusion-weighted imaging aids in differentiation between benign and malignant subtypes of vascular tumors.
- MR angiography separates low-flow from high-flow lesions and help in the peri-interventional assessment.

INTRODUCTION

Soft tissue vascular anomalies are malformations and tumors that result from errors of vascular embryogenesis and include a wide range of a complex heterogeneous group of pathologies of the circulatory system that can influence any sort of lymphatic and/or hematic vessels of diverse anatomic locations. The global incidence of vascular tumors in children less than 3 years is 6% to 8% and of vascular malformations is 1.2%.[1] Vascular anomalies represent the foremost common congenital and neonatal abnormalities and predominantly happen in the head and neck region in around 4.5% of children.[2]

The extreme variability of tissue types and districts involved by these lesions determines a wide heterogeneity of clinical manifestations that necessitate the establishment of multidisciplinary teams for managing such lesions. Furthermore, vascular anomalies can be expressed as a part of complex syndromes or rare malformations. In these cases, the clinical approach, diagnosis, and treatment will be more specific and may require genetic analysis. Diagnostic imaging has an important role in both the diagnosis and management of vascular lesions of the head and neck. Imaging confirms the diagnosis, maps the lesion, and monitors disease progression and/or response to therapy.[3] Additionally, imaging provides a means of direct treatment for some vascular abnormalities. With advances in imaging technology, including multiplanar and cross-sectional techniques, imaging offers detailed information on the relationship with neighboring vital

[a] Department of Diagnostic Radiology, Mansoura University Faculty of Medicine, Elgomhoria Street, Mansoura 35512, Egypt; [b] Department of Vascular Surgery, Mansoura University Faculty of Medicine, Elgomhoria Street, Mansoura 35512, Egypt; [c] Marian University, Head and Neck Radiology, ProScan Imaging, Carmel, IN, USA
[†] Deceased
* Corresponding author.
E-mail address: sureshmukherji@hotmail.com

Magn Reson Imaging Clin N Am 30 (2022) 199–213
https://doi.org/10.1016/j.mric.2021.07.005

structures and associated anomalies that may result in the diagnosis of a clinical syndrome.[4]

METHODS OF EXAMINATION
Computed Tomography Scan and Ultrasound Examination

Gray-scale ultrasound examination coupled with color Doppler imaging and spectral analysis is the initial screening imaging modality for the diagnosis of vascular malformations. Ultrasound imaging is widely available, easy to use, noninvasive, has a low cost, and usually does not require sedation. However, the value of ultrasound imaging may be limited in deep and complex lesions.[5] Contrast-enhanced ultrasound examination has been suggested for the evaluation of congenital venous malformations (CVMs) and has been used for monitoring response to therapy, including microcirculatory changes.[6]

Contrast-enhanced computed tomography (CT) scans or CT angiography is useful in the assessment of vascular malformations. Multidetector CT scans help to evaluate for vascular anatomy, enhancement, calcification, thrombus, phleboli, and the involvement of adjacent structures. CT scans provide high temporal resolution and are relatively easy to interpret. However, a CT scan has an overall limited usefulness, because it provides less information on the flow dynamics, and is associated with exposure to ionizing radiation. Hence, ultrasound examination and MR imaging are the primary noninvasive imaging modalities for the evaluation of vascular malformations.[7]

MR Imaging

Routine MR imaging has proven advantageous to differentiate high-flow from low-flow lesions owing to its reproducibility and ability to reliably delineate the extent of these lesions. Owing to these benefits, coupled with the lack of ionizing radiation and multiplanar capabilities, MR imaging has become the first-line imaging modality in the assessment of vascular anomalies.[8–10]

Diffusion-weighted imaging added to the scanning protocol of vascular anomalies can provide additional information to conventional MR imaging examination, such as the prediction of intravascular coagulopathy[11] within venous malformation and discrimination between hemangioma and malignant tumors.[12,13] Moreover, the apparent diffusion coefficient (ADC) values can differentiate between venous malformations, hemangioma, and other soft tissue tumors.[14,15] Based on its ability to quantitatively measure intralesional flow, arterial spin labeling has been used to differentiate between high- and low-flow

vascular anomalies and to evaluate the hemodynamics of soft tissue vascular anomalies especially after treatment.[16,17]

MR angiography (MRA) is considered a key diagnostic tool for evaluating vascular anomalies. Unfortunately, conventional MRA temporal resolution does not achieve satisfactory results. MRA using time-resolved postcontrast sequences such as time-resolved imaging of contrast kinetics has a higher temporal resolution. Time-resolved MRA provides a valuable hemodynamic assessment of vascular anomalies and proper characterization of the vascular lesion components, not only helping in the classification of vascular anomalies, but also guiding surgeons or interventional radiologists for treatment roadmap.[18–20] Four-dimensional flow MRA is another technique that yields quantitative measurements about the flow inside the vascular anomaly allowing better discrimination between high and low flow lesions and providing follow-up data for staged therapy, such as sclerotherapy of venous malformations.[21]

CLASSIFICATION

A commonly agreed terminology is crucial for the appropriate evaluation and patient management. In the last century, a wide range of terms has been used to describe vascular anomalies. Many classifications used anatomic labels or descriptive terms, regardless of the biological behavior of the different pathologies. This approach in classification caused clinical confusion and consequently clinical and therapeutic errors. The literature has been abundant with confusing terms such as cavernous hemangioma, which truly are venous vascular malformations. Other terms were used like capillary hemangioma instead of hemangioma and cystic hygroma or lymphangioma instead of lymphatic malformation. It is important to understand which terms are interchangeable and to move toward more consistent terminology.

The classification system described by Mulliken and Glowacki[22] separates the lesions into 2 groups: those that are vascular malformations, with normal endothelial cell turnover, and those that are vascular tumors, with high endothelial cell turnover. The first International Society for the Study of Vascular Anomalies (ISSVA) Classification dated 1996[1] distinguished vascular anomalies in relation to their hemodynamic characteristics in 2 main subtypes, namely, "fast flow" and "slow flow." Fast flow malformations were the arteriovenous ones; the slow flow as capillary, venous, and lymphatic malformations.

The ISSVA provides the most standardized and accepted classification. The ISSVA classification was first introduced in 1997 and most recently

Table 1
Classification of vascular malformations

Simple	Combined
Low flow	CM–VM
VM	CM–LM
LM	LM–VM
CM	CM–AVM
High flow	CM–LM–AVM
AVM	
AVF	

Abbreviations: CM, Capillary malformation; LM, lymphatic malformation; VM, venous malformation.

updated in 2018.[23,24] Currently, it is the prevailing classification system routinely used by multidisciplinary teams that diagnose and manage patients with vascular anomalies, particularly among pediatric subspecialties and interventional radiologists. ISSVA classification emphasizes the known genetic mutations associated with CVM, reflecting a growing interest in the genetic basis of vascular malformations.[25] This classification divides vascular anomalies into 2 major categories: (1) vascular malformations (**Table 1**), and (2) vascular tumors, which are vascular lesions with a proliferative behavior (**Table 2**). This classification divides vascular tumors into benign, intermediate, and malignant grades. Some vascular lesions, for which is still debated the "reactive" rather than "neoplastic" nature, are grouped within benign tumors. Malformations of major named vessels involve any large caliber vessel and consist of anomalies in the origin, course, number, length, diameter (aplasia, hypoplasia, ectasia/aneurysm), or valves.[23]

VASCULAR MALFORMATIONS

Vascular malformations (VMs) are considered the second major category of vascular anomalies. However, in stark contrast with vascular tumors, they do not regress or enlarge; they grow at the same rate as the child.[26] The latest version of the

ISSVA classifies CVMs into 4 groups: simple malformations, combined malformations, malformations of major named vessels, and malformations associated with other anomalies (syndromic vascular malformation). Simple vascular malformations are composed of a single type of vessel (capillaries, lymphatics, or veins). The exception to this rule is arteriovenous malformations (AVMs), which are composed of arteries, veins, and nidus with capillaries. Based on their flow characteristics, simple vascular malformations are further differentiated into high-flow lesions and low-flow lesions.[23]

Capillary Malformations

Capillary malformations are low-flow vascular lesions that usually referred to as a port wine stain, which are found in 0.5% of the population and affect the skin capillaries; however, they pose a risk of transmission to Sturge–Weber syndrome when they involve 25% of 1 side of the face and 33% involving both sides.[27]

MR imaging is beneficial in the diagnosis and the lesions may appear as subtle signal abnormality within the subcutaneous fat with skin thickening[28] (**Fig. 1**). It also might detect the associated gyral atrophy, gyral enhancement, enhancement of ipsilateral choroid plexus, and cortical calcification. Abnormal cortical veins and contrast stasis can be seen on cerebral angiography.[29]

Venous Malformations

Venous malformations (VMs) are the most common vascular malformations. VMs result from errors in the development of the venous network, leading to dilated and dysfunctional veins that are deficient in muscle cells. They are commonly seen in the head and neck region. Clinically, superficial venous malformations appear as a nonpulsatile, compressible region of soft tissue swelling with no changes in skin temperature, bruit, or thrill. They commonly increase in size and coloration during a Valsalva maneuver. A blue-to purple hue or superficial veins can be seen in cases

Table 2
Classification of vascular tumors

Vascular Tumors			
Benign	Benign (Reactive)	Locally Malignant	Malignant
Infantile hemangioma	Epithelioid hemangioma	Kaposiform	Angiosarcoma
Congenital	Lobular capillary	Hemangioendothelioma	Epithelioid
hemangioma	hemangioma	Retiform	Hemangioendothelioma
	Tufted Hemangioma	hemangioendothelioma	Infantile fibrosarcoma
	Spindle cell hemangioma		

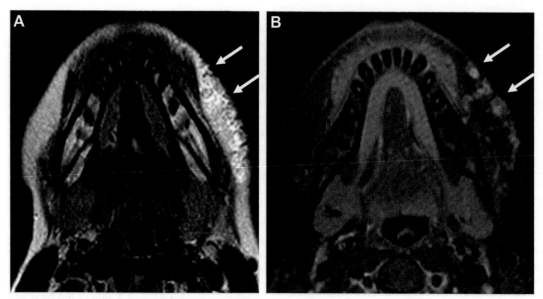

Fig. 1. Capillary malformation. (*A*) Axial T2-weighted images shows an ill-defined area of increased T2 signal involving the subcutaneous tissues overlying the body of the mandible (*arrows*). (*B*) Fat-suppressed contrast-enhanced T1-weighted images demonstrates ill-defined enhancement in this superficial low-flow vascular malformation (*arrows*).

associated with skin involvement. Lesions enlarge owing to hormonal changes during puberty, pregnancy, and oral contraceptive use or internal thrombosis after trauma. Pain consider as a sign of intralesional thrombosis.[30,31]

VMs display heterogeneous echotexture on ultrasound examination and are hypoechoic relative to the surrounding soft tissues. The superficial VMs are compressible when the pressure is applied to the transducer, whereas the diffuse lesions manifest as multiple varicosities infiltrating different tissue planes with the monophasic flow on spectral Doppler analysis.[26] Nevertheless, the flow may not be detected in some lesions with internal thrombosis or very slow flow. CT scans and conventional radiography have limited to detection of phleboliths related to intralesional thrombosis and calcifications[2,32] (**Fig. 2**).

Venous malformations display intermediate to low signal intensity on T1-weighted MR imaging and high signal intensity on T2-weighted images and short T1 inversion recovery sequences. A relatively high signal intensity might be detected on T1-weighted images owing to thrombosis or hemorrhage, whereas T1-weighted and T2-weighted hypointense foci may correspond with thrombi, phleboliths, and areas of previous treatment or vascular septa. Furthermore, fluid levels are not commonly seen with VMs. Contrast-enhanced T1-weighted imaging of VMs exhibits a variable degree of enhancement based on acquisition timing, ranging from early homogenous

enhancement to delayed heterogeneous enhancement.[30,32] When distinguishing between hemangiomas and VMs, T2 signal of hemangiomas is moderately higher compared with skeletal muscle, but significantly lower than that of cerebrospinal fluid and less than the relatively hypocellular VM or lymphatic malformation.[4] Perilesional edema or the presence of an enhancing soft tissue component should prompt consideration of biopsy to evaluate for malignancy[13] (**Fig. 3**).

Time-resolved MRA is valuable to assess lesion flow patterns and the type of venous drainage. VMs are classified based on the type of venous drainage into (i) type I, which is an isolated malformation without venous drainage; (ii) type II, which drains into normal veins; (iii) type III, which drains into dysplastic veins; and (iv) type IV, which are lesions that consist of venous ectasia.[33,34] Identifying the various types of VMs has important implications regarding management planning and prognosis. Sclerotherapy is the recommended therapy for type I and II VMs with a lower number of treatment sessions, whereas types III and IV are associated with more complications.[35]

Venous malformations show higher ADC values in comparison with hemangiomas and other soft tissue tumors. The mean ADC value in VMs ($1.85 \times 10^{-3} mm^2/s$) is higher compared with hemangioma ($1.22 \times 10^{-3} mm^2/s$).[14] The mean ADC value of nonthrombosed intraorbital VMs ($2.80 \times 10^{-3} mm^2/s$) is higher compared with other soft tissue tumors ($1.18 \times 10^{-3} mm^2/s$).[15]

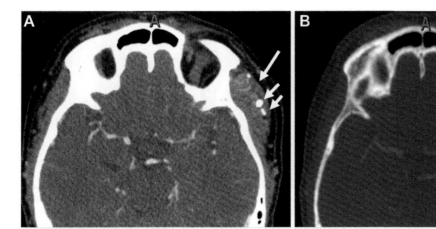

Fig. 2. Venous malformation. (*A*) Axial contrast-enhanced CT scan shows a slightly enhancing mass involving the let temporalis muscle (*long arrow*) that contains focal areas of increase attenuation (*short arrows*). (*B*) Bone windows confirm the presence of phleboliths (*short arrows*). The combination of an intramuscular mass containing phleboliths is suggestive of a venous malformation.

Additionally, ADC value $1.454 \times 10^{-3} \text{mm}^2/\text{s}$ was used as a cut-off value to predict intravascular coagulopathy within VMs.[11]

Sclerotherapy is the treatment of choice for VM and lymphatic malformation with surgical resection being the second-line therapy. Sclerosing agents include STS, polidocanol, and absolute alcohol. Capillary malformations are commonly treated with ablative treatment such as a pulsed dye laser (**Fig. 4**). Surgery is reserved for lesions that are refractory to ablative treatment or are causing significant disfigurement.[29] Imaging is important for response to the therapy and monitoring patients after therapy.

Glomuvenous Malformation

Glomuvenous malformation, previously referred to as glomangioma, is a developmental hamartoma of glomus body origin, and is categorized as a VM subtype by the 2018 ISSVA classification.[23] Glomuvenous malformations may be sporadic or demonstrate an autosomal-dominant inheritance. Lesions present as clustered purple or blue tender vascular nodules, cutaneous and subcutaneous in location. Glomuvenous malformations may be solitary, or multiple and plaque-like, demonstrating a "pebbly" or cobblestone appearance, which helps to differentiate this entity from common VMs.[36–39]

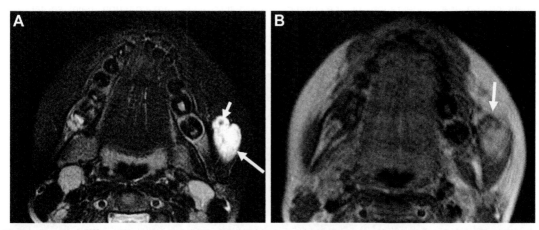

Fig. 3. Venous malformation. (*A*) Axial T2-weighted images show an expansile high signal mass involving the right master muscle (*long arrow*). The focal area of decreased signal is suspicious for a phlebolith. (*B*) Contrast-enhanced T1-weighted images show the mass to be enhancing (*arrow*). Dynamic imaging showed delayed enhancement (not shown) that was consistent with venous pooling and helped confirm the diagnosis of venous malformation.

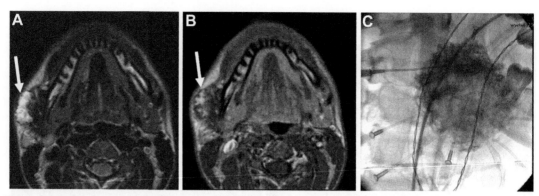

Fig. 4. Venous malformation treated with sclerotherapy. (*A*) Axial T2-weighted images shows an ill-defined high signal mass involving the right masseter muscle (*arrow*). (*B*) Postcontrast–enhanced T1-weighted images shows delayed ill-defined enhancement (*arrow*). (*C*) The mass was confirmed to be a low-flow venous malformation and was treated with sclerotherapy.

Imaging is important to detect its extent, because a deep subfascial extension of the lesions is common. Lesions usually appear as a multilobulated, septated mass of low signal intensity on T1-weighted imaging and highly bright signal intensity on T2-weighted imaging with delayed heterogenous filling after contrast administration. Dynamic time-resolved MRA demonstrates patchy enhancement in the arterial phase and possible early venous shunting. However, the absence of dilated feeding arteries or draining veins helps to differentiate this entity from an AVM.[2,39]

Lymphatic Malformations

Lymphatic malformations consist of cystic dilated lymphatic channels and spaces without a connection to the lymphatic system. They are described as macrocystic, microcystic, or combined, depending on the appearance of the cystic spaces. Lymphatic malformations are usually apparent at birth or by 2 years of age; they also grow with the child and can affect any part of the body, most commonly the head and neck (approximately 70%).[40]

Macrocystic lymphatic malformations typically appear as multiple, anechoic cystic spaces with thin internal septations (**Fig. 5**). Varying degrees of internal floating echoes can be seen in the cystic spaces if the lesion is complicated with hemorrhage or infection. Heterogeneous echogenic clots as well as fluid–fluid levels in the lesion can be related to intralesional hemorrhage but are not pathognomonic to lymphatic malformations and can be seen with VMs and other vascular lesions[2,28] (**Fig. 6**).

These lesions show intermediate to low signal intensity on T1-weighted MR images and high signal intensity on T2-weighted images and short T1 inversion recovery sequences (see **Fig. 5**). Fluid–fluid levels are common. Faint septal and capsular enhancements are noted after

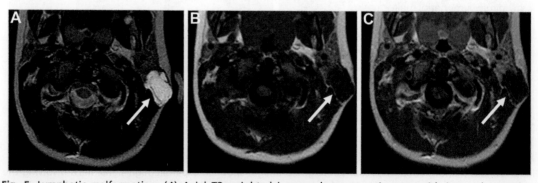

Fig. 5. Lymphatic malformation. (*A*) Axial T2-weighted images shows a cystic mass with internal septations involving the posterior portion of the parotid gland that abuts the anterior border of the trapezius muscle (*arrow*). (*B*) Noncontrast T1-weighted image shows the lesion to be low signal nonenhancing on the contrast-enhanced images (*C*) (*arrows*).

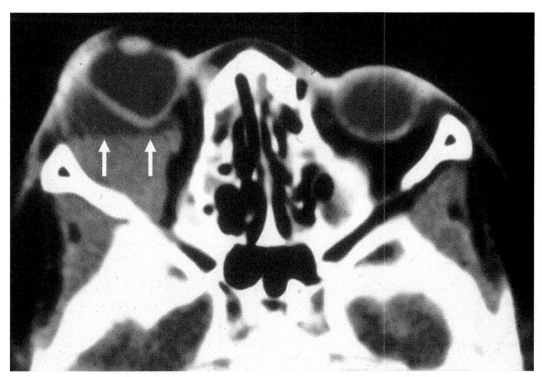

Fig. 6. Lymphatic malformation with hemorrhage. Axial noncontrast CT scan obtained through the orbits shows a large retrobulbar lymphatic malformation with a blood–fluid level indicative of recent hemorrhage that has result in deforming the globe ("tension globe").

intravenous contrast administration. Microcystic lymphatic malformations may simulate a solid enhancing mass; however, this appearance is due to the aggregate enhancement of the cyst walls and septa that are in close vicinity.[2,26,41]

The diagnosis of lymphatic malformations may overlap with other pediatric tumors, especially low-grade well-circumscribed tumors that grow very slowly or aggressive tumors when they are necrotic and predominantly cystic with bleeding inside and fluid–fluid levels.[42] Neoplasms that can mimic lymphatic malformations in neonates and infants include teratoma, rhabdomyosarcoma, and lipoblastoma, whereas synovial sarcoma, angiomatoid fibrous histiocytoma, and epithelioid sarcoma mimic lymphatic malformations in older children.[41] Conventional MR imaging signs as the presence of solid enhancing component and internal vascularity or diffusion restriction on diffusion-weighted imaging aid in the differentiation between lymphatic malformations and neoplastic masses.

Arteriovenous Malformations

AVMs or arteriovenous fistulas form one-third of vascular malformations and result from an abnormal connection or channel formation between arteries and veins. In arteriovenous fistulas, single or multiple direct communication is present between arteries and veins without an intervening capillary bed, whereas in AVMs there is a low-resistance nidus connected to feeding arteries and draining veins.[5,43] The majority of AVM growth is expected to occur during childhood; however, sudden accelerated AVM growth may be triggered by trauma or a hormonal effect during adult life.

On ultrasound examination, AVMs appear as conglomerates of tortuous and enlarged vascular channels characterized by pulsatile flow with high velocities in the draining vein, and turbulent flow at the connecting channel.[28] A CT scan may be helpful in the diagnosis of AVM because it appears as a serpiginous vascular mass with dilated arterial feeder and early venous shunting.[35] (**Fig. 7**).

MR imaging is the imaging modality of choice to assess the extensions of AVM and secondary changes in the adjacent tissue. Increased signal intensity on T1-weighted images indicate fibrofatty proliferation, whereas a high signal on T2-weighted imaging denotes perilesional edema. High-flow vessels appear as flow voids on spin echo sequences and hyperintense foci on gradient

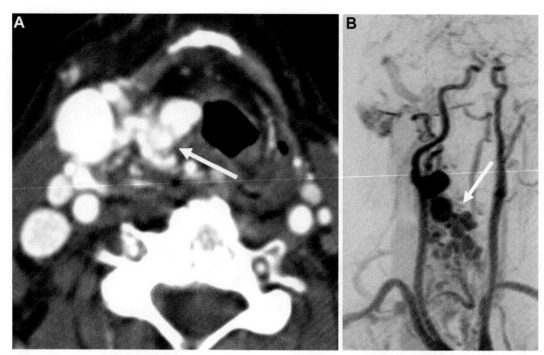

Fig. 7. AVM. (*A*) Axial contrast-enhanced CT scan shows multiple dilated enhancing vessels involving the right aryepiglottic fold associated with draining veins extending through the thyrohyoid membrane (*arrow*). (*B*) Contrast-enhanced MRA performed in the same patient shows the extensive AVM involving the right neck (*arrow*).

echo sequences. Contrast-enhanced T1 imaging should not demonstrate an enhancing soft tissue mass; however, enhancement of the surrounding soft tissues may be seen in the setting of complications, such as ischemia, infection, or hemorrhage.[2]

Dynamic contrast MRA is useful in showing the high-flow nature of the malformation with early venous filling and aid in identifying the feeding artery, draining veins, and nidus as a tangle of vessels (see **Fig. 7**). Based on the angioarchitectures, Yakes classified AVMs and suggested possible treatment strategies.[44]

- A type I AVM is a direct AVF that can be occluded with mechanical devices such as plugs or coils.
- A type IIa AVM has typical nidus supplied by multiple inflow arteries with direct artery to arteriolar and vein to venule communication.
- ype IIb AVM similarly has multiple inflow arteries, which supplies a typical nidus that drains into an aneurysmal draining vein. The treatment of type II AVMs should target nidus obliteration, either through a transarterial approach or direct injection.
- ype IIIa AVM features multiple artery-to-arteriole communications into an enlarged

central vein where the vein the wall serves as the nidus. Type IIIa AVM therapy demands transarterial embolization of the nidus coupled with direct puncture and obliteration of the outflow veins.
- ype IIIb AVM features multiple arteries to arterioles that drain into an aneurysmal central vein with multiple, usually dilated, outflow veins. They are treated through a transarterial approach to embolize the inflow artery combined with direct puncture occlusion of the aneurysmal venous outflow and embolization of the other outflow veins by coils or plugs.
- ype IV AVM has multiple small arteriolar to venule communications that diffusely infiltrate tissues. The recommended treatment is superselective ethanol (50%) injection through a transarterial or direct puncture approach.

Findings on follow-up MR imaging after AVM treatment include nidus thrombosis and decreased or absent early venous filling related to shunting. Thrombosis after sclerotherapy of the CVMs leads to heterogeneous signal intensity on both T1- and T2-weighted images and absent contrast enhancement with progressive shrinkage of the VMs. Peripheral high T2 signal intensity with marked postcontrast enhancement may be observed if the follow-up MR imaging is performed early in the post-treatment phase. These features are a result of inflammatory changes and may persist for up to 3 months.[45] More recently, 4-dimensional flow MRA is used to assess the flow inside intracranial AVM and decrease of flow after endovascular or radiation therapy.[46]

Combined Vascular Malformations

In combined-type vascular malformation, there are 2 or more simple vascular malformations incorporated in 1 lesion. Capillary–lymphatico–venous malformations are the most common complex combined vascular malformation. An example is an angiokeratoma, which is characterized by a combination of capillary and lymphatic. In newborns, angiokeratoma may be confused with the more frequent segmental infantile hemangioma (IH) in its prodromal phase.[1] MR imaging can aid in the classification of these lesions, particularly to determine the presence of a high-flow component[47] (**Fig. 8**).

VASCULAR TUMORS
Infantile Hemangioma

Infantile, juvenile, or cellular hemangioma is considered the most common benign vascular tumor of neonates and early childhood. IH has an estimated prevalence of 3% to 10%; 60% arise in the head and neck regions and are seen frequently in low birth-weight, premature infants, Caucasians, and females.[48–50] IHs are histologically positive for glucose-transporter GLUT-1. It presents at birth as a telangiectatic stain or ecchymotic patch or within the first few weeks of life as a solitary cutaneous lesion on the cervicofacial area.

In most cases, IH follows a consistent natural course that consists of 3 phases of growth patterns. The first phase is the proliferative phase, which is characterized by rapid growth within the first year of life, followed by a second rapid growth phase. The involution phase generally begins around 6 to 18 months of age and completes by age 4 to 5 years. Up to 50% of IHs will leave residual anetoderma, telangiectasia, scarring, or redundant skin after involution.[50,51] Approximately 24% of patients with IH develop complications, most commonly ulceration. Based on the lesion characteristics and its relation to other vital structures, other complications may include visual impairment, hearing impairment, bleeding, and airway obstruction.[4] The first line of treatment options for HI is beta blockers, and less common corticosteroids (intralesional or systemic) or surgery.[52]

Based on the level of skin involvement,[51] IH can be subclassified into 3 categories: (i) superficial lesions, which only involve the outer skin layers and will often appear and involute earlier in age, they appear as bright red lesions; (ii) deep lesions, which are subcutaneous and grow into the adipose tissue, they often exhibit a bluish hue and commonly overlying telangiectasias; and (iii) mixed lesions, which display both superficial and deep features. According to the anatomic configuration, IH can be classified into focal, segmental, facial segmental, indeterminate, and multifocal lesions. Focal tumors arise from a single local point and are round, popular, or nodular. Segmental lesions are plaque-like and involve a larger region of skin. Facial segmental IH can be defined as frontotemporal, maxillary, mandibular, and/or frontonasal. However, facial segmental hemangiomas are present and affect a skin area designated as V3. This

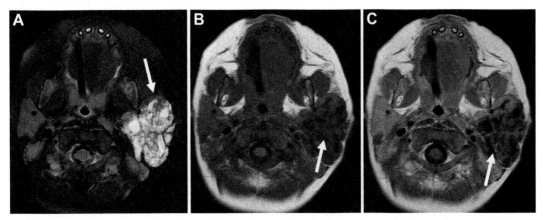

Fig. 8. Capillary–lymphatic malformation. (*A*) Axial T2-weighted images show a high signal mass replacing the left parotid gland with multiple internal septations (*arrow*). The high T2 signal mass is indicative of a lymphatic component. Axial precontrast (*B*) and postcontrast (*C*) T1-weighted images show enhancement of the septa (*arrow*) suggestive of a capillary component. The combination is indicative of a capillary lymphatic malformation.

area encompasses the mandibular and preauricular region, chin, inferior lip, neck, and sometimes the breastbone. Indeterminate IH is classified into this category when the lesion cannot be determined definitively as either focal or segmental. Multifocal tumors are classified by multiple IH lesions, typically 5 or more. Rarely, IHs are associated with other abnormalities, as it happens in syndromic forms.

Imaging features of IH differ according to the growth phase. IH in the proliferative phase display an isointense signal to muscle on T1-weighted imaging and a moderately high signal on T2-weighted imaging with homogenous intense enhancement after contrast administration. Flow voids may be visualized within and around the mass reflecting the high vascularity of the proliferative phase (**Fig. 9**). There is a decrease in the hemangioma size and decreased enhancement during the involutional phase when compared with initial scans. The absence of flows is also indicative of the involution (**Fig. 10**). The lesion may show fibrofatty or fatty changes as a bright signal on T1-weighted imaging. Imaging findings during the involution phase may be limited to localized tissue distortion without a detectable mass lesion or by persistent facial asymmetry owing to prolonged hyperemia and overgrowth of the nearby bony structures.[50–55]

MR imaging may also be used to determine the extent of a lesion and to detect any nearby anomalies. Hemangiomas in the neck can extend to the aerodigestitial tract, subsequently compromising the related airway that may indicate rapid intervention. Facial IHs may be associated with intraorbital extension or are linked to intracranial abnormalities.[4] MR imaging and MRA of the brain are useful in evaluating the anomalies associated with PHACES syndrome,[56] which characterized by posterior fossa abnormalities (P), infantile type of hemangiomas (H), segmental arterial anomalies, especially aorta (A), cardiovascular anomalies (C), eye anomalies IHs, and sternal clefting, and/or supraumbilical raphe (S).

Owing to high incidence and rapidly growing pattern of IHs, they are frequently misdiagnosed as malignant soft tissue tumors. Diffusion-weighted imaging is useful in discriminating IHs from malignant soft tissue tumors. The ADC values of IH are higher than those of malignant soft tissue tumors.[12,13] A biopsy is mandatory whenever other aggressive or malignant lesions are suspected clinically, as rhabdomyosarcoma, angiosarcoma, and kaposiform hemangioendothelioma (KHE).

Congenital Hemangioma

Congenital hemangiomas are presented in utero and already visible at birth; hence, prenatal ultrasound examination and fetal MR imaging might play a vital role in the diagnosis and planning for delivery and postnatal care[57] (**Fig. 11**). They represent about 3% of the overall incidence of hemangiomas and rarely involve the head and neck region. In most cases, they arise in the skin and underlying subcutaneous soft tissue as red to purple plaques and as superficial telangiectasia when fully developed. Eventually, they evolve into a grayish color spot, with a pale peripheral halo. The discrimination between IHs and congenital hemangiomas is mainly based on their clinical course and histologically by the absence of GLUT-1 protein expression.[4,55]

MR imaging findings are mainly similar to those of IHs; however, unlike IHs, a greater proportion of congenital hemangiomas display more heterogeneous signal intensity and postcontrast enhancement. The borders of congenital hemangiomas

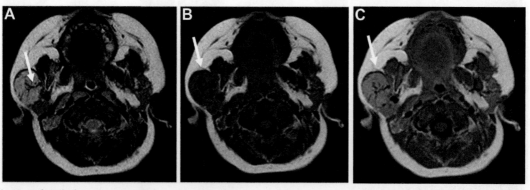

Fig. 9. Infantile hemangioma (IH) proliferative phase. (*A*) Axial T1-weighted images shows a large high signal mass involving the right parotid glad. The mass contains multiple internal serpiginious flow voids (*arrow*). Axial precontrast (*B*) and postcontrast (*C*) T1-weighted images shows homogeneous enhancement of the IH. The large internal flow voids are characteristic of the proliferative phase.

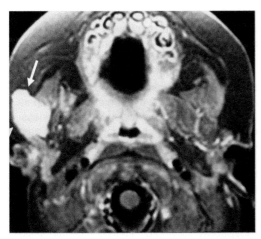

Fig. 10. Infantile hemangioma (IH) involuting phase. Axial fast-suppressed postcontrast T1-weighted images shows a homogeneously enhancing hemangioma without the flow voids. The absence of the flow void is indicative of the involuting phase.

tend to be less sharply marginated than IH. Congenital hemangiomas may exhibit areas of calcifications, whereas none of the IHs had visible calcification.[50,52,54] Additionally, venous thrombosis was also more common in congenital hemangiomas.[4]

Based on the pattern of involution, congenital hemangiomas are subclassified into 3 categories:

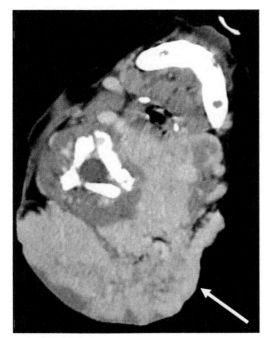

Fig. 11. Congenital hemangioma. Axial contrast-enhanced CT scan shows an extensive hemangioma in a newborn (*arrow*).

(i) rapidly involving congenital hemangioma (RICH), which regresses rapidly within 1 year of age; (ii) noninvoluting congenital hemangioma, which does not regress and surgical treatment is necessary; (iii) and partial involuting congenital hemangiomas, which is a rare type that partially regresses. On MR imaging, RICH are frequently displaying homogenous enhancement and flow voids compared with noninvoluting congenital hemangioma, whereas noninvoluting congenital hemangioma show heterogeneous enhancement and fat stranding of the nearby soft tissue.[58] RICH has a higher incidence of complication, because it is known to be associated with mild transient thrombocytopenia and consumption coagulopathy, which typically self-resolves within a few weeks. Although rare, RICHs have been associated with (Kasabach–Merritt phenomenon) or high-output cardiac failure owing to arteriovenous or portovenous shunting.[59] In the first few months of life, RICH can more commonly ulcerate and bleed specifically during the involution phase.[48]

Epithelioid Hemangioma

Epithelioid hemangioma or angiolymphoid hyperplasia with eosinophilia is a rare, distinct, slowly progressive vascular neoplasm with no specific age or location prediction; however, the head and neck region is a common site.[1,51] Epithelioid hemangioma arises from the skin, subcutaneous soft tissue, and bone. In up to 50% of cases, it may occur multifocally. Three histologic subtypes of epithelioid hemangioma are identified: conventional, cellular, and angiolymphoid hyperplasia with eosinophilia.[60] Local recurrence is reported in 30% of cases and spontaneous regression has been reported. The optimal treatment is complete excision.

Epithelioid hemangioma is not typically part of the radiology differential diagnosis of vascular tumors because of its rarity, nonspecific imaging appearance, and variable locations and presenting ages. Usually, the pathologist is the first to diagnose this tumor. Osseous lesions usually are lytic, expansile, and have internal septa, whereas soft tissue lesions display low to similar signal intensity to muscle on T1-weighted imaging and higher signal intensity than muscle on T2-weighted imaging.[60]

Lobular Capillary Hemangioma (Pyogenic Granuloma)

Lobular capillary hemangioma/pyogenic granuloma is an acquired benign vascular neoplasm of the skin and mucosa. It has an estimated prevalence of 1% and often occurs in the head and neck, most commonly in the oral cavity and lip. The lesion consists of a capillary proliferation secondary to minor trauma or possibly the result of a hormonal effect. Clinically, it manifests as localized pedunculated vascular bright red nodules that commonly bleed because of its friable surface.[61]

Lesions appear as a well-circumscribed mass with similar imaging characteristics to proliferating IHs. They demonstrate isointense signals to muscles on T1-weighted imaging and bright signal intensity on T2-weighted images with intense homogenous enhancement after contrast administration.[62] Pedunculated lesions can be treated by ligation, whereas other forms are best treated by surgical intervention.

Kaposiform Hemangioendothelioma and Tufted Angioma

KHE is a rare locally aggressive vascular tumor, usually present at birth. Histologically, lesions are GLUT-1 negative and composed of irregular nodular areas of compressed vessels, simulating capillary vascular malformation, and Kaposi sarcoma. Unlike Kaposi sarcoma, there is a lack of periodic acid-Schiff–positive globules. Tufted hemangioma belongs to the spectrum at the benign end. In contrast with IH, spontaneous regression without therapy is uncommon.[1,51] KHE may be associated with Kasabach–Merritt syndrome, which is characterized by the combination of a rapidly progressive vascular tumor, microangiopathic hemolytic anemia, and coagulopathy secondary to profound thrombocytopenia.[59] Surgical excision, occasionally combined with radiation, is the treatment of choice for the localized cutaneous lesions. In many cases, surgery is inappropriate technically because of local invasion and coexisted life-threatening thrombocytopenia secondary to Kasabach–Merritt syndrome.[4]

The imaging characteristics of KHE are similar to other proliferative vascular tumors. On MR imaging, it appears as a T2 hyperintense lesion in subcutaneous tissue. The lesion aggressiveness is demonstrated by irregular borders, the signs of skin infiltration, and the involvement of different tissue planes. The tumor margins are occasionally obscured by perilesional edema. Large lesions tend to display a destructive aggressive behavior with internal flow voids and hemorrhagic foci that show blooming on gradient echo or susceptibility-weighted images. Small lesions have nonspecific imaging features, but may grow suddenly and show aggressive behavior. After contrast administration, KHE demonstrates early avid contrast enhancement, small feeding arteries, and draining veins. The tumor has a very low malignant potential, but regional nodal metastases can be seen rarely. KHE tends to have infiltrative borders and displays diffuse heterogeneous enhancement after contrast injection compared with tufted hemangioma.[51,63]

Angiosarcoma

Angiosarcoma is a rare aggressive vascular tumor with a poor to lethal prognosis. It has a high incidence of local recurrence and metastatic disease and more frequent in males (4:3). Angiosarcoma makes up 0.5% of all pediatric sarcomas. When they do occur during childhood, they demonstrate more aggressive behavior than those that present during adulthood.[2,51,64]

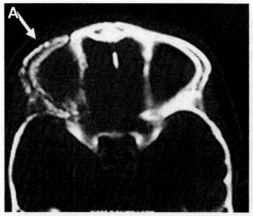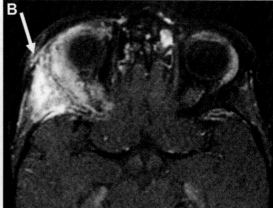

Fig. 12. Angiosarcoma. (*A*) Bone windows show an aggressive and permeative process involving the rook of the right orbit (*arrow*). (*B*) Fat-suppressed contrast-enhanced T1-weighted image shows a hypervascular aggressive mass involving the lateral wall of the right orbit extending laterally into the temporalis muscle and medially into the orbital vault.

Angiosarcoma appears on MR imaging as an aggressive heterogeneous mass with contrast pooling and prominent edema of nearby tissues and lymphedema. They exhibit an isointense signal on T1-weighted imaging, although hyperintensity and fluid–fluid levels may be present in the presence of hemorrhage, and T2-weighted imaging hyperintensity. Similar to KHE, flow voids if present is indicative of high-flow arterial vessels. After contrast administration demonstrate homogenous brisk enhancement of the soft tissue mass, with nonenhancing cystic areas indicative of necrosis.[64,65] A wide range of ADC values have been reported, likely related to the angiosarcoma's heterogeneous composition (**Fig. 12**). Metastatic or synchronous lesions at other anatomic locations, more commonly in the lungs, and to a lesser extent in the liver, soft tissues, bones, and lymph nodes, may be present at initial diagnoses.[65]

Epithelioid Hemangioendothelioma

Epithelioid hemangioendothelioma is a malignant endothelial vascular tumor with a wide range of age distribution; however, children are rarely affected. It may arise at any anatomic site including the head and neck region. There is a high probability of lymph node metastases and very rarely, a lymph node can be the primary origin.[66,67]

Epithelioid hemangioendothelioma of the head and neck appears as a hypointense mass on T1 images and hyperintense on T2 images with avid enhancement and central nonenhancing degeneration after contrast administration. Because there are no distinctive radiologic features, this tumor can only be definitively diagnosed with histopathologic analysis. Nevertheless, MR imaging remains important, as it can be used for initial staging, planning of biopsy, and therapy.[67]

CLINICS CARE POINTS

- Imaging is essential to proper characterize the various types of vascular malformation.
- The treatment of vascular malformations can be properly triaged based on imaging.
- Correct diagnosis will result in improved patient outcomes.

REFERENCES

1. Moneghini L, Sangiorgio V, Tosi D, et al. Head and neck vascular anomalies. A multidisciplinary approach and diagnostic criteria. Pathologica 2017;109:47–59.
2. Green JR, Resnick SA, Restrepo R, et al. Spectrum of imaging manifestations of vascular malformations and tumors beyond childhood: what general radiologists need to know. Radiol Clin North Am 2020; 58:583–601.
3. Mulliken JB, Burrows PE, Fishman SJ. Mulliken & Young's vascular anomalies: hemangiomas and malformations. New York: Oxford University Press; 2013.
4. Steinklein JM, Shatzkes DR. Imaging of vascular lesions of the head and neck. Otolaryngol Clin North Am 2018;51:55–76.
5. Nosher JL, Murillo PG, Liszewski M, et al. Vascular anomalies: a pictorial review of nomenclature, diagnosis and treatment. World J Radiol 2014;6: 677–926.
6. John P. Vascular anomalies. In: Temple M, Marshalleh FE, editors. Pediatric interventional radiology: hand book of vascular and non-vascular interventions. New York: Springer; 2014. p. 177–224.
7. Wiesinger I, Jung W, Zausig N, et al. Evaluation of dynamic effects of therapy-induced changes in microcirculation after percutaneous treatment of vascular malformations using contrast-enhanced ultrasound (CEUS) and time intensity curve (TIC) analyses. Clin Hemorheol Microcirc 2018;69: 45–57.
8. Bashir U, Shah S, Jeph S, et al. Magnetic resonance (MR) imaging of vascular malformations. Pol J Radiol 2017;82:731–41.
9. Mohammad SA, AbouZeid AA, Fawzi AM, et al. Magnetic resonance imaging of head and neck vascular anomalies: pearls and pitfalls. Ann Pediatr Surg 2017;13:116–24.
10. Flors L, Leiva-Salinas C, Norton PT, et al. Ten frequently asked questions about MRI evaluation of soft-tissue vascular anomalies. AJR Am J Roentgenol 2013;201:W554–62.
11. Razek AA, Ashmalla GA. Prediction of venous malformations with localized intravascular coagulopathy with diffusion-weighted magnetic resonance imaging. Phlebology 2019;34:156–61.
12. Saito M, Kitami M, Takase K. Usefulness of diffusion-weighted magnetic resonance imaging using apparent diffusion coefficient values for diagnosis of infantile hemangioma. J Comput Assist Tomogr 2019;43:563–7.
13. Mamlouk MD, Nicholson AD, Cooke DL, et al. Diffusion-weighted imaging for cutaneous vascular anomalies. Clin Imaging 2017;46:121–2.
14. Dong MJ, Zhou GY, Sun Q, et al. [Evaluation of MR diffusion-weighted imaging (MR-DWI) between head and neck hemangioma and venous malformation in children]. Shanghai Kou Qiang Yi Xue 2010; 19:378–82.

15. Kalin-Hajdu E, Colby JB, Idowu O, et al. Diagnosing distensible venous malformations of the orbit with diffusion-weighted magnetic resonance imaging. Am J Ophthalmol 2018;189:146–54.

16. Boulouis G, Dangouloff-Ros V, Boccara O, et al. Arterial spin-labeling to discriminate pediatric cervicofacial soft-tissue vascular anomalies. AJNR Am J Neuroradiol 2017;38:633–8.

17. Ramachandran S, Delf J, Brookes J, et al. Novel use of arterial spin labelling in the imaging of peripheral vascular malformations. BJR Case Rep 2020;6: 20200021.

18. Schicchi N, Tagliati C, Agliata G, et al. MRI evaluation of peripheral vascular anomalies using time-resolved imaging of contrast kinetics (TRICKS) sequence. Radiol Med 2018;123:563–71.

19. Higgins LJ, Koshy J, Mitchell SE, et al. Time-resolved contrast-enhanced MRA (TWIST) with gadofosveset trisodium in the classification of soft-tissue vascular anomalies in the head and neck in children following updated 2014 ISSVA classification: first report on systematic evaluation of MRI and TWIST in a cohort of 47 children. Clin Radiol 2016;71:32–9.

20. Razek AA, Gaballa G, Megahed AS, et al. Time resolved imaging of contrast kinetics (TRICKS) MR angiography of arteriovenous malformations of head and neck. Eur J Radiol 2013;82:1885–91.

21. Lee JY, Suh DC. Visualization of soft tissue venous malformations of head and neck with 4D flow magnetic resonance imaging. Neurointervention 2017; 12:110–5.

22. Mulliken JB, Glowacky J. Hemangiomas and vascular malformations in infant and children: a classification based on endothelial characteristics. Plast Reconstr Surg 1982;69:412–22.

23. Monroe EJ. Brief description of ISSVA classification for radiologists. Tech Vasc Interv Radiol 2019;22: 100628.

24. ISSVA Classification of Vascular Anomalies _2018 International Society for the Study of Vascular Anomalies. Available at: issva.org/classification. Accessed August 19, 2021.

25. Hoeger PH. Genes and phenotypes in vascular malformations. Clin Exp Dermatol 2020. https://doi.org/10.1111/ced.14513.

26. Hussein A, Malguria N. Imaging of vascular malformations. Radiol Clin North Am 2020;58:815–30.

27. Colletti G, Valassina D, Bertossi D, et al. Contemporary management of vascular malformations. J Oral Maxillofac Surg 2014;72:510–28.

28. Johnson CM, Navarro OM. Clinical and sonographic features of pediatric soft-tissue vascular anomalies part 1: classification, sonographic approach and vascular tumors. Pediatr Radiol 2017;47:1184–95.

29. Cox JA, Bartlett E, Lee EI. Vascular malformations: a review. Semin Plast Surg 2014;28:58–63.

30. Olivieri B, White CL, Restrepo R, et al. Low-flow vascular malformation pitfalls: from clinical examination to practical imaging evaluation–part 2, venous malformation mimickers. AJR Am J Roentgenol 2016;206:952–62.

31. Lowe LH, Marchant TC, Rivard DC, et al. Vascular malformations: classification and terminology the radiologist needs to know. Semin Roentgenol 2012; 47:106–17.

32. Dubois J, Alison M. Vascular anomalies: what a radiologist needs to know. Pediatr Radiol 2010;40:895–905.

33. Grossberg JA, Howard BM, Saindane AM. The use of contrast-enhanced, time-resolved magnetic resonance angiography in cerebrovascular pathology. Neurosurg Focus 2019;47:E3.

34. Abdel Razek AAK, Albair GA, Samir S. Clinical value of classification of venous malformations with contrast-enhanced MR angiography. Phlebology 2017;32:628–33.

35. Snyder E, Puttgen K, Mitchell S, et al. Magnetic resonance imaging of the soft tissue vascular anomalies in torso and extremities in children: an update with 2014 International Society for the Study of Vascular Anomalies classification. J Comput Assist Tomogr 2018;42:167–77.

36. Heiberg Brix AT, Tørring PM, Kamaleswaran S, et al. Glomuvenous malformations. Ugeskr Laeger 2019; 181. V10180740.

37. Wortsman X, Millard F, Aranibar L. Color Doppler ultrasound study of glomuvenous malformations with its clinical and histologic correlations. Actas Dermo-sifiliogr 2018;109:e17–21.

38. Shaikh R, Alomari AI, Mulliken JB, et al. Subfascial involvement in glomuvenous malformation. Skeletal Radiol 2014;43:895–7.

39. Flors L, Norton PT, Hagspiel KD. Glomuvenous malformation: magnetic resonance imaging findings. Pediatr Radiol 2015;45:286–90.

40. Navarro OM. Magnetic resonance imaging of pediatric soft-tissue vascular anomalies. Pediatr Radiol 2016;46:891–901.

41. White CL, Olivieri B, Restrepo R, et al. Low-flow vascular malformation pitfalls: from clinical examination to practical imaging evaluation–part 1, lymphatic malformation mimickers. AJR Am J Roentgenol 2016;206:940–51.

42. Keenan S, Bui-Mansfield LT. Musculoskeletal lesions with fluid-fluid level: a pictorial essay. J Comput Assist Tomogr 2006;30:517–24.

43. Fujima N, Osanai T, Shimizu Y, et al. Utility of noncontrast-enhanced time-resolved four-dimensional MR angiography with a vessel-selective technique for intracranial arteriovenous malformations. J Magn Reson Imaging 2016;44:834.

44. Griauzde J, Wilseck ZM, Chaudhary N, et al. Endovascular treatment of arteriovenous malformations of the head and neck: focus on the Yakes

classification and outcomes. J Vasc Interv Radiol 2020;31:1810–6.

45. Sadick M, Overhoff D, Baessler B, et al. Peripheral vascular anomalies - essentials in periinterventional imaging. Rofo 2020;192:150–62.

46. Li CQ, Hsiao A, Hattangadi-Gluth J, et al. Early hemodynamic response assessment of stereotactic radiosurgery for a cerebral arteriovenous malformation using 4D flow MRI. AJNR Am J Neuroradiol 2018;39: 678–81.

47. Clemens RK, Pfammatter T, Meier TO, et al. Combined and complex vascular malformations. Vasa 2015;44:92–105.

48. Hoff SR, Rastatter JC, Richter GT. Head and neck vascular lesions. Otolaryngol Clin North Am 2015; 48:29–45.

49. Flucke U, Karanian M, Broek RWT, et al. Soft tissue special issue: perivascular and vascular tumors of the head and neck. Head Neck Pathol 2020;14: 21–32.

50. Tomà P, Esposito F, Granata C, et al. Up-to-date imaging review of paediatric soft tissue vascular masses, focusing on sonography. Radiol Med 2019;124:935–45.

51. Eberson SN, Desai SB, Metry D. A basic introduction to pediatric vascular anomalies. Semin Intervent Radiol 2019;36:149–60.

52. Sadick M, Müller-Wille R, Wildgruber M, et al. Vascular anomalies (part i): classification and diagnostics of vascular anomalies. Rofo 2018;190: 825–35.

53. Benzar I. A diagnostic program of vascular tumor and vascular malformations in children according to modern classification. Acta Med 2017;60:19–26.

54. Griauzde J, Srinivasan A. Imaging of vascular lesions of the head and neck. Radiol Clin North Am 2015;53:197–213.

55. Flors L, Park AW, Norton PT, et al. Soft-tissue vascular malformations and tumors. Part 1: classification, role of imaging and high-flow lesions. Radiologia 2019;61:4–15.

56. Luu M, Frieden IJ. Infantile hemangiomas and structural anomalies: PHACE and LUMBAR syndrome. Semin Cutan Med Surg 2016;35:117–23.

57. Kolbe AB, Merrow AC, Eckel LJ, et al. Congenital hemangioma of the face-Value of fetal MRI with prenatal ultrasound. Radiol Case Rep 2019;14:1443–6.

58. Gorincour G, Kokta V, Rypens F, et al. Imaging characteristics of two subtypes of congenital hemangiomas: rapidly involuting congenital hemangiomas and non-involuting congenital hemangiomas. Pediatr Radiol 2005;35:1178–85.

59. Mahajan P, Margolin J, Iacobas I. Kasabach-Merritt phenomenon: classic presentation and management options. Clin Med Insights Blood Disord 2017;10. 1179545X17699849.

60. Errani C, Zhang L, Panicek DM, et al. Epithelioid hemangioma of bone and soft tissue: a reappraisal of a controversial entity. Clin Orthop Relat Res 2012;470:1498–506.

61. Ginat DT, Stein SL, McCann S, et al. Neuroimaging of vascular skin lesions and related conditions. In: Ginat D, editor. Neuroradiological imaging of skin diseases and related Conditions. Cham (Switzerland): Springer; 2019. p. 171–96.

62. Loftus WK, Spurrier AJ, Voyvodic F, et al. Intravenous lobular capillary haemangioma (pyogenic granuloma): a case report and a review of imaging findings as reported in the literature. J Med Imaging Radiat Oncol 2018;62:217–23.

63. Gong X, Ying H, Zhang Z, et al. Ultrasonography and magnetic resonance imaging features of kaposiform hemangioendothelioma and tufted angioma. J Dermatol 2019;46:835–42.

64. Merrow AC, Gupta A, Patel MN, et al. 2014 revised classification of vascular lesions from the International Society for the Study of Vascular Anomalies: radiologic-pathologic update. Radiographics 2016; 36:1494–516.

65. Gaballah AH, Jensen CT, Palmquist S, et al. Angiosarcoma: clinical and imaging features from head to toe. Br J Radiol 2017;90:20170039.

66. Hettmer S, Andrieux G, Hochrein J, et al. Epithelioid hemangioendotheliomas of the liver and lung in children and adolescents. Pediatr Blood Cancer 2017; 64(12). https://doi.org/10.1002/pbc.26675.

67. Epelboym Y, Engelkemier DR, Thomas-Chausse F, et al. Imaging findings in epithelioid hemangioendothelioma. Clin Imaging 2019;58:59–65.

Moving?

Make sure your subscription moves with you!

To notify us of your new address, find your **Clinics Account Number** (located on your mailing label above your name), and contact customer service at:

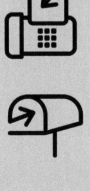

Email: journalscustomerservice-usa@elsevier.com

800-654-2452 (subscribers in the U.S. & Canada)
314-447-8871 (subscribers outside of the U.S. & Canada)

Fax number: 314-447-8029

Elsevier Health Sciences Division
Subscription Customer Service
3251 Riverport Lane
Maryland Heights, MO 63043

Moving?

Make sure your subscription moves with you!

To notify us of your new address, find your Clinics Account Number (located on your mailing label above your name), and contact Customer Service at:

Email: journalscustomerservice-usa@elsevier.com

800-654-2452 (subscribers in the U.S. & Canada)
314-447-8871 (subscribers outside of the U.S. & Canada)

Fax number: 314-447-8029

Elsevier Health Sciences Division
Subscription Customer Service
3251 Riverport Lane
Maryland Heights, MO 63043

To ensure uninterrupted delivery of your subscription, please notify us at least 4 weeks in advance of move.

Printed and bound by CPI Group (UK) Ltd, Croydon, CR0 4YY

08/05/2025

01864700-0009